Female Transcervical Sterilization

PARFR Series on Fertility Regulation

Proceedings of an International Workshop on Non-Surgical Methods for Female Tubal Occlusion June 22 to 24, 1982, Chicago, Illinois, sponsored by the Program for Applied Research on Fertility Regulation Northwestern University, Chicago, Illinois

Female Transcervical Sterilization

edited by

Gerald I. Zatuchni, M.D., M.Sc.

Professor, Department of Obstetrics and Gynecology
Northwestern University Medical School;
Director of Technical Assistance,
Program for Applied Research on Fertility Regulation
Northwestern University, Chicago, Illinois

James D. Shelton, M.D., M.P.H.

Office of Population
Agency for International Development
Washington, D.C.

Alfredo Goldsmith, M.D., M.P.H.

Assistant Professor, Department of Obstetrics and Gynecology
Northwestern University Medical School;
Head, Research Project Development,
Program for Applied Research on Fertility Regulation
Northwestern University, Chicago, Illinois

John J. Sciarra, M.D., Ph.D.

Professor and Chairman, Department of Obstetrics and Gynecology
Northwestern University Medical School;
Program Director, Program for Applied Research on Fertility Regulation
Northwestern University, Chicago, Illinois

Prepared with the technical assistance of Carolyn K. Osborn

With 53 contributors

HARPER & ROW, PUBLISHERS

PHILADELPHIA

Cambridge *New York* *Hagerstown* *San Francisco* *London* *Mexico City* *São Paulo* *Sydney*

1817

Acquisitions Editor: Lisa A. Biello
Sponsoring Editor: Sanford J. Robinson
Manuscript Editor: Mary K. Smith
Indexer: Julia Schwager
Art Director: Maria S. Karkucinski
Production Assistant: Charles W. Field
Compositor: Waldman Graphics, Inc.
Printer/Binder: Haddon Craftsmen

 Printed in the United States of America. For information write Harper & Row, Publishers, Inc., East Washington Square, Philadelphia, Pennsylvania 19105

Library of Congress Cataloging in Publication Data
Main entry under title:

Female transcervical sterilization.

(PARFR series on fertility regulation)
Proceedings of the International Workshop on Non-Surgical Methods for Female Tubal Occlusion, held June 22–24, 1982, in Chicago, sponsored by the Program for Applied Research on Fertility Regulation, Northwestern University.
Bibliography: p.
Includes index.
1. Tubal sterilization—Congresses. 2. Hysteroscopic sterilization—Congresses. 3. Quinacrine—Congresses. 4. Mecrylate—Congresses. 5. Adhesives in surgery—Congresses. 6. Silicones in surgery—Congresses. I. Zatuchni, Gerald I., 1933– . II. International Workshop on Non-Surgical Methods for Female Tubal Occlusion (1982 : Chicago, Ill.) III. Northwestern University (Evanston, Ill.). Program for Applied Research on Fertility Regulation. IV. Title. V. Series. [DNLM: 1. Sterilization, Tubal—Methods—Congresses. WP 660 I608f 1982]
RG138.F45 1983 618.1 83-106

ISBN 0-06-14-2904-X

The authors and publisher have exerted every effort to ensure that drug selection and dosage set forth in this text are in accord with current recommendations and practice at the time of publication. However, in view of ongoing research, changes in government regulations, and the constant flow of information relating to drug therapy and drug reactions, the reader is urged to check the package insert for each drug for any change in indications and dosage and for added warnings and precautions. This is particularly important when the recommended agent is a new or infrequently employed drug.

Preface

Since 1972, the Program for Applied Research on Fertility Regulation (PARFR) has constituted a research program aimed at the development of new methods of fertility control, and the application of research technology to the solution of clinical problems in the field of contraceptive research.

One important part of the PARFR program over the years has been an annual workshop targeted at a very specific area of high research interest, bringing together leaders in the field for a scholarly interchange of ideas. Ten such workshops have been offered, and have been intended to aid in defining the state of the art in a given area and in arriving at some conclusions that might help PARFR, the United States Agency for International Development, and other international funding agencies to determine the best direction for future research and for clinical trials.

The subject of the workshop on which this volume is based, the non-surgical or transcervical methods for tubal occlusion, holds great interest for the contraceptive research community in general, and for PARFR investigators in particular, because of the importance of voluntary sterilization in international family planning programs.

Over the past decade, several of the PARFR workshops have dealt directly with female sterilization; the first such workshop, in 1973, covered the then-new topic of hysteroscopic sterilization. In 1975, a PARFR workshop addressed the Advances in Female Sterilization, and at that meeting a number of researchers first reviewed their work with quinacrine, with methyl cyanoacrylate, and with Silastic, looking at these compounds as potential agents for tubal occlusion.

Because of the increasing worldwide interest in sterilization in the mid-1970s, another conference, held in 1977, was devoted to the reversal of sterilization. Then in 1980, at a workshop in Mexico City, participants discussed new methods of female sterilization, including mechanical devices and pharmacologically active agents. Thus, PARFR has had an ongoing interest in and commitment to the development of such new methods of sterilization.

Interest in transcervical methods of female sterilization is growing, not only in the research community but among the potential users of such methods. Thus, in June, 1982, some 66 investigators and family planning specialists from 13 countries met in Chicago to participate in a program designed to comprehensively consider the laboratory, animal, and clinical studies with quinacrine and methyl cyanoacrylate, and to review the current status of hysteroscopic tubal occlusion with both mechanical devices and with Silastic plugs. The participants looked critically at these new and exciting methods, from the most simple to the most complex, considering their shortcomings and their advantages.

This volume provides a compendium of the reports and discussions presented at the meeting, and suggests that transcervical methods hold considerable promise, and should be welcome to the many women throughout the world for whom a simple, safe, nonsurgical means of fertility regulation would be a highly attractive option.

Gerald I. Zatuchni, M.D., M.Sc.
James D. Shelton, M.D., M.P.H.
Alfredo Goldsmith, M.D., M.P.H.
John J. Sciarra, M.D. Ph.D.

Acknowledgments

The editors wish to acknowledge the significant contribution of Diane Krier-Morrow, M.B.A., Director of Administration of the Program for Applied Research on Fertility Regulation, in the coordination and implementation of this international conference. Her administrative skills played an important part in the effectiveness and ease with which the meeting was run.

Carolyn K. Osborn expresses her gratitude and appreciation to Ruvenia Thomas, who provided tireless, steady, and dependably excellent secretarial assistance in the preparation of the manuscript.

The following organizations provided generous support in the development of the International Workshop on Non-Surgical Methods for Female Tubal Occlusion:

BioNexus, Inc.

United States Agency for International Development

Finally, the editors and PARFR thank the authors for their diligence in preparing excellent manuscripts on time, and the participants for their valuable presentations and informed discussion.

The discussion summaries were prepared by Carolyn K. Osborn.

Contents

Female Transcervical Sterilization

PARFR Series on Fertility Regulation

1

The Need for Nonsurgical Sterilization

JAMES D. SHELTON

J. JOSEPH SPEIDEL

The years since 1960 have witnessed a widely recognized contraceptive revolution throughout the world. Perhaps less well appreciated, in the years since 1970, a revolution has occurred in the use of voluntary sterilization. Largely as a result of new techniques and widespread availability, voluntary sterilization has become by far the most prevalent method of contraception in the world today. Although the changes in the past decade have been dramatic, there is considerable evidence that a large unsatisfied demand for sterilization services remains. Good techniques for nonsurgical female sterilization have a number of potential major advantages over current techniques and thereby offer considerable potential to help meet that unsatisfied need.

DEMAND FOR STERILIZATION SERVICES

Estimates of worldwide use of contraceptive methods adapted by the authors from several sources are shown in Table 1-1.* [1,3,4,5,9,10] Since 1970, the estimated use of sterilization services has increased dramatically. In fact, we estimate that in 1982, sterilization accounted for approximately one third of overall contraceptive use and was roughly equal to the use of oral contraceptives and the IUD combined (Table 1-2). This increase in use of sterilization was associated with the introduction of new techniques, such as laparoscopy and minilaparotomy. These techniques greatly improved the practicality, acceptability, and safety of female sterilization procedures by allowing an inpatient procedure carried out under general anesthesia to be performed more quickly and with less debility on an outpatient basis using local anesthesia. Use of sterilization also increased during this period because donors of international population assistance and medical facilities in both developed and developing countries increased the availability of sterilization services. The Agency for International Development (AID), for example, increased funding for sterilization activities from a few thousand dollars in fiscal year 1970 to over $25 million in fiscal year 1981.

Although these technologies have had considerable impact, there is good evidence for a large unmet demand in developing countries for sterilization services. In Table 1-3 data from 33 developing countries are presented de-

*Piotrow PT: Population Information Program. Personal communication, May 1982.

TABLE 1-1. Estimated Number of Couples Using Contraception Worldwide by Method, Selected Years (Millions)

	1970	1977	1982
Voluntary sterilization	20	80	110
Developed world		16	28
Developing world		64	82
Oral contraceptives	30	54	52
Developed world		28	27
Developing world		26	25
Condom	25	35	40
Developed world		23	25
Developing world		12	15
IUD	15	45	60
Developed world		10	11
Developing world		35	49
Other methods	60	65	70
Total	150	279	332

rived from the World Fertility Survey (WFS) and Contraceptive Prevalence Surveys (CPS).[4,7,8] Of particular interest is the percent of currently married women of reproductive age who indicate they want no more children. In most countries surveyed this proportion approaches or exceeds 50%. Clearly, the proportion of women who say they want no more children is only one indication of the demand for sterilization services, and not all these women would actually wish a sterilization procedure. Nevertheless, the very high proportion of such women in almost every country, and the wide divergence with the proportion actually currently using sterilization or any other method, is powerful evidence that a vast unsatisfied need continues to exist (Table 1-3).

POTENTIAL ADVANTAGES AND DISADVANTAGES OF NONSURGICAL STERILIZATION

Since the role of any fertility control modality in a setting results from a complex interplay of factors, the potential of a new technology such as nonsurgical sterilization cannot be accurately predicted. These factors include

TABLE 1-2. Percent Distribution of Estimated Contraceptive Users Worldwide by Method, Selected Years

	1970	1977	1982
Voluntary sterilization	13	29	33
Oral contraceptives	20	19	16
Condom	17	13	12
IUD	10	16	18
Other methods	40	23	21
Total	100	100	100

TABLE 1-3. Selected Survey Responses by Currently Married Women of Reproductive Age in Selected Countries

	PERCENT WHO WANT NO MORE CHILDREN	PERCENT CURRENTLY USING STERILIZATION	PERCENT USING ANY METHOD OF CONTRACEPTION
Brazil (Piaui, CPS—1979)	70	15	31
Brazil (São Paulo, CPS—1978)	66	16	64
Colombia (CPS—1978)	70	8	48
Costa Rica (CPS—1978)	52	14	65
El Salvador (CPS—1978)	60	18	34
Guatemala (CPS—1978)	47	6	18
Jamaica (CPS—1979)	67	10	55
Mexico (CPS—1978)	56	8	41
Panama (CPS—1979, 80)	65	30	61
Dominican Republic (WFS—1975)	52	14	36
Guyana (WFS—1975)	55	9	35
Haiti (WFS—1977)	46	0	20
Paraguay (WFS—1979)	32	2	41
Peru (WFS—1977)	61	3	36
Trinidad & Tobago (WFS—1977)	47	4	56
Venezuela (WFS—1977)	55	8	52
Bangladesh (CPS—1979)	56	3	12
Korea (CPS—1979)	74	20	54
Thailand (CPS—1978)	65	16	53
Fiji (WFS—1974)	50	18	46
Indonesia (WFS—1976)	39	0	33
Malaysia (WFS—1974)	45	4	36
Nepal (WFS—1976)	30	2	3
Pakistan (WFS—1975)	43	1	7
Philippines (WFS—1978)	54	6	39
Sri Lanka (WFS—1975)	61	11	35
Kenya (WFS—1977)	17	1	8
Lesotho (WFS—1977)	15	1	7
Senegal (WFS—1978)		0	4
Sudan (North, WFS—1978)	17	0	5
Tunisia (Jendouba, CPS—1979)	50	16	32
Jordan (WFS—1976)	42	2	29
Syria (WFS—1978)	37	0	23
Turkey (WFS—1978)	57	0	45

CPS, Contraceptive Prevalence Surveys; WFS, World Fertility Survey.

safety, cost, ease of delivery of services, and individual and social acceptability.[9]

A number of the advantages of nonsurgical sterilization are interrelated and draw on the potential technical simplicity of these techniques, as opposed to conventional procedures. These include the need for less training of personnel; improved geographic availability; and decreased cost, complexity, and time required prior to, during, and after the procedure. Other potential advantages include improved safety and side-effects, and, very importantly, freedom from the negative psychological and cultural factors related to surgery itself and from fear of "operations." These potential advantages apply, to a greater or lesser extent, to the various techniques under development.

SIMPLICITY AND PRACTICALITY

An important reason for the rapid increase in use of voluntary sterilization in the decade of the 1970s was the advance in sterilization technology that made sterilization practical in many settings where previously it was not. Further simplification of techniques is likely to result in further increases in use of the procedure.

The need for less technical training of personnel would be a compelling advantage for nonsurgical sterilization, particularly in developing countries. Almost all developing countries have a severe lack of physicians.[12] Furthermore, while current methods of female sterilization are simple enough in principle to be performed by general practitioners and even paramedical personnel, in actual practice these procedures draw primarily on the skills of more specialized surgeons and obstetricians/gynecologists, who are in even shorter supply in developing countries. For example, in 1978 there were only nine specialists in obstetrics and gynecology working in Nepal, a country of 14 million people.[6] Any procedure that could easily utilize nonspecialist physicians and nonphysicians could make sterilization services much more available. The geographic availability of services also relates to the distribution of physicians. There is a major imbalance in physician distribution in developing countries, and rural areas are particularly neglected. For example, in India, up to four fifths of the physicians are in urban areas, which include only one fifth of the population.[12] Also related to the geographic imbalance of service availability is the concentration of hospitals and other fixed health facilities in urban areas. Insofar as nonsurgical sterilization can be freed from hospitals and relatively sophisticated health facilities, these services could be much more accessible, particularly to people in rural areas, who are potentially in the greatest need of services.

Several other advantages of nonsurgical sterilization relate to potential simplicity. If a nonsurgical procedure could approach the technical simplicity of an IUD insertion, it could offer major advantages in terms of decreased time, decreased cost, and fewer of the materials, supplies, and equipment required for current methods. This is particularly true for developing countries where financial resources are scarce and logistical supply systems are notoriously poor.[11] In developing countries the general admonition to keep things simple must be considered a fundamental axiom.

SAFETY

Although female sterilization is one of the safest methods of contraception,[13] it does have an associated mortality risk. One recent analysis of sterilization-attributable deaths in Bangladesh identified anesthesia overdosage, tetanus,

TABLE 1-4. Reasons Not Interested in Sterilization of Currently Married Women Aged 15–44 Who Do Not Want More Children—Selected Surveys, Latin America (Percent Distribution)

REASONS	EL SALVADOR (1978)	GUATEMALA (1978)	SÃO PAULO STATE, BRAZIL (1978)	PANAMA (1979)	PIAUI STATE, BRAZIL (1979)	NORTHEAST BRAZIL* (1980)
Fear of operation	20.4	40.8	24.0	32.1	52.2	36.7
Fear of side-effects	10.0	5.6	7.8	3.6	25.3	21.1
Menopausal/subfecund	11.4	11.6	10.1	12.2	6.4	†
"Thinks she can't get pregnant anymore"	10.3	3.9	†	3.8	1.6	6.9
Prefers temporary method of contraception	4.7	7.6	25.3	7.9	0.4	5.1
Religious reasons	12.1	5.7	1.5	3.3	4.7	7.3
Husband doesn't permit	9.8	11.0	†	4.9	1.9	3.1
"Does not want/like"	11.8	2.9	6.9	13.9	†	6.5
Other reasons	9.5	10.9	24.4	18.3	7.5	13.3
Total	100.0	100.0	100.0	100.0	100.0	100.0

*Includes the States of R.G. do Norte, Paraiba, Pernambuco, and Bahia.
†Included in other reasons.

intraperitoneal hemorrhage, and other infections, in decreasing order of importance, as the primary causes of death in the cases studied.[2] While the various methods of nonsurgical sterilization have potential associated risks, they clearly also have considerable potential for obviating the current risks of conventional surgical procedures.

FEAR OF SURGERY

As with many other decisions, the decision of whether to undergo sterilization is influenced by many factors. Although current female sterilization procedures are quite simple, they are ultimately viewed essentially as a form of surgery and carry with them the major emotional and intellectual connotations of an "operation." While it is difficult to evaluate the importance of this factor, some survey information indicates that it is a substantial impediment. Responses of Latin American women in six surveys who wanted no more children are presented in Table 1-4.* Asked why they were not interested in sterilization, the women in all six surveys indicated that fear of the operation and fear of side-effects, taken together, were the most important reasons. It is reasonable to believe that these factors also have a significant influence on the decision of many other women as to whether to undergo sterilization.

*Morris L: Unpublished data.

REVERSIBILITY

While most of this chapter has dealt with potential advantages of nonsurgical sterilization, one disadvantage of these methods, with the exception of the tubal plug approaches, is the fact that they are permanent methods with little chance of reversal. In principle, current methods of surgical sterilization should be undertaken by women who definitely want no more children. Nevertheless, methods using the tubal ring, clip, or Pomeroy techniques offer much better potential for reversal than the primary nonsurgical methods now under development.

CONCLUSION

In the interest of voluntarism and free choice, couples should be provided with the opportunity to select from the widest variety of options among contraceptive methods, including both male and female sterilization.

There is considerable evidence in the field of family planning services that improving the availability, accessibility, and acceptability of contraceptive services will markedly increase their use. This has already been demonstrated in the case of current surgical female contraceptive technology. Nonsurgical female sterilization offers some major advantages in these same parameters. Given the very large demand for voluntary sterilization that apparently still remains, techniques for nonsurgical female sterilization could have a major impact on family planning programs.

REFERENCES

1. GREEN CP: Voluntary sterilization: World's leading contraceptive method. Popul Rep [M], No. 2, 1978
2. GRIMES DA, PETERSON HB, ROSENBERG MJ et al: Sterilization: Attributable deaths in Bangladesh. Int J Gynaecol Obstet 20:149–154, 1982
3. KOLS A, RINEHART W, PIOTROW PT et al: Oral contraceptives in the 1980s. Popul Rep [A], No. 6, 1982
4. LIGHTBOURNE R, SINGH S, GREEN CP: The world fertility survey: Charting global childbearing. Popul Bull 37:1–54, 1982
5. LISKIN L: IUDs: An appropriate choice for many women. Popul Rep [B], No. 4, 1982
6. MARSH EM: Observations and Recommendations Concerning Voluntary Surgical Contraception in Nepal. Consultant Report, American Public Health Association, 1978
7. MORRIS L, LEWIS G, POWELL DL et al: Contraceptive prevalence surveys: A new source of family planning data. Popul Rep [M], No. 5, 1981
8. NATIONAL INSTITUTE FOR POPULATION RESEARCH AND TRAINING: Bangladesh contraceptive prevalence survey report—1979. Dacca, Bangladesh, June 1981
9. SPEIDEL JJ, RAVENHOLT RT: The potential of reversible sterilization in family planning programs. In Sciarra JJ, Zatuchni GI, Speidel JJ (eds): Reversal of Sterilization. Hagerstown, MD, Harper & Row, 1978
10. STEPHAN J, KELLOGG EH, PIOTROW PT: Legal trends and issues in voluntary sterilization. Popul Rep [E], No. 6, 1981
11. TIETZE C, BONGAARTS J, SCHEARER B: Mortality associated with the control of fertility. Fam Plann Perspect 8:6–14, 1976
12. WORLD HEALTH ORGANIZATION: Sixth Report on the World Health Situation. Geneva, 1980
13. WORLD HEALTH ORGANIZATION: Report on WHO meeting on health research. Lancet 1:1177–1178, 1982

2

Anatomic and Physiologic Factors Affecting the Development of Transcervical Sterilization Techniques

CARLTON A. EDDY

CARL J. PAUERSTEIN

Birth is the culmination of a series of complex physiologic events, many of which occur within the oviduct. The male and female determinants of each new person are first brought together within the oviduct. Therefore the oviduct is a logical target for methods designed to prevent this union.

The uterus and tubes link the peritoneal cavity, into which the ovum is released, and the vagina, into which spermatozoa are deposited. As understanding of reproductive physiology and medical technology have improved, this direct and accessible area of communication, the oviduct, offers an ever more tempting site for contraceptive intervention.

The widely accepted concepts that tubal patency denotes fertility and that lack of patency is synonymous with infertility attest that the anatomic complexity and functional diversity of the oviduct have been underestimated. Tubal sterilization techniques, particularly those designed to obliterate the tubal lumen, must confront the oviduct's complex anatomy and physiology.

This chapter will focus on tubal anatomy and physiology as related to the development of tubal sterilization techniques using "nonsurgical" transcervical approaches. We will also consider some practical aspects of tubal sterilization procedures, including reversibility.

THE ANATOMY OF THE OVIDUCT

The oviducts are paired, hollow, seromuscular organs that extend from the superior-lateral aspect of the uterine fundus to the ovaries (Fig. 2-1). Each oviduct is supported throughout its length by a peritoneal fold, the mesosalpinx, and is bordered anteriorly by the round ligament and posteriorly by the ovarian ligament and mesovarium. The oviduct is attached medially to the uterine fundus and laterally to the infundibular pelvic ligament and ovary by way of an elongated mucosal fold, the fimbria ovarica.[2,29]

The extrauterine oviduct is sheathed throughout its length by a serosal covering consisting of a layer of loose connective tissue covered by a single layer of mesothelium continuous with the mesosalpinx. Beneath the mesothelial layer, smooth muscle fibers, distinct from those of the tubal muscularis,

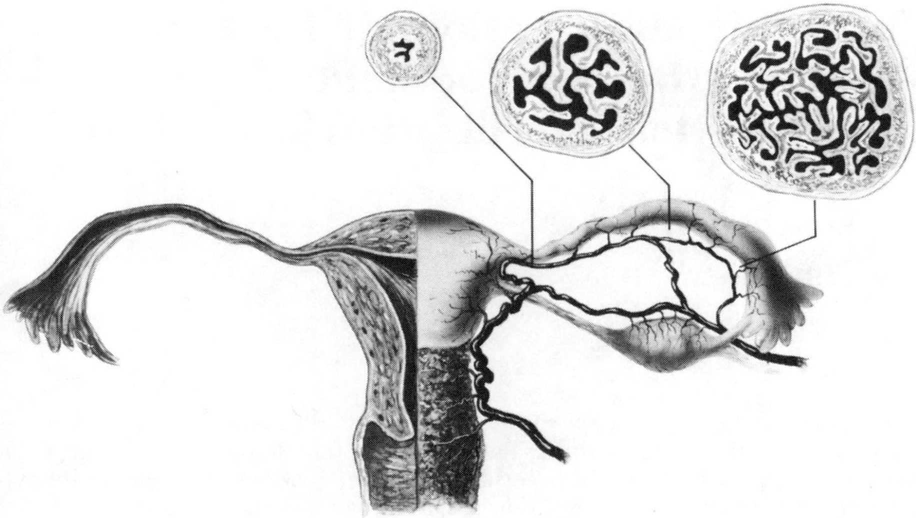

FIG. 2-1. Female internal genitalia. (*Left*) Morphology of the tubal lumen demonstrating its confluence with the uterus, cervix, and vagina. (*Right*) Arterial blood supply to the oviduct. (*Above*) Representative cross sections of the oviduct at various levels.

are present. The connective tissue is highly vascular and contains numerous lymphatic vessels. These originate primarily along the mesosalpingeal border, extend parallel to the oviduct, and branch extensively, penetrating into the muscular and mucosal layers of the oviduct.

The middle muscular layer, the myosalpinx, consists of smooth muscle arranged in layers, the orientation of which approximates their planes of contraction. The layers are not always clearly delineated from each other. Toward the uterine end of the oviduct, three muscle layers are present: (1) an outer longitudinal layer, (2) a prominent middle circular layer, and (3) an inner longitudinal layer. The outer longitudinal and middle circular layers can be distinguished throughout the length of the oviduct. In contrast, the inner longitudinal layer becomes discontinuous within the distal two thirds of the oviduct, where it persists as scattered muscle bundles within and at the base of the mucosa.[20]

The mucosa, or endosalpinx, lines the tubal lumen. It is composed of an epithelial layer resting on a core of lamina propria. The lamina propria consists of loose connective tissue interspersed with numerous blood vessels and lymphatic spaces bound within a collagen fiber matrix.[2] The mucosa is thrown into folds that project into the lumen. The height and complexity of the folds vary among the segments of the oviduct. The epithelium is made up predominantly of ciliated and secretory cells. The relative proportion of the cell types varies within different regions of the oviduct. Ciliated cells predominate in the distal oviduct and decrease toward the uterus, whereas the inverse is true of secretory cells. Two additional cell types are seen occasionally. Wedge- or cone-shaped "peg" cells may represent depleted secretory or ciliated cells.[19] Round "basal" cells may be the precursors of epithelial cells. The latter two cell types collectively represent less than 2% of the epithelial cell population.

The length of the oviduct varies from 6 cm to 15 cm, with 11 cm being average.[21] Length may also vary according to the organ's state of contractility, blood flow, and lymphatic drainage, all of which may change in response to the organ's endocrine status. On the basis of its anatomy, the oviduct is divided into the infundibulary, ampullary, isthmic, and intramural segments.

The infundibulum is the short trumpet-shaped distal enlargement of the ampulla containing the fimbriated tubal abdominal ostium. This portion of the oviduct constitutes the normal functional connection between the ovary and oviduct and is responsible for ovum pickup. It contains the largest luminal diameter of any segment, up to 2 cm at its widest diameter. The cone-shaped ostium opens into the abdominal cavity. The epithelium is densely ciliated; the relative distribution of ciliated cells approaches 70% in fertile women.[3] Ciliary beat is toward the uterus, as it is in cilia throughout the oviduct. The mucosa is complexly folded and completely fills the lumen. The myosalpinx is extremely thin.

The ampulla is the longest portion of the oviduct, constituting approximately two thirds of its length. The lumen varies in diameter from 2 cm at its distal end to from 1 mm to 2 mm at its junction with the isthmus. The endosalpinx is extensively folded. Numerous longitudinally oriented folds, together with extensive secondary folds, collectively fill the entire lumen, rendering it a potential space. Ciliated cells predominate in the distal ampulla and gradually decrease in number toward the isthmus. The thin myosalpinx is easily distended and easily collapsed. Peritubal adhesions, even if mild, may functionally occlude the lumen.

The isthmus makes up the remaining one third of the extrauterine oviduct. The isthmic lumen is narrow, ranging in diameter from 1 mm to 2 mm at its junction with the ampulla to 0.1 mm at the uterine junction. The endosalpinx is composed of numerous low primary folds that run longitudinally. They describe a cruciform cross section near the uterine end and undergo transition rather abruptly into the extensively folded endosalpinx at the ampullary-isthmic junction. Secretory cells predominate over ciliated cells. The isthmus is the most densely muscular segment of the extrauterine oviduct, with well-developed longitudinal and circular muscle layers, as described above.

The interstitial segment of the oviduct traverses the uterine wall and is surrounded by thick myometrium. The longitudinal and circular muscle layers of the isthmus continue into the uterus. Vascular rings accompanied by uterine muscle bundles surround the intramural portion of the oviduct. An additional inner layer of musculature is arranged in spirals that encircle the intramural portion.[27] This segment varies in length from 1 cm to 3.5 cm. It has a narrow lumen, variously described as ranging from "hairlike" to several millimeters in diameter.[22,25] The path described may be straight or tortuous.

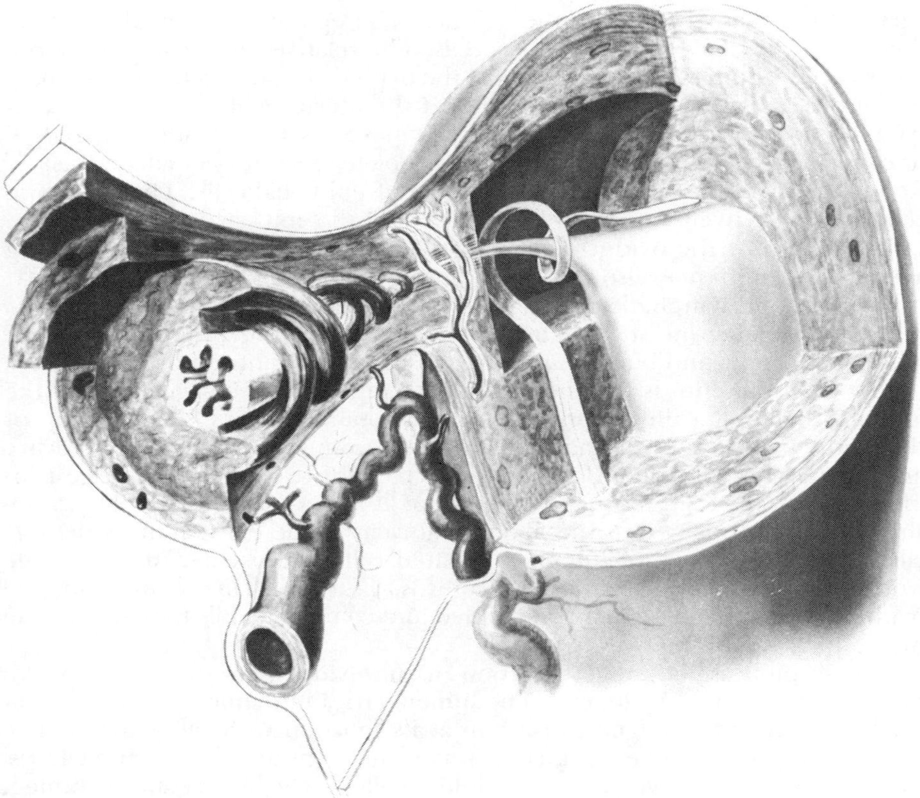

FIG. 2-2. Semidiagrammatic representation of the uterotubal junction. The intramural oviduct is composed of longitudinally and circularly arranged muscle fibers within a matrix of spirally arranged fibers of the autochthonous layer of myometrium that encircle the tubal lumen. Numerous anatomical features complicate the free passage of material intraluminally. See text and other figures for details.

As the endometrial cavity is approached, the lumen enlarges to terminate in the funnel-shaped uterine ostium. The mucosa lining this segment is more densely ciliated than that of the isthmus and is of a type intermediate between that of the endometrium and that of the oviduct. Mucosal folds are few, are longitudinally arranged, and become continuous with the endometrial mucosa (Fig. 2-2).

BLOOD SUPPLY

The oviduct is a well-vascularized organ. The blood supply is derived from the uterine and ovarian arteries. A major branch of each artery anastomoses, giving rise to reduplicated vascular arcades. The magnitude of the contribution of the ovarian and uterine blood vessels to the oviduct may vary between individuals. The most commonly described pattern is one in which the uterine artery and its branches perfuse the interstitial and medial two thirds of the oviduct,[25] whereas the ovarian artery supplies the distal oviduct.[10] The ability of the tube to autoregulate its blood supply can lead, under extreme instances, to either the ovarian or uterine artery alone supplying the entire oviduct. Venous drainage follows the arterial supply. Venous plexuses are present in the endosalpinx, myosalpinx, and serosal layers. The three plexuses become confluent in the serosa and drain into extrinsic veins associated with the ovarian and uterine arteries.

LYMPHATIC DRAINAGE

The oviduct contains a well-developed system of lymphatic vessels that is more extensive in the isthmic region than in the ampullary segment. Lymphatic networks drain the endosalpinx, the myosalpinx, and the serosa. On emerging from each region, the lymphatic vessels combine to enter the mesosalpinx and to drain into the para-aortic nodes.[11,12]

TUBAL PHYSIOLOGY

The primary function of the oviduct is transportation; initially it simultaneously conveys the ovum and spermatozoa in opposite directions, and then it transports the developing embryo into the uterus. A second important function is provision of an appropriate milieu for gamete survival, fertilization, and early embryo development.

Gamete transport through the oviduct is a complex physiological process that involves the conversion of metabolic energy into mechanical energy by smooth muscle and ciliated and secretory cells. The relative importance of each of these components is not known. It is probable that there are regional differences in the contribution and importance of each. In the infundibulum and ampulla with their thin myosalpinx, large lumen, and complex, densely ciliated mucosal folds, ciliary activity may be of major importance in ovum transport, with contractile activity a subordinate effector. In contrast, transport through the isthmus, with its prominent myosalpinx, narrow lumen, and sparsely ciliated endosalpinx, appears to result primarily from contractile activity.

TUBAL CONTRACTILITY

Because of the arrangement of muscle fibers in layers oriented in circular and longitudinal fashion, the oviduct is capable of generating a variety of contractile patterns, including peristaltic, antiperistaltic, and segmental contractions. Unlike the alimentary tract, the oviduct does not generate regular peristaltic contractions. Instead, it demonstrates segmental contractions that propagate simultaneously in opposite directions over short distances. Ovum transport, therefore, assumes a discontinuous pattern of reciprocal movements in which the ovum is forced out of areas of contraction into inactive regions. Thus, ovum transport appears to occur in a series of random movements that, over several days, acquire a gradual net bias toward the uterus.

The role of tubal contractility in sperm transport is less clear. Spermatozoa are motile and may actively participate in their transport through the female tract. The segmental contractions of the myosalpinx may compartmentalize the oviduct, randomly moving its contents throughout the tube. This mechanism, in concert with the inate motility of spermatozoa, may result in the transportation of the spermatozoa to the vicinity of the newly ovulated ovum.

The oviduct exhibits continuous, spontaneous activity. Complete quiescence never occurs. Even during pregnancy, when the uterus is largely quiescent, owing to high levels of circulating progesterone, the oviducts remain spontaneously active, although at a reduced rate similar to that seen in the late luteal or early proliferative phases of the menstrual cycle.[5] Two peaks of contractility occur: one at the time of ovulation, when estrogen levels are highest; the other during menstruation, when progesterone levels are lowest. The relative refractoriness of the oviduct to the inhibitory influence of progesterone may be important to ensure that gamete transport can proceed despite rising progesterone levels after ovulation.

SECRETORY ACTIVITY

The tube furnishes the environment for gamete survival, fertilization, and early embryo development. Tubal fluid is a complex product derived primarily from hormone-dependent secretory activity of the tubal epithelium and selective transudation from the blood with varying contributions from the uterus, the peritoneal cavity, and, in the postovulatory interval, the ovarian follicle. Tubal secretory activity, a predominantly estrogen-dependent phenomenon, is antagonized by progesterone and is maximal at the time of maximum estrogen production.

Tubal secretory cells undergo morphologic changes during the ovarian cycle. During the early proliferative stage, under low-estrogen conditions, the tubal mucosa is thin, exhibiting a low cuboidal profile. Secretory activity is largely absent at this time. As the cycle progresses, rising estrogen levels result in progressive mucosal thickening. Secretory cells increase in height and become domed. Following the preovulatory estrogen peak, the mucosal epithelium attains maximal thickness. The domed, microvilli-covered apices of secretory cells protrude into the lumen above the tips of the ciliated cells, rendering their cilia relatively inconspicuous. At ovulation, the secretory cells discharge their contents into the lumen. During the late luteal and menstrual phases of the cycle, the mucosa again thins and secretory activity stops.

Quantitative differences in secretion exist in different segments of the oviduct.[1] The major volume of secretions is produced by the isthmus. Qualitative differences have also been demonstrated. Histochemical studies indicate that regionalization of glycoprotein secretion also occurs.[9,17] The isthmus is the primary site of production of mucin, a product that may be of importance in sperm and ovum transport.

CILIARY ACTIVITY

The ciliated cell is characterized by the presence of 250 to 300 elongated, regularly arranged kinocilia at the cell apex. As noted above, ciliated cells predominate at the level of the fimbria. Their number diminishes somewhat in the ampulla and significantly declines in the isthmus. As the tube enters the uterus, there is a transient increase in the number of ciliated cells.[7] However, this general pattern of distribution of ciliated and secretory cells may be interrupted in certain highly localized areas in which one or the other cell type predominates. In general, ciliated cells tend to be found in greatest numbers on the apex and sides of mucosal folds, whereas secretory cells occupy a more basal position.

Cilia exhibit a highly organized and synchronized pattern of contractility in which a propulsive power stroke is followed by a nonpropulsive retracting stroke. The cilia within individual cells are arranged in rows. The beating of cilia proceeds row by row within individual cells. Moreover, adjacent ciliated cells exhibit synchronized metachronal integration with each other so that waves of ciliary beating proceed in orderly fashion across large areas of endosalpinx. The rate of ciliary beating is relatively constant, except for a transient increase during the postovulatory period.[6]

Physiologists disagree about specific changes in the morphology and distribution of ciliated cells during the menstrual cycle. Human tubal epithelium does not appear to undergo marked cyclic, estrogen-driven ciliogenesis. Some changes, such as increase in cell size and subcellular organization, may occur as the cycle progresses. Some renewal of ciliated cells does occur, but there is little evidence for cyclic deciliation/reciliation or for the regular transformation of ciliated into secretory cells.[28]

MECHANISM OF GAMETE TRANSPORT

We have integrated the above observations into a tentative schema of the mechanism of gamete transport. Following ovulation, ovum pickup occurs by way of contractile and ciliary activity involving the ovarian and tubal mesenteries that bring the surface of the ovary and the fimbria into proximity. Concurrently, spermatozoa, present in the upper vagina, have colonized the cervix, the uterine crypts, and possibly the proximal isthmus. In response to segmental contractility of the isthmus and their own flagellar movements, sperm ascend the oviduct. Estrogen-induced secretory activity of the isthmic mucosa and the increased height of the secretory cells protect the sperm from the pro-uterine ciliary beat. The production of thick mucin aids this process by agglutinating the cilia and by filling the isthmic lumen. The mucin plug may also enhance sperm transport in a manner analogous to that of midcycle cervical mucus. The ovum, slowly traveling down the ampulla, where secretory activity is sparse but ciliary beating is prominent, encounters the spermatozoa and is fertilized. During the fertilized ovum's 3-day sojourn in the oviduct, increasing progesterone levels clear the isthmic lumen of mucin and cause retraction of the secretory cells, enabling the pro-uterine accelerated beat of the isthmic cilia to assist the pro-uterine segmental contractions of the tube in propelling the developing embryo through the isthmus into the uterus.

PRACTICAL CONSIDERATIONS

Techniques of nonsurgical, transcervical sterilization seek either to induce localized trauma leading to closure of the oviduct or to insert intraluminal occluding devices to achieve a similar end. Because of the oviduct's anatomy and function, these can be formidable tasks.

We know now that the human reproductive tract has evolved functional redundancy, which allows fertility to be maintained in the face of considerable anatomical and functional modification. The ability of the oviduct to recanalize and to heal itself is quite remarkable and contributes to the difficulty in developing tubal sterilization techniques that are technically simple, that avoid extensive destruction of the oviduct, and that are associated with low morbidity.

ANATOMY

The oviduct is a hollow organ, the hydraulics of which influence the delivery of occlusive agents or devices. The diameter of the tubal lumen undergoes a reduction of up to 95% from 2 cm at the abdominal ostium to 100μ within the uterus. The thickness of the myosalpinx is greatest in areas where the luminal diameter is smallest. This relationship reaches an extreme at the level of the intramural segment, in which a threadlike lumen is surrounded by a massive thickness of muscle. Thus, if one seeks to deliver drugs or tissue adhesives in volumes adequate to traumatize the entire luminal circumference of a length of oviduct sufficient to ensure sterilization, spillage into the peritoneal cavity with resultant chemical peritonitis would be difficult to avoid. The constricted lumen and limited compliance of the intramural segment of the oviduct mean that delivery of a sufficient volume of material through this segment, particularly if the material is viscous or begins to polymerize or adhere rapidly, may require unacceptably high pressures. Rapid injection at high pressure could lead to embolization of the material into the dense vascular plexuses surrounding the intraluminal segment of oviduct.

The lumen of the intramural portion of the tube may describe any of a variety of pathways through the wall of the uterus; sometimes these are straight, curved, or tortuous (Fig. 2-3). When such pathways are long and incorporate abrupt angulations, passage of material from the endometrial cavity into the lumen of the oviduct may be difficult.

The uterotubal junction may function as a physiological sphincter regulating the passage of ova and spermatozoa between the oviduct and uterus. Although no anatomical sphincter is present, the arrangements of blood vessels and muscle fibers favor the possibility of active closure of the lumen under appropriate conditions. The blood vessels that encircle the oviduct in the vasomuscular layer are surrounded by perivascular muscular sheaths with fibers that are oriented parallel to the long axis of the blood vessels. Conges-

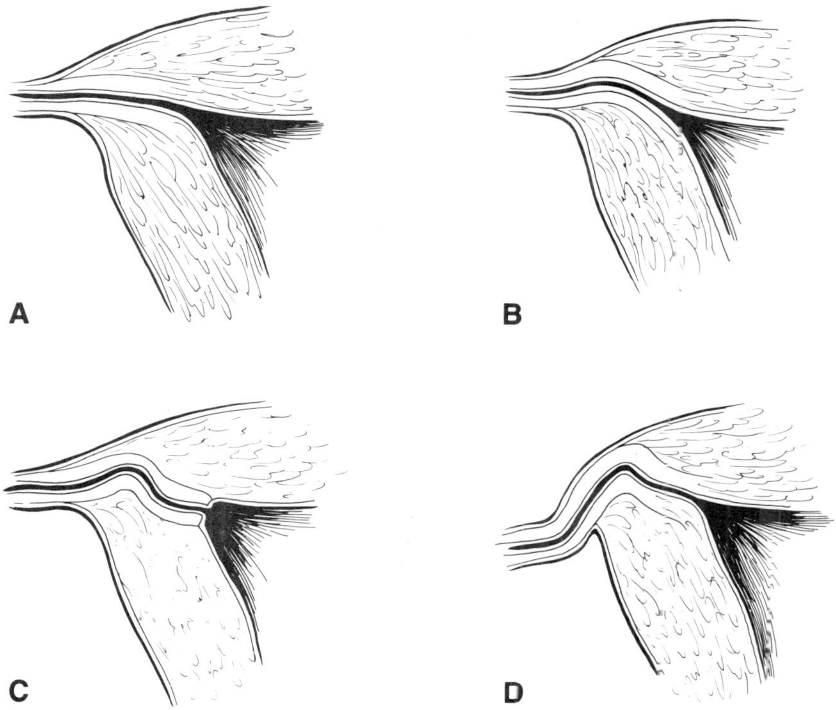

FIG. 2-3. Typical pathways described by the intramural oviduct. (*A*) Straight. (*B*) Convex. (*C*) Tortuous (*D*) Angulated.

tion of these vessels with blood or contraction of their perivascular muscle fibers could result in constriction of the tubal lumen (Fig. 2-4). Similarly, contraction of the autochthonous spiral muscle fibers that surround the intramural portion of the tube effectively closes down the lumen (Fig. 2-5). Contraction of the intrinsic inner longitudinal fibers of the oviduct could also create transient acute angulation and closure of the lumen. Thus, during periods of spontaneous muscle activity or vascular distention, the intramural lumen may be physiologically narrowed and resistant to the passage of material. Attempts to force material through this area under pressure might induce more spasm and edema.[14]

COMPLIANCE

Compliance is the designation given to the ability of the oviduct to yield to intraluminal pressure by expanding or distending. For small deformations, the tube responds to radial stresses with radial compliance or ballooning. The mucosa, as well as the muscularis, yields in response to an ovum or fluid, for example. Cross sections of a distal oviduct with and without an ovum are shown in Figures 2-6 and 2-7. In the absence of the ovum, the lumen is

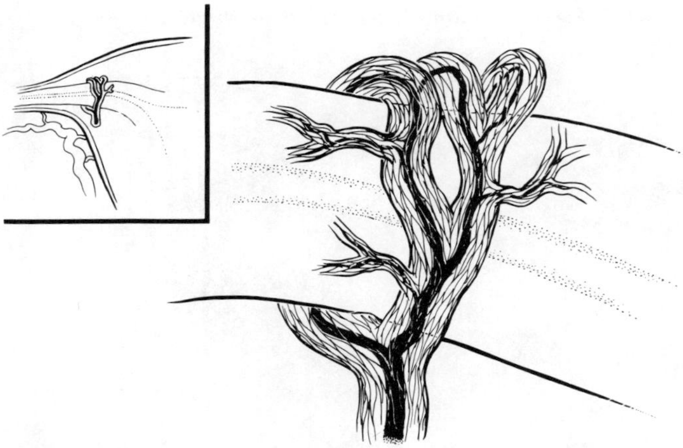

FIG. 2-4. Arrangement of blood vessels within the vascular layer of the intramural oviduct. (*Insert*) Anatomical orientation and location.

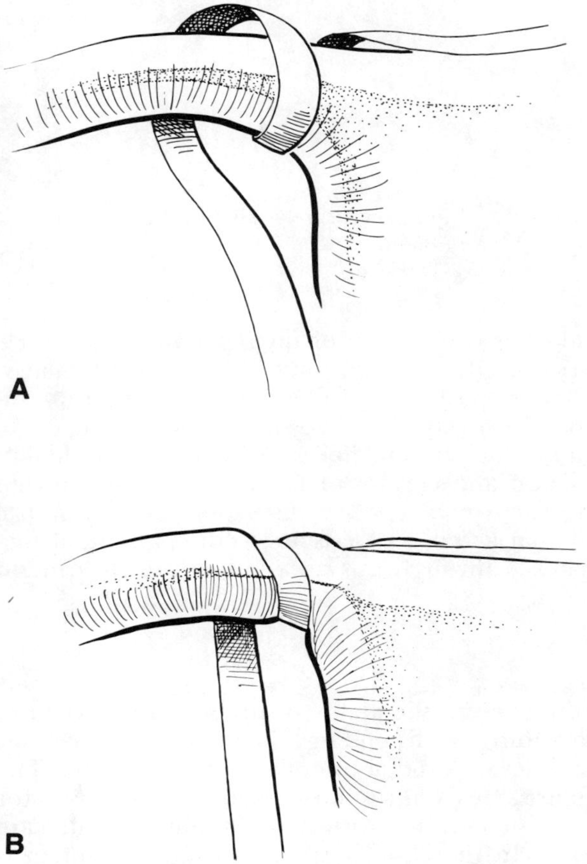

FIG. 2-5. Occlusion of the intramural oviduct through contraction of spiral muscle fibers. (*A*) Relaxation. (*B*) Contraction.

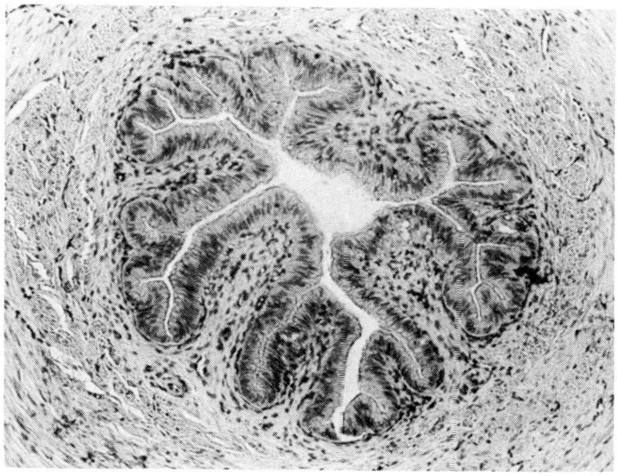

FIG. 2-6. Cross section of rabbit oviduct showing lumen occupied by endosalpingeal folds.

largely a potential space occupied by folds of endosalpinx. When the ovum is present, many of these folds have been displaced. When intraluminal pressure is increased, the lumen expands and the cross section becomes more circular as mucosal folds are obliterated. The radial compliance of the oviduct wall is greater than that of ova. When ova larger than the tubal lumen are present, distention of walls, rather than compression of the ova, occurs. When mucosal compliance is maximal and additional stress is applied, further luminal distention occurs as the myosalpinx expands. The effective compliance of the muscle layer is small compared with that of the endosalpinx. However, the two are physically in series, that is, the more compliant mucosa first accommodates increased intraluminal pressure and the muscle then complies.[4]

Compliance is a function of muscle wall thickness. The ampulla, with its thin myosalpinx, is highly compliant. It may be passively distended to three or four times its normal diameter without a concomitant increase in intra-

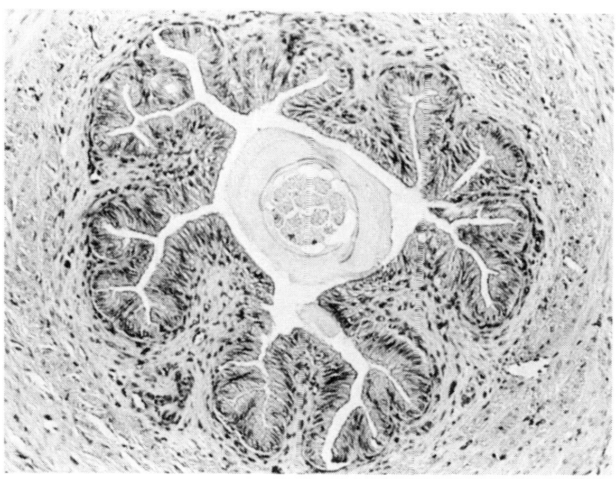

FIG. 2-7. Cross section of rabbit oviduct in the presence of an ovum. The endosalpinx has been displaced in order to accommodate the ovum.

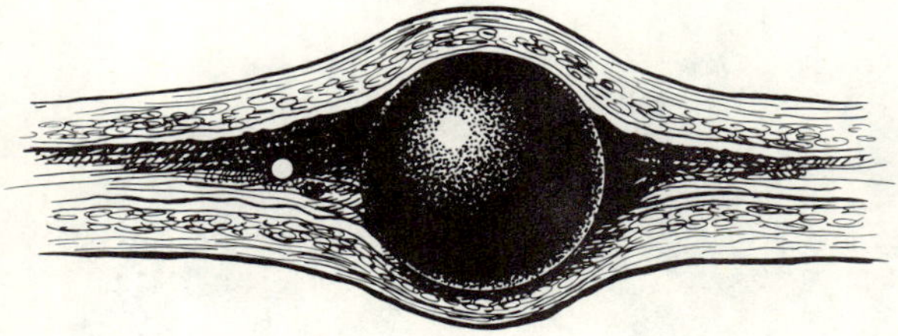

FIG. 2-8. Rabbit isthmus containing a 1200μ diameter Silastic sphere lodged in the lumen. Despite the presence of such an object occluding the lumen, pregnancy was consistently achieved. White object to the left is the comparative size of an ovum.

luminal pressure.[29] In contrast, the isthmus and intramural segments, with a thick myosalpinx, are less compliant. The physiological arrest of the ovum at the ampullary isthmic junction appears to be a function of luminal diameter; the isthmic lumen is too small to accommodate the ovum until tubal contractility or other propulsive, pressure-generating forces push the ovum into the isthmus, thereby dilating its walls. Compliance of the oviduct wall appears to be hormonally controlled, since opening pressure during transuterine insufflation differs according to the stage of the menstrual cycle.[23]

To be effective, occlusive intraluminal material or devices must totally occlude the lumen and remain in place. Tubal compliance works against this. The elasticity of the tubal wall cannot be relied on to anchor an intraluminal plug or device unless the plug or device occupies a long segment of oviduct. If a tight seal is made, there is risk of inducing tissue erosion if the plug or occlusive device is rigid. Ideally, the lumen should be maximally stretched by the device to anchor it and to seal off the lumen.

Introduction of plastic or Silastic spheres 1200μ to 1300μ in diameter into the abdominal ostia of rabbit oviducts resulted in their transport through the ampulla. They were arrested at the ampullary isthmic junction owing to the inability of the tube to distend sufficiently to accommodate them (Fig. 2-8). Despite tubal distention by an object whose diameter was three times that of the tubal lumen, 21 of 28 animals with these spheres lodged in their oviducts became pregnant.[15] Fertilization required that spermatozoa bypass the spheres in order to reach the ova. More remarkably, the fertilized ova had to squeeze past the spheres to reach the uterus. This study demonstrates the remarkable persistence of fertility and suggests that drastic procedures are necessary for interference with pregnancy by way of intratubal plugs.

TRAUMA AND HEALING

Successful occlusion of the tube requires trauma sufficient to destroy the tissue parenchyma so that it is replaced by nonfunctional scar tissue, which occludes the lumen. Tissue repair entails replacement of dead cells and damaged tissue by new parenchyma or connective tissue. Resolution of any injury depends on the nature and duration of exposure to the causative agent, on the extent of tissue destruction, and on the type of tissue injured.

The initial trauma that damages or destroys cells is followed by an inflammatory phase characterized by vascular permeability, edema, fibrin forma-

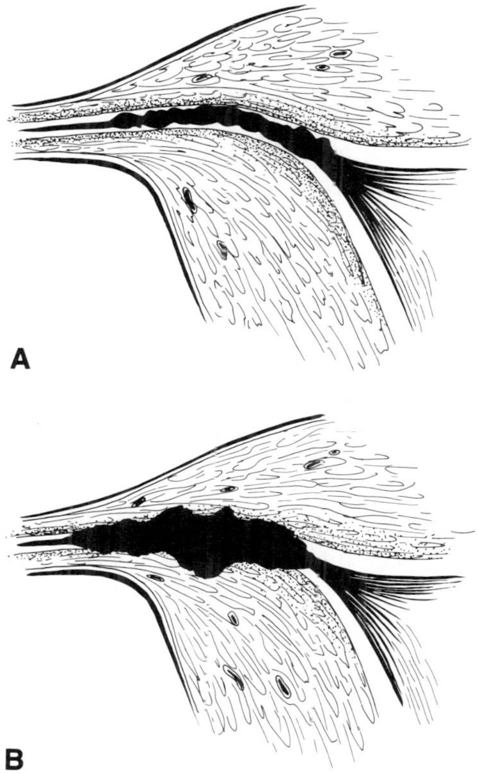

FIG. 2-9. Types of intraluminal trauma commonly achieved in transcervical sterilization attempts. (*A*) Trauma involving only the epithelium. Such trauma is repaired through epithelial proliferation and regeneration, which may restore normal function. (*B*) More extensive trauma leading to destruction of the epithelium with muscle involvement. Healing generally entails replacement of functional tissue with granulation tissue. The resultant scarring may totally occlude the lumen, leading to sterility. Partial occlusion may predispose to ectopic pregnancy.

tion, and infiltration of tissue with leukocytes. Healing then begins. If the trauma is mild, the inflammation resolves in a short time through proteolysis of fibrin, debridement by macrophages, and regeneration of functional tissue. Following moderately extensive tissue destruction, chronic inflammation occurs. This prolongs healing because a large quantity of dead and damaged cells must be phagocytized and removed from the area before repair can be completed. If the offending agent, such as a tubal plug or chemical irritant, cannot be removed, fibrinolysis is ineffective and healing is further delayed. After very extensive trauma, resolution by repair is not possible and healing occurs by fibroblastic proliferation and formation of nonfunctional scar tissue.[18,26]

The type of tissue injured and its regenerative ability are important. In general, the more highly specialized the tissue is, the less the capacity for regeneration. Cells that continue to multiply throughout life have the best regenerative capacity. The myosalpinx is in the former group, whereas the endosalpinx is in the latter.

Mild and extensive trauma to the intramural segment of the oviduct is shown in Figure 2-9. In the first example, trauma is essentially limited to the epithelium. There has been little loss of tissue, and healing will occur by first intention by way of epithelialization. This type of trauma is characteristic of

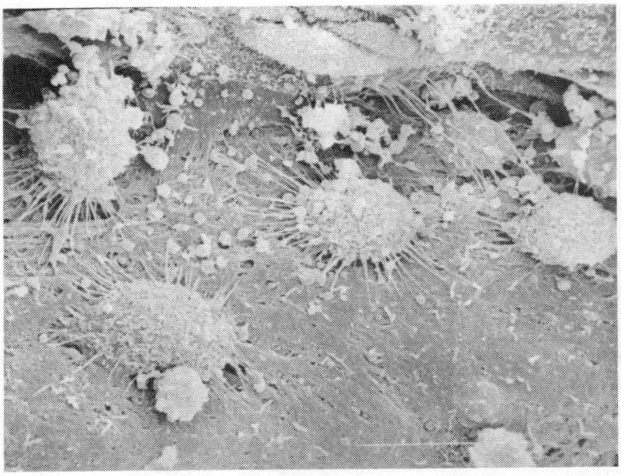

FIG. 2-10. Epithelialization following mechanical trauma to the oviduct. Numerous migrating epithelial cells are seen in transit from an intact zone to an area of lamina propria denuded of epithelium. Pseudopodia conveying locomotion are seen, and the cells appear to be engaged in phagocytosis of cellular debris (SEM, rabbit oviduct, 24 hours post anastomosis, ×2200).

mild chemical and physical injury of brief duration. Within hours, epithelial cells begin migrating into the area to bridge the gap and to ingest and digest fibrin and other material within the wound. Other epithelial cells undergo multiplication to replace lost cells and finally undergo maturation to restore function. In Figure 2-10, individual epithelial cells migrating across an exposed area of lamina propria are shown. Pseudopodia conveying locomotion are evident, and the cells appear to be engaged in phagocytosis of cellular debris. In the case of extensive tubal trauma represented in Figure 2-9, widespread destruction has occurred. The epithelium has disappeared and much of the myosalpinx has been destroyed. Healing will occur by second intention and will entail formation of granulation tissue, leading to gross defects in oviduct architecture and loss of function. Concurrent epithelialization may occur to varying degrees, conferring some residual function. This type of trauma is more characteristic of corrosive substances or electrocautery currents of high wattages applied for long duration.

The anatomy of the oviduct tends to minimize trauma and to promote healing. The oviduct, particularly the intramural segment, is highly vascular. Thermal trauma induced cryosurgically or by cautery requires a prolonged exposure to overcome the buffering of tissue temperature resulting from blood flow, which tends to keep tissue temperature normal. Since delivery tips of instruments must be sufficiently small to enter the uterine tubal ostium to destroy the intramural segment without extensive endometrial and myometrial destruction, the establishment of an appropriate thermal gradient to achieve appropriate depth of coagulation necrosis poses a problem. The rich vascularization also supports rapid growth, healing, and restoration of function.

Finally, the well-developed lymphatic system provides efficient removal of excess interstitial fluid, macromolecules, debris, and cells. Following injury, the lymphatics dilate and become more permeable, aiding in increased lymph flow and uptake of cellular debris.

FAILURE OF STERILIZATION ATTEMPTS

Current hysteroscopic techniques result in bilateral tubal closure rates of 16% to 100%.[24] Patients must employ additional contraceptive techniques for several months after operation, presumably until luminal obliteration and scarring are completed. Pregnancy may occur as a result of any of the following conditions subsequent to attempted hysteroscopic sterilization:

The oviduct remains undamaged and fully functional.

The oviduct sustains minimal damage consistent with maintenance or early return of function and patency.

The severely damaged and occluded oviduct undergoes delayed spontaneous recanalization.

Unilateral closure may result when an occluding agent is blindly introduced into the endometrial cavity under pressure and flows into only one oviduct, owing to differential opening pressures. Alternatively, failure to visualize the uterine tubal ostium and to confirm correct placement of sterilizing instruments can lead to maintenance of function. If the trauma is inadequate, the oviducts may sustain mild damage that involves the epithelium only superficially. Finally, in severely traumatized oviducts, chronic inflammation may lead to reestablishment of patency through delayed formation of tubouterine fistulas. Pregnancies that occur soon after failure of mid-tubal sterilization are associated with a lower ectopic rate than are pregnancies that occur after failure of late sterilization.[13] This may indicate minimal damage and maintenance or rapid reestablishment of a relatively normal lumen immediately after sterilization but chronic damage and loss of tubal function in oviducts that later become patent through fistula formation. This same temporal distribution in poststerilization pregnancy appears following transcervical hysteroscopic sterilization.[24] The patient who has been so sterilized is thus at increased risk for ectopic pregnancy. The causes of tubal gestation are obscure and may include the invasiveness of human trophoblastic tissue, the ability of the blastocyst to implant in and use substrate at extrauterine sites, the failure of tubal transport mechanisms within the oviduct and, most significantly, partial occlusion of the oviduct inconsistent with passage of the developing blastocyst. A disproportionate number of ectopic pregnancies that follow hysteroscopic sterilization are cornual. These are more difficult to diagnose and treat, and they carry the threat of a disastrous outcome.

Some investigators have suggested that damage to the muscle of the intramural portion of the oviduct, or alteration in the oviduct's ability to effect gamete transport, is the basis for the apparent efficacy of sterilization techniques in which tubal patency is maintained.[8,16]

REVERSIBILITY

Reversibility of hysteroscopic sterilization is contingent on the extent of tubal destruction. The achievement of long-term bilateral tubal closure seems inconsistent with reversibility, if one accepts that effective sterilization requires an insult sufficient to discourage tissue regeneration.

Intraluminal plugs offer a promise of reversibility. The destruction of a localized segment of oviduct associated with such devices may not preclude reversal, since a major portion of the tube remains intact. Ideally, if such devices totally occluded the lumen without inducing significant tissue damage, removal would result in reestablished fertility without the need for surgical repair.

REFERENCES

1. BAJPAI VK, SHIPSTONE AC, GUPTA DN et al: Differential response of the ampullary and isthmic cells to ovariectomy and estrogen treatment: An ultrastructural study. Endokrinologie 69:11, 1977
2. BECK LR, BOOTS LR: The comparative anatomy, histology and morphology of the mammalian oviduct. In Johnson AD, Foley CW (eds): The Oviduct and its Functions, p 1. New York, Academic Press, 1974
3. BROSENS IA, VASQUEZ G: Fimbrial microbiopsy. J Reprod Med 16:171, 1976
4. CHATKOFF ML: A biophysicist's view of ovum transport. Gynecol Invest 6:105, 1975
5. COUTINHO EM, MAIA H JR, MATTOS CER et al: Contractility of the fallopian tube. Gynecol Invest 6:146, 1975
6. CRISTOPH FN, DENNIS KJ: The cellular composition of the human oviduct epithelium. Br J Obstet Gynaecol 84:219, 1977
7. FADEL HE, BERNS D, ZANEVELD LJD et al: The human uterotubal junction: A scanning electron microscope study during different phases of the menstrual cycle. Fertil Steril 27:1176, 1976
8. FALK RD, LOWER BR, CROWLEY JP et al: Transcervical fallopian tube blockage with gelatin-resorcinol-formaldehyde (GRF). In Sciarra JJ, Droegemueller W, Speidel JJ (eds): Advances in Female Sterilization Techniques, p 208. Hagerstown, MD, Harper & Row, 1976
9. FREDRICSSON B: Histochemistry of the oviduct. In Hafez ESE, Blandau RJ (eds): The Mammalian Oviduct, p 311. Chicago, University of Chicago Press, 1969
10. GATSALOV MD: The intraorganic venous bed of the human fallopian tube. Arkh Anat 2:87, 1963
11. GATSALOV MD: The lymphatic system of the mucous membrane of the human fallopian tube. Akush Ginek (Sofiia) 5:85, 1963
12. GATSALOV MD: The lymphatic system of the serous membrane of the fallopian tube in humans. Sborn Nauch Trud Severo-Ostetinsk Med Inst 11:166, 1964
13. GRUNERT GM: Late tubal patency following tubal ligation. Fertil Steril 35:406, 1981
14. HAFEZ ESE, BLACK DL: The mammalian uterotubal junction. In Hafez ESE, Blandau RJ (eds): The Mammalian Oviduct: Comparative Biology and Methodology, p 85. Chicago, University of Chicago Press, 1967
15. HEESCH CM, HODGSON BJ: Medicated intratubal silastic spheres do not prevent pregnancy in rabbits. Contraception 13:497, 1976
16. ISRANGKUN C, PHAOSAVASDI S: Hysteroscopic sterilization: Complications in 196 cases. In Sciarra JJ, Droegemueller W, Speidel JJ (eds): Advances in Female Sterilization Techniques, p 148. Hagerstown, MD, Harper & Row, 1976
17. JANSEN RPS: Cyclic changes in the human fallopian tube isthmus and their functional importance. Am J Obstet Gynecol 136:292, 1980
18. MULLER HK: Handbook of Inflammation, Vol III, Mechanisms of Clearing Injured Tissues. Amsterdam, Elsevier, 1981
19. NOVAK E, EVERETT HS: Cyclical and other variations in the tubal epithelium. Am J Obstet Gynecol 16:743, 1928
20. PAUERSTEIN CJ, ALEXANDER RW, MOBLEY JA et al: Comparative anatomy of the inner longitudinal muscle layer of the oviductal isthmus. Obstet Gynecol 35:504, 1970
21. PAUERSTEIN CJ, HODGSON BJ, KRAMEN MA: The anatomy and physiology of the oviduct. In Wynn RM (ed): Obstetrics and Gynecology Annual 1974, p 137. New York, Appleton-Century-Crofts, 1974
22. ROCKER I: The anatomy of the uterotubal junction area. Proc R Soc Med 57:707, 1964
23. RUBIN IC: Most favorable time for transuterine insufflation to test tubal patency. JAMA 84:661, 1925

24. SCIARRA JJ, DROEGEMUELLER W, SPEIDEL JJ (EDS): Advances in Female Sterilization Techniques. Hagerstown, MD, Harper & Row, 1976
25. SWEENEY WJ III: The interstitial portion of the uterine tube—its gross anatomy, course, and length. Obstet Gynecol 19:3, 1962
26. TROWBRIDGE HO, EMLING RC: Inflammation: A Review of the Process. Bristol, Distribution Systems, 1978
27. VASEN LCLM: The intramural part of the fallopian tube. Int J Fertil 4:399, 1959
28. VERHAGE HG, BAREITHER ML, JAFFE RC et al: Cyclic changes in ciliation, secretion, and cell height of the oviductal epithelium in women. Am J Anat 156:505, 1979
29. WOODRUFF JD, PAUERSTEIN CJ: The Fallopian Tube Structure, Function, Pathology, and Management. Baltimore, Williams & Wilkins, 1969

3
The Use of Chemical Agents in Female Sterilization

RALPH M. RICHART

Vasectomy is a simple technique that can readily be applied to large populations using an outpatient approach. Although it is a surgical procedure, male sterilization does not require entering the abdominal cavity and the incision and surgical manipulation are not associated with a high degree of risk. Because the procedure and the anatomy of the vas are relatively straightforward, paramedical technicians can be trained to perform vasectomies and significant numbers of male sterilizations have been performed by nonmedical teams in a number of countries.

In contrast, conventional female sterilization using any of the standard surgical approaches requires abdominal entry because the fallopian tubes are located within the abdominal cavity. A woman who is in the postpartum period or is thin and cooperative can be sterilized surgically through a relatively small incision, as with laparoscopic tubal sterilization. Even in highly favorable cases using state-of-the-art technology, however, a surgeon's skills are required in most settings because vital internal structures are close to the area being treated and may inadvertently be injured. The procedure is highly skill dependent and must be performed in a relatively protected environment.

Sterilization requires of the patient only a single motivation, following which it is, in demographic terms, the most effective family planning procedure in the cafeteria of contraceptive methods. As a surgical procedure, however, it is essentially unavailable to much of the developing world, owing to an inadequate number of physicians, particularly trained surgeons, in rural areas where most of the population lives; further, the surgically trained physicians who do practice in rural areas are overwhelmed with other problems, which to them are more pressing than elective sterilization. Even in the developed countries and even with the use of new technologies, female sterilization is an expensive procedure and absorbs a significant part of the available health funds.

Clearly a female sterilization procedure that is simple, inexpensive, nonmorbid, and nonsurgical would be a useful adjunct to the delivery of family planning services, particularly in the rural areas of developing countries.

Investigators have made a number of attempts to develop a nonsurgical female sterilization technique using cryotherapy, electrocoagulation, mechanical plugs, the instillation of hot water, and chemical materials to produce local epithelial necrosis and fibrosis, and obliteration of the lumen through scarring. The physical methods, such as cryotherapy and silicone rubber instillation, and certain chemical applications, are discussed elsewhere in this volume. It is the purpose of this chapter to review, principally from a historical perspective, the work with those agents not considered in more detail in other chapters.

STRONG CAUSTIC AGENTS

Strong caustic agents, including silver nitrate, zinc chloride, copper sulfate, and formaldehyde, were all studied extensively in animals, and with the exception of copper sulfate, each was also studied in humans (Table 3-1). All these agents produce significant local necrosis when applied topically to any epithelial surface with accompanying acute and chronic inflammation and edema. Their action is produced in part by protein coagulation, and the depth and extent of injury is dependent on the amount of material applied and the concentration of the active ion. The extent of the injury with these agents is difficult to control, and the tissue necrosis may be so extensive as to produce significant morbidity and even mortality in small animals.

In most of the animal experiments and in some of the human applications as well, massive tubal necrosis of the epithelium, the lamina propria, and even the muscularis, was described for silver nitrate, zinc chloride, and copper sulfate. Formaldehyde also produced necrosis but appeared to be more easily controlled. Despite extensive tubal damage, however, the common experience among investigators studying these potential tube-closing agents was that tubal regeneration was routine following a single acute application. It would appear that the acute insult left behind islands of epithelium that were capable of regenerating rapidly and recovering the luminal surfaces before they were

TABLE 3-1. Strong Caustic Agents

CHEMICAL	TYPE OF STUDY	SOURCE
Silver nitrate	Rabbit	Richart et al[43]
		Omran & Hulka[33]
	Monkey	Neuwirth et al[32]
	Pig	Omran & Hulka[33]
	Human	Richart et al[41]
		Ringrose[44]
		Babcock[2]
		Froriep[18]
Zinc chloride	Rabbit	Richart et al[43]
	Monkey	Neuwirth et al[32]
	Rat	Zipper et al[54]
	Human	Babcock[2]
Copper sulfate	Rabbit	Schenker & Polishuk[46]
	Rat	Zipper et al[49]
Formaldehyde (alone or with ethanol)	Rat	Zipper et al[51]
	Rabbit	Schenker & Polishuk[46]
	Human	Davis (in men)[8]

TABLE 3-2. Clinical Trials With Ethanol-Formalin

SOURCE	NO. PATIENTS	NO. APPLICATIONS	CUMULATIVE BILATERAL CLOSURE RATE (%)*
Zipper et al (1972)[51]	8	1	0
	18	2	12
	21	3	35
	30	4	76
	12	5	93
	4	6	95
Total	93		

*After 2 years' follow-up, 8.7% of patients who had a diagnosis of tubal closure had become pregnant.

scarred closed. Even when massive injuries using high concentrations of silver nitrate were produced, a significant proportion of the fallopian tubes remained open, despite major systemic reactions in the animals or humans treated with the substance. It became clear that chronicity was important in producing closure, even with highly active chemicals, and attempts were made to improve the closure rate either by multiple lavages, in the case of formaldehyde; by combining one of these agents with another agent, such as formaldehyde with ethanol; or by suspending an active agent in a vehicle that would prolong the release rate and the epithelial exposure.

In the case of formaldehyde, Zipper and his associates used the substance alone and with ethanol, with repeated applications, and reported a significant increase in the closure rates as the number of applications was increased (Table 3-2). The number of applications to produce a high degree of closure was unacceptable clinically, however, and despite the benign response of the patients to repeated doses of ethanol-formalin, the approach was eventually abandoned. Other investigators combined silver nitrate with a bland carrier and reported good closure rates in animals and in humans, but at higher concentrations there were significant clinical sequelae, including severe chemical pelvic peritonitis,[44] and the silver nitrate–dermabase cream combination was abandoned as not being appropriate for human use.

Our group continued to study silver nitrate because of its good tube-closing properties in a slow-release form and, in collaboration with Gregor and his colleagues,[19] devised a thixotropic silver acetate–alginate system that appeared to be promising. Experiments in primates, however, were unsatisfactory, since even in a slow-release vehicle, the silver acetate could not be controlled with sufficient precision to ensure a lack of unacceptable clinical side-effects.

STRONG ACIDS AND BASES

Strong acids and bases produce an immediate acute inflammatory response and tissue necrosis, accompanied by severe inflammation and edema. Investigations of their use in animals and humans are listed in Table 3-3. The tissue response is similar to that found with other highly polar groups. As with strong caustic agents there is no specificity in the response to strong

TABLE 3-3. Strong Acids and Bases

CHEMICAL	TYPE OF STUDY	SOURCE
Sulfuric acid	Rabbit	Richart et al[43]
Salicylic acid	Rabbit	Richart et al[43]
Phenol	Rabbit Human	Richart et al[43] Salgado[45] People's Republic of China[39]
Sodium hydroxide	Rabbit	Richart et al[43]

acids and bases and their application leads to widespread damage, which is dose related. Sodium hydroxide, sulfuric acid, and salicylic acid have not been applied to the human fallopian tubes, since the experience in animals was unsatisfactory. Although tubal damage could be produced, tubal closure was difficult to secure after an acute injury, the agents were difficult to control, and systemic effects and pelvic chemical peritonitis were common. In contrast, phenol has been used in a slow-release carrier by investigators from the People's Republic of China, who have reported good results. Their experience is detailed in Chapters 17 through 19.

SCLEROSING AGENTS

Various sclerosing agents are used by vascular surgeons to produce venous thrombosis in the treatment of varicosities. Three representatives of this group of drugs—sodium morrhuate, sodium tetradecyl sulfate (Sotradecol), and sodium lauryl sulfate—have been applied to the fallopian tube, but as single agents they produce little or no effect on the tubal epithelium and they fail to produce tubal closure. Sodium morrhuate has been used in humans in association with tubal ligation but appears otherwise not to be clinically useful in producing tubal closure (Table 3-4).

GRANULOMA-PRODUCING AGENTS

Many agents produce granulomas when placed subcutaneously in animals (Table 3-5). The beryllium compounds are particularly active in this regard and rapidly produce very large nodules when injected subcutaneously. Tal-

TABLE 3-4. Sclerosing Agents

CHEMICAL	TYPE OF STUDY	SOURCE
Sodium morrhuate	Rabbit Human	Richart et al[43] Dieckmann & Harrod[13] Pitkin[34]
Sodium tetradecyl sulfate	Rabbit	Richart et al[43]
Sodium lauryl sulfate	Rabbit	Schenker & Polishuk[46]

TABLE 3-5. Granuloma-producing Agents*

CHEMICAL	TYPE OF STUDY
Talc	Rabbit Human†
Asbestos	Rabbit Monkey
Cellobiose	Rabbit Monkey
Silica	Rabbit Monkey
Diatomaceous earth	Rabbit Monkey
Beryllium nitrate	Rabbit Monkey
Quartz	Monkey
Plant cells	Monkey

*Richart RM, Taylor HC, Neuwirth RS: Experimental studies of fallopian tube occlusion. In Richart RM, Prager D (eds): Human Sterilization, pp 360–367. Springfield, IL, Charles C Thomas, 1972.

†Ringrose C: Office tubal sterilization. Obstet Gynecol 42:151, 1973.

cum powder has produced granulomas in the peritoneal cavity, and asbestos is a classic granuloma-producing agent at any site. When these substances are infiltrated into the myometrium in the region of the interstitial fallopian tube, however, relatively small granulomas are produced, and they enlarge only slowly over a prolonged period. Even beryllium nitrate produces only microscopic granulomas after 9 months *in situ.* None of the granulomas produced by any agents reached sufficient size to close the interstitial fallopian tube mechanically. Except for Ringrose's use of talc as a potentiating agent along with silver nitrate,[22,44] the granuloma-producing agents have not been applied chemically and appear to offer no potential for human use in producing tubal blockade.

CYTOTOXIC AGENTS

A variety of cytotoxic agents exist and have been tested for their tube-closing abilities (Table 3-6). These include thioTEPA, colchicine, cadmium, podophyllin, and quinacrine. The use of quinacrine is discussed in detail in other portions of this volume. The other cytotoxic agents produce focal epithelial necrosis but not to a sufficient degree to ablate the epithelium. More importantly, they fail to produce fibrosis and tubal blockade and appear to have no potential for human use. In addition, most cytotoxic agents are mutagenic

TABLE 3-6. Cytotoxic Agents

CHEMICAL	TYPE OF STUDY	SOURCE
ThioTEPA	Rat	Zipper et al[52]
Quinacrine	Rat	Zipper et al[53]
	Rabbit	Zipper et al[50]
		Richart et al[43]
	Human	Zipper et al[54]
		Davidson & Wilkins[7]
		Benoit et al[3]
		Israngkun et al[24]
		Mehtaji et al[26]
		Bhatt et al[4]
		Alvarado et al[1]
Colchicine	Rat	Zipper et al[52]
Cadmium	Rat	Zipper et al[52]
Podophyllin	Rat	Zipper et al[52]

and have distant cellular effects, even when applied locally, and thus would not be suitable for human use even if they closed tubes.

TISSUE ADHESIVES

Tissue adhesives, principally from the cyanoacrylate series, have also been studied extensively and are treated in greater detail in other sections of this volume. Gelatin resorcinol formalin (GRF) was fabricated by Battelle Memorial Institute and was studied extensively in animals but was apparently difficult to control, was inconsistent in producing tubal closure, and was abandoned prior to instituting clinical trials (Table 3-7).

TABLE 3-7. Tissue Adhesives

CHEMICAL	TYPE OF STUDY	SOURCE
Methyl cyanoacrylate	Rabbit	Corfman et al[5]
		Richart et al[43]
	Monkey	Neuwirth et al[32]
	Pig	Omran & Hulka[33]
	Human	Stevenson & Taylor[48]
		Neuwirth et al[31]
Ethyl cyanoacrylate	Rabbit	Richart et al[43]
	Monkey	Richart et al[43]
Isobutyl cyanoacrylate	Rabbit	Richart et al[43]
	Pig	Omran & Hulka[32]
Gelatin resorcinal formalin (GRF)	Rabbit	Grode et al[21]
		Falb et al[17]
	Mouse	Davis et al[11]

OTHER AGENTS

Silicone rubber instillation and intratubal devices have been used to mechanically block the fallopian tube of rabbits[9,11,14,21] and both have reached the stage of clinical trial.[15,34–36] Droegemueller and associates have used cryosurgery to occlude the fallopian tubes of baboons and also of women.[13,18]

Moulding and his collaborators have reported the use of hot water applied to the fallopian tubes of rabbits through a cannula to produce tubal necrosis and fibrosis,[26–28] but the method appears to be difficult to control and clinical trials have not been undertaken.

CLINICAL TRIALS

Clinical trials have been performed with silver nitrate (Table 3-8), ethanol-formalin (see Table 3-2), phenol-mucilage (Tables 3-9 and 3-10), methyl cyanoacrylate (MCA) (Table 3-11), and quinacrine. These trials have used a variety of delivery systems, ranging from simple lavage, to a hysteroscopically guided tubal cannulation,[24,37] to a blind delivery system using a soft rubber balloon as a piston to force the material into the fallopian tubes.[42]

In addition to these systems, Corfman and Taylor described a handheld cannula,[6] the Battelle group fashioned a tube-finding triangulation device,[16]

TABLE 3-8. Clinical Trials With Silver Nitrate ($AgNO_3$) in Hydrophilic Cream

SOURCE	YEAR	NO. PATIENTS	CLOSURE RATE	PREGNANCIES	COMMENTS
Richart et al[41]	1971	14	100%	None	Culdoscopic delivery of 10% $AgNO_3$. Pelvic tenderness and low-grade fever were noted.
Ringrose[44]	1973	100	50%	5	Blind cannula delivery of 10% $AgNO_3$ in dermabase cream.
		100	70%	1	Blind cannula delivery of 15% $AgNO_3$ in dermabase cream.
		60	Not stated	Not stated	Blind cannula delivery in 20% $AgNO_3$ in dermabase cream.
					Patients suffered major complications particularly with higher doses, including two cases of paralytic ileus and other untoward effects. Talc was added to some preparations.

TABLE 3-9. Clinical Trials in 3940 Patients Treated With Phenol-Mucilage, 1979*

% BILATERAL OCCLUSION	COMMENTS
Ranged from 77.6% to 93.5%	A series of compounds was used in which active agent was phenol. In some, salicylic acid was added. No data were given for composition of formulation in each of 7 series, but rate continued to improve until last series reached 93.5%.

*Research Group of Tubal Occlusion by Drugs: Sterilization by occlusion of the fallopian tubes with mucilago phenol: A seven years' clinical observation. Chinese J Obstet Gynecol 14:79, 1979.

TABLE 3-10. Relationship Between Tubal Filling Length and Pregnancy Rate With Phenol-Mucilage

LENGTH OF FILLED TUBE (CM)	PREGNANCY RATE (%)
1–2	7.1
2–4	3.3
4	1.1
Ampulla	0.08
Fimbria	0.0

*Adapted from data in Research Group of Tubal Occlusion by Drugs: Sterilization by occlusion of the fallopian tubes with mucilago phenol: A seven years' clinical observation. Chinese J Obstet Gynecol 14:79, 1979.

TABLE 3-11. Results of Clinical Trials With MCA

SOURCE	YEAR	NO. PATIENTS	BILATERIAL CLOSURE (%)	COMMENTS
Stevenson & Taylor[48]	1972	12		Prehysterectomy application
Stevenson[47]	1976	34	66	Hysterosalpingography at 8 weeks
		11	90	Reapplication of MCA
Neuwirth et al[31]	1980	131	72	Closure rates of 54% to 78% in three series with various volumes of MCA (0.4–0.65)
		19	74	Reapplication of MCA
Richart & Neuwirth*	1981	180	80	0.6 ml MCA; modified FEMCEPT device
		19	98	Reapplication of MCA following patency detected by hysterosalpingography

*Unpublished data.

and Moulding and associates attempted to isolate the cornua with a balloon to facilitate tubal injection.[29] These methods were largely unsuccessful.

There are a number of factors that constrain the design of a delivery system for caustic chemicals to the fallopian tubes. The principal one among these is that any substance toxic to the tubal epithelium will also be toxic to the peritoneal cavity. Thus, the system must reproducibly deliver the tubal sclerosing agent to the tubal lumen without producing an intraperitoneal spill. This constraint has been met in the FEMCEPT/MCA system by carefully controlling the volume and viscosity and by the precision of the blind delivery system. In the case of quinacrine, the drug appears not to produce significant side-effects when delivered to the peritoneal cavity, but the constraint has also been met by using delivery systems that diffuse the drug slowly into the fallopian tube, minimizing the quantity that reaches the peritoneal cavity. Other more caustic agents have been difficult to apply in a clinically acceptable fashion and have largely been abandoned. These considerations have been discussed in greater detail elsewhere.[39]

DISCUSSION

Attempts to close the fallopian tubes by the use of caustic chemicals date back to 1849, when Froriep used a nitric acid-coated probe to cauterize the tubal lumen.[17] Babcock also used a chemical contraceptive approach in 1924.[2] Other attempts at an outpatient-oriented sterilization approach used principally hot cautery until the early 1960s, when systematic studies directed toward a chemical cauterization technique were undertaken. Large numbers of chemical agents from virtually every class of compound that might be appropriate candidates for this procedure were screened, but most were found wanting.

At present, only three chemical agents are actively being pursued in clinical trials: quinacrine, phenol, and methyl cyanoacrylate. The efficacy of these three compounds is comparable, but they differ significantly in their modes of delivery. The phenol-based system apparently requires a high degree of skill in blindly placing a cannula at the tubal ostium. It is not clear to what degree this skill is transferable to large numbers of operators. The quinacrine investigators have yet to settle on a delivery mode, but the newer approaches to delivery, using IUD vectors or slow-release pellets, will provide great simplicity, if the experiments produce acceptable closure rates. The FEMCEPT system is more complex in its engineering and is a more expensive delivery system than a reusable cannula or an IUD vector, but it has produced increasingly satisfactory bilateral closure rates, and the delivery technique appears to be readily transferable, since most of the fourteen investigators who have used the system obtain comparable closure rates.

The nonchemical mechanical tubal blockade systems, including the intratubal devices and the silicone rubber technique, use hysteroscopy to identify the tubal ostia and to administer the tube-blocking device. Hysteroscopy is a highly sophisticated, mechanically complex technique that requires great skill for its application and service accessibility. It is not clear whether any system that uses a hysteroscope for delivery will be widely applicable, particularly in the developing countries. Whether any or all of these outpatient-directed female sterilization techniques will gain widespread application must await the results of fertility trials under field use in a variety of settings.

The acceptability of one or more of these techniques depends, however, not only on the clinical results but on the context in which they are introduced and the context in which the data are compared with other family planning techniques. Surgical tubal ligation is a definitive procedure in which the tubes are physically identified and physically closed by coagulation, segmental excision, or application of a variety of occluding appliances. These techniques have an extremely low failure rate. However, they have significant morbidity and some mortality and are essentially unavailable to most of the world, owing to a lack of surgeons and operative support facilities. Intrauterine contraceptive devices, steroidal contraceptives, and barrier techniques all have a high failure rate and a high discontinuation rate, and the IUDs and steroidal contraceptives are associated with a variable degree of side-effects.

The outpatient female sterilization techniques should be thought of as lying someplace between the IUD and surgical sterilization in terms of acceptability to users. They will never achieve the high degree of reliability that has come to be associated with surgical sterilization, but they are nonoperative, they do not require extensive surgical support facilities, they do not require surgical skills, and they can readily be applied to large numbers of women. The FEMCEPT/MCA system, for example, is applied with about the same ease as is an IUD insertion. There is clearly a trade-off between expensive, complex, highly available procedures on the one hand and inexpensive, simple, but less reliable procedures on the other. As long as a woman understands the trade-offs, then she should be free to choose among the techniques.

In areas in which surgical sterilization is, for all practical purposes, unavailable to the majority of the population, the introduction of these simple, rapid, inexpensive outpatient-oriented techniques should fill a significant gap in the armamentarium of family planning procedures. From a demographic point of view, the small number of failures should be unimportant in proportion to the high success rate, provided the women using these outpatient techniques are not led to believe that they are the equivalent of conventional surgical sterilization and also are not led to expect a 100% success rate.

Strategically, a variety of protocols can be constructed using an outpatient-oriented sterilization program, with the choice again representing a trade-off between expense and success rate. In some settings, for example, the choice may be to make a single application, to detect the failures as pregnancies, and to abort those women with failed procedures and then resterilize them using a second application or a conventional technique. In other settings it may be appropriate to treat each woman twice, thus lowering the failure rate but increasing the cost. In the most medically sophisticated areas, a single treatment followed by a hysterosalpingogram to identify the failures may be chosen.

Whichever route is chosen, there are sufficient data now to predict that these techniques can potentially be applied to large numbers of women in a short period of time with low morbidity and a high degree of demographic effectiveness. Whether they will in fact prove acceptable to the women who must use them must await field trials, but the results to date are encouraging.

REFERENCES

1. ALVARADO A, QUINONES R, AZNAR R: Tubal instillation of quinacrine under hysteroscopic control. In Sciarra JJ, Butler JC Jr, Speidel JJ (eds): Hysteroscopic Sterilization, pp 85–94. New York, Intercontinental Book Corporation, 1974
2. BABCOCK WW: Chemical hysterectomy. Am J Obstet Gynecol 7:693–696, 1924
3. BENOIT A, MELANCON J, GAGNON M: Chemically-induced tubal occlusion in the human female using intrauterine instillation of quinacrine. Contraception 12:95, 1975
4. BHATT RV, PATHAK ND, CHAUHAN LN et al: A study of transcervical instillation of quinacrine before hysterectomy to test tubal blockage. Bombay, India Fertility Research Program, September 1977, p 171
5. CORFMAN PA, RICHART RM, TAYLOR HC: Response of the rabbit oviduct to a tissue adhesive. Science 148:1348, 1965
6. CORFMAN PA, TAYLOR HC: An instrument for transcervical treatment of the oviducts and uterine cornua. Obstet Gynecol 27:800, 1966
7. DAVIDSON OW, WILKINS C: Chemically-induced tubal occlusion in the human female following a single instillation of quinacrine. Contraception 7:333, 1973
8. DAVIS JE: New methods of vas occlusion. In Zatuchni GI, Labbok MH, Sciarra JJ (eds): Research Frontiers in Fertility Regulation, pp 252–261. Hagerstown, Md, Harper & Row, 1980
9. DAVIS RH, ERB R, KYRIAZIS GA et al: Fallopian tube occlusion in rabbits with silicone rubber. J Reprod Med 14:56, 1975
10. DAVIS RH, MCDONALD J, KYRIAZES G et al: Effect on fertility of intrauterotubal injection of gelatin. Obstet Gynecol 42:446, 1973
11. DAVIS RH, MOONKA EK, PLATT HA et al: Chronic occlusion of the rabbit fallopian tube with silicone rubber. Obstet Gynecol 6:142, 1978
12. DIECKMANN WJ, HARROD JP JR: Tubal ligation (sterilization) by a modified Madlener method. Am J Obstet Gynecol 68:897–902, 1954
13. DROEGEMUELLER W, GREER BE, DAVIS JR et al: Cryocoagulation of the endometrium at the uterine cornua. Am J Obstet Gynecol 131:1, 1978
14. ERB RA, DAVIS RH, KYRIAZES G et al: Device and technique for blocking the Fallopian tubes. Contemp OB/GYN, February 1974, p 92
15. ERB RA, REED TP: Hysteroscopic oviductal blocking with formed-in-place silicone rubber plugs: I. Method and apparatus. J Reprod Med 23:65–68, 1979
16. FALB RD, LOWER BR, CROWLEY JP et al: Transcervical fallopian tube blockage with gelatin-resorcinol-formaldehyde (GRF). In Sciarra JJ, Droegemueller W, Speidel JJ (eds): Advances in Female Sterilization Techniques, pp 208–215. Hagerstown, Md, Harper & Row, 1976
17. FRORIEP R: Zur vorbeugung der notwendigkeit des kaiserschnitts und der perforation. Notizen Nat Neilkd 211:9–10, 1849
18. GREER BE, DROEGEMUELLER W, BINGHAM PE et al: Uterine cryosurgery in baboons. In Sciarra JJ, Droegemueller W, Speidel JJ (eds): Advances in Female Sterilization Techniques, pp 231–238. Hagerstown, Md, Harper & Row, 1976
19. GREGOR HP, HSIA HT, PALEVSKY S et al: Fallopian tube cauterization by silver ion-polymer gels. In Paul DR, Harris FW (eds): Controlled Release Polymeric Formulations. New York, ACS Symposium Series #33, 1976
20. GRODE GA, PAVKOV KL, FALB RD: Feasibility study on the use of a tissue adhesive for the nonsurgical blocking of fallopian tubes. Fertil Steril 22:552, 1971
21. HEFNAWI F, FUCHS A-R, LAURENCE KA: Control of fertility by temporary occlusion of the oviduct. Am J Obstet Gynecol 99:421, 1967
22. IMLACH A: Edmonton gynecologist at legal odds with provincial college. Can Med Assoc J 112:1345–1355, 1975
23. ISRANGKUN C, PHAOSAVASDI S, NEUWIRTH RS et al: Clinical evaluation of quinacrine hydrochloride for sterilization of the human female. Contraception 14:75–80, 1976
24. LINDEMANN H-J, MOHR J: Review of clinical experience with hysteroscopic sterilization. In Sciarra JJ, Droegemueller W, Speidel JJ (eds): Advances in Female Sterilization Techniques, pp 153–161. Hagerstown, Md, Harper & Row, 1976
25. MEHTAJI S, JADWANI K, GOYAL V; Chemical sterilization with quinacrine. Fourth Transaction of Scientific Papers. Bombay, Indian Fertility Research Program, September 1977, p 167
26. MOULDING T, NORTON W, ORR W: Preliminary studies for achieving transcervical oviduct occlusion by hot water or low pressure steam. Adv Plann Parent 12:79–85, 1977

27. MOULDING T, SIROTTA P: Hot water as a tubal occluding agent. Contraception 19:433–442, 1979
28. MOULDING T, SIROTTA P: Hot water as a tubal occluding agent: Studies in detail. National Technical Information Service, PB293382
29. MOULDING T, STRAW W, THOMPSON H: The contrast pressure technique for female sterilization. Contraception 13:547–557, 1976
30. NEUWIRTH RS, RICHART RM, STEVENSON TC et al: An outpatient approach to female sterilization with methylcyanoacrylate. Am J Obstet Gynecol 136:951–956, 1980
31. NEUWIRTH RS, RICHART RM, TAYLOR HC: Chemical induction of tubal blockade in the monkey. Obstet Gynecol 38:51–54, 1971
32. OMRAN KF, HULKA JF: Tubal occlusion: A comparative study. Int J Fertil 15:226, 1970
33. PITKIN RM: Sodium morrhuate for tubal sterilization. Obstet Gynecol 28:680, 1966
34. RAKSHIT B: Attempts at chemical blocking of the Fallopian tube for female sterilisation. J Obstet Gynaecol India 20:618, 1970
35. REED TP, ERB RA: Hysteroscopic oviductal blocking with formed-in-place silicone rubber plugs: II. Clinical studies. J Reprod Med 23:69–72, 1979
36. REED TP, ERB RA: Tubal occlusion with silicone rubber. J Reprod Med 25:25–28, 1980
37. REED TP, ERB RA, DEMAEYER J: Tubal occlusion with silicone rubber: An update. Presented at Lankenau Hospital, January 1980
38. Research Group of Tubal Occlusion by Drugs. Sterilization by occlusion of the Fallopian tubes with mucilago phenol: A seven years' clinical observation. Chin J Obstet Gynecol 14:79, 1979
39. RICHART RM: Female sterilization using chemical agents. In Zatuchni GI (ed): Research Frontiers in Fertility Regulation, vol 1, no 5, December 1981. Chicago, Program for Applied Research of Fertility Regulation
40. RICHART RM, GUTIERREZ-NAJAR AJ, NEUWIRTH RS: Transvaginal human sterilization: A preliminary report. Am J Obstet Gynecol 111:108–110, 1971
41. RICHART RM, NEUWIRTH RS: Unpublished data
42. RICHART RM, NEUWIRTH RS, BOLDUC L: Single application fertility regulating device: Description of a new instrument. Am J Obstet Gynecol 127:86–90, 1977
43. RICHART RM, TAYLOR HC, NEUWIRTH RS: Experimental studies of fallopian tube occlusion. In Richart RM, Prager D (eds): Human Sterilization, pp 360–367. Springfield, IL, Charles C Thomas, 1972
44. RINGROSE C: Office tubal sterilization. Obstet Gynecol 42:151, 1973
45. SALGADO C: Sterilisation induced by intrauterine caustic injections. An Brasil Genet, June 1941
46. SCHENKER JG, POLISHUK JG: Regeneration of rabbit endometrium following intrauterine instillation of chemical agents. Gynecol Invest 4:1–13, 1973
47. STEVENSON TC: Methylcyanoacrylate (MCA) for tubal occlusion In Sciarra JJ, Droegemueller W, Speidel JJ (eds): Advances in Female Sterilization Techniques, pp 216–224. Hagerstown, MD, Harper & Row, 1976
48. STEVENSON TC, TAYLOR DS: The effect of methylcyanoacrylate tissue adhesive on the human fallopian tube and endometrium. J Obstet Gynecol 79:1028, 1972
49. ZIPPER J, MEDEL M: Human fertility control through the use of endouterine metal antagonisms of trace elements. In Control of Human Fertility. Nobel Symposium 15, Stockholm, Almqvist & Wiksell, 1970
50. ZIPPER J, INSUNZA S: Pharmacological agents that potentiate or inhibit the occlusive action of quinacrine in the rabbit tube and rat uterus. In Duncan GW, Falb RD, Speidel JJ (eds): Female Sterilization: Prognosis for Simplified Outpatient Procedures, pp 131–149. New York, Academic Press, 1972
51. ZIPPER J, MEDEL M, PASTENE L et al: Intrauterine instillation of chemical cytotoxic agents for tubal sterilization and treatment of functional metrorrhagias. Int J Fertil 14:289, 1969
52. ZIPPER J, MEDEL M, PRAGER R: Alterations in fertility induced by unilateral intrauterine instillation of cytotoxic compounds in rats. Am J Obstet Gynecol 101:971, 1968
53. ZIPPER J, PRAGER R, MEDEL M: Biological changes induced by unilateral intrauterine instillations of quinacrine in the rat and their reversal by either estrogen or progesterone. Fertil Steril 24:48, 1973
54. ZIPPER JA, STACHETTI E, MEDEL M: Human fertility control by transvaginal application of quinacrine on the fallopian tube. Fertil Steril 21:581, 1970

4

Evaluation of the Acceptability of Nonsurgical Sterilization

ROCHELLE N. SHAIN

SUSAN C. M. SCRIMSHAW

Physicians and reproductive physiologists engaged in contraceptive research seldom have formal training in social science. Yet the hard-won products of their work must ultimately be used by people—people who may not perceive the contraceptive as the researcher had intended or hoped, people who might even reject it. Clinical trials may go poorly because of the "human element," and the researcher trained only in biology may not suspect the extent to which individual preferences have affected results. Ideally, the researcher should have access to social science information on potential acceptability of a method, with attention paid to all its attributes, as it is being developed.[6,7] At the very least, clinical trials, even very early ones with small samples, should be accompanied by data collection instruments designed to measure acceptability.

This chapter presents a sample data collection instrument for assessing the acceptability of nonsurgical methods of sterilization, either before their introduction (potential acceptability) or during clinical trials (actual acceptability). The model questionnaire presented in Appendix 4-1 is based on quinacrine or methyl cyanoacrylate (MCA) occlusion, but the accompanying discussion is intended to facilitate adaptation of the questionnaire to other methods. The questionnaire is itself an adaptation of one used to assess the potential acceptability of reversible sterilization.[10] Data analysis is also briefly discussed.

BACKGROUND

CONTRACEPTIVE ACCEPTABILITY

The development of new contraceptives during the 20th century has been characterized first and foremost by the search for safe and effective methods. The concept of method acceptability was something of a luxury. However, researchers have since discovered that good (but not yet perfect) technical solutions are not necessarily universally embraced. This failure to use the products of science can be attributed both to variations in individual perceptions of a method and to cultural norms that influence acceptability.

Grateful acknowledgment is made to Drs. Harold D. Dickson and Gerald I. Zatuchni for their advice regarding statistical analysis and the description of chemical occlusion, respectively.

On the individual level, with the growth of the consumer movement in the United States, there has been a corresponding change in the individual from passive acceptor to reactor to both physicians and medical technology.[1] This has been well documented in the medical sociology literature. For example, Friedson discusses the trapped feeling physicians have as they are caught between patient demands and their own feelings about optimal care.[2] While there has not been the same consumer activism in medicine internationally, most individuals still do not accept new technology without question.

Cross-culturally, there has been wide variation in preferred contraceptive methods.[5,7,8] Polgar and Marshall provide an analysis that clarifies acceptability from both the individual and the cross-cultural perspective.[5,7] In their key article, "The Search for Culturally Acceptable Fertility Regulating Methods," they describe the points of intervention in the human reproductive cycle and how some of these are perceived in different societies.[7] They also delineate attributes of the various methods, with examples of how these affect acceptability. As discussed by Marshall in another paper,[5] fertility regulation methods are viewed as clusters of attributes, not simply as material objects. These attributes include actual facts about the method (*e.g.*, it is a female method) as well as perceived attributes that may not be based on reality (*e.g.*, using it will make one weak). The decision to use a given contraceptive will be based on weights given to the positive and negative attributes, as well as on the intensity of the desire to postpone or prevent another pregnancy. Of course, the assessment of a given method will vary somewhat from individual to individual and will reflect cultural perspectives as well. The measurement of the perception of both real and perceived attributes will help the researcher understand more precisely which aspects of a method are most attractive and which make it less likely to be used.

Until very recently, most acceptability research was conducted *post facto*, after problems had developed with specific methods or programs. We emphasize that methods should be evaluated at earlier stages in their development. There are limitations to this approach; for example, as noted by Keller, people change and may eventually accept methods they previously thought they would not use.[4] Nonetheless, the resultant data serve important functions, particularly when all the attributes of a given method are known. In the earliest stages of method development, research provides insight into individual characteristics that are so unacceptable that they should be minimized or eliminated and those that are so highly desirable that they should be given additional emphasis. At the time a method is introduced, acceptability research adds credibility to clinical trials. Although subjects of clinical trials are atypical, since they are self-selected, often paid, and receive considerable attention, knowing and understanding their reactions to a specific method is essential.[4] Lastly, acceptability data can be used to guide actual programs in terms of the methods offered, the amount and type of educational material provided, and the explanations and support appropriate to the method.

It is not enough for social scientists to measure acceptability on the one hand and for biomedical researchers to develop new methods and improve existing ones on the other hand. The two must work together for optimum results: good, acceptable contraceptive methods that are widely used. The protocol presented in the remainder of this chapter is offered as a step toward the goal of appropriate integration of biomedical and social research.

EVALUATION OF THE ACCEPTABILITY OF REVERSIBLE STERILIZATION

In 1977–1978, a study was undertaken to assess the potential importance of reversibility on selection of tubal sterilization. Despite increasing biomedical research in this area and positive feelings among professionals concerning its importance, there were *no* baseline data on how much more acceptable sterilization might be if it were reversible. If overall receptivity to new technology could be determined before it achieved its final form, women could be provided with a voice in contraceptive development and scientists could obtain the kind of information that could lead to maximizing acceptance of that technology. Although it appeared self-evident that reversibility would significantly enhance sterilization acceptability, a fundamental question demanded an answer: if sterilization retained its basic character, would the appeal of reversibility be overshadowed and perhaps be eliminated by the prospect of two surgical procedures?

In order to focus on the attribute of reversibility, all other characteristics of current methods, such as surgery, costs, and effectiveness were held constant. Study participants were told to make the following asssumptions about reversible sterilization: it would be as effective as current techniques in preventing pregnancy; it would cost the same as an initial ligation; it would be reversible 95% of the time; and each operation, the one to tie women's tubes and the one to untie them, would be a relatively simple procedure involving surgery performed in the hospital under general anesthesia. If, under such circumstances, significantly more women believed they would undergo sterilization if it were reversible, reversibility could be identified as a singularly important variable.

Completed questionnaires were obtained from 1074 randomly selected obstetric and gynecology patients in offices and clinics throughout San Antonio. Current attitudes and intentions toward permanent sterilization were compared with what women believed their attitudes and intentions would be toward hypothetically reversible sterilization. Results indicated a highly significant increase in selection of reversible surgical sterilization over all other existing contraceptive methods.[10] Interestingly, however, of the women objecting to permanent sterilization, 14% did so primarily because of its surgical character. Even more important, unnecessary surgery was the most prominent objection to reversible surgical sterilization: 43% of subjects who rejected the procedure did so primarily because of its surgical requirements.[9] These data indicate that there may be a sizable proportion of women for whom nonsurgical sterilization may be the ideal contraceptive method.

In order to evaluate potential and actual acceptability of nonsurgical sterilization, the questionnaire and methodology of the prior study have been adapted to current purposes. As already noted, the model questionnaire appearing in Appendix 4-1 is based on chemical (quinacrine or MCA) occlusion. Quinacrine and MCA were selected because many of their characteristics are already known and can be described to potential acceptors. Because decisions made by study subjects regarding potential acceptability will have been based on full information about chemical sterilization, results can be expected to correspond better to actual behavior than do those of the previous study.

ADAPTATION OF THE RESEARCH INSTRUMENT

The most important overall principle in adapting the basic questionnaire to this and other studies is use of appropriate language. Vocabulary and sentence structure must be sufficiently simple so that the questionnaire is fully understandable to non–high school graduates but not so simple that it is offensive to better educated women. Where literacy levels are low, the questionnaire should be available in the subject's preferred language and should be administered by an interviewer who is fluent in the given language.

The structure of the model questionnaire is almost identical to that of its predecessor: section I provides an explanation of the study, section II elicits sociodemographic information, section III elicits attitudes and intentions toward current methods of surgical sterilization, and section IV elicits attitudes and intentions toward the type of sterilization under study, in this case quinacrine or MCA occlusion. The current questionnaire contains an additional section (section V) for use only during clinical trials. It will be discussed briefly in a separate section toward the end of this chapter.

It should be noted that, although men play a role in deciding for or against female sterilization, the research instrument is directed toward women. The questionnaire has been adapted and employed to study couple decisions regarding reversible male and female sterilization. However, in the interest of simplicity (subject recruitment, data analysis, and interpretation), only the female version has been adapted to current purposes.

SECTION I—EXPLANATION

The explanation page defines birth control, describes current methods of male and female sterilization and provides a description appropriate to either quinacrine or MCA occlusion. This description is based on what the characteristics of chemical occlusion are likely to be at the time these procedures are made publicly available. The importance of providing a clear and thorough description of the study procedure cannot be overemphasized. Results are highly suspect in the absence of appropriate explanation. Negative as well as positive differences between the study procedure and the method with which it is being directly compared should be delineated. Similarities between the new procedure and existing contraceptive methods should be noted where appropriate. Because adequate explanation is so critical to the success of any study, the following paragraph describing quinacrine or MCA sterilizaton is included within the text. It provides information on type and duration of treatment, overall characteristics, permanence, effectiveness, site of treatment in terms of hospital versus doctor's office, surgery and anesthesia requirements, side-effects, and costs:

> Research is being conducted to develop various types of sterilization procedures for men and women that do not require surgery. In this questionnaire, we are

> concerned with *one* method of nonsurgical sterilization for women. It would involve inserting a chemical into the mouth of the uterus (womb) through the vagina, followed by another treatment, 1 month later. This would cause the tubes to close within 6 to 12 weeks. During this time other contraceptive methods should be used to prevent pregnancy. In this questionnaire we will refer to this method of nonsurgical sterilization as having one's tubes blocked or closed. Such a procedure could *never* be undone or reversed. We expect that, when first introduced, it will not be as successful as surgical sterilization in preventing pregnancy. We expect it will be successful in 95% of cases, compared with close to 100% for the surgical procedure. Your tubes would be blocked in the doctor's office, without need for anesthesia. There should not be any short- or long-term effects, except for some mild cramping pain at the time of treatment. We estimate that this procedure will cost much less than surgical sterilization.

This paragraph can serve as a model for describing other methods of nonsurgical sterilization.

SECTION II—SOCIO-DEMOGRAPHIC QUESTIONS

This section elicits information on the following independent variables: age, marital status, ethnicity, religion, education, employment status, total family income, pregnancy status, fecundity, health problems during pregnancy, parity, intended parity, intention to have more children, status of last pregnancy (in terms of being wanted or unwanted), willingness to consider a future abortion, prior abortion experience, use of contraceptives, current contraceptive behavior, contraceptive method, satisfaction with contraceptive method, and previous discontinuation of a method because of dissatisfaction.

SECTION III—RECEPTIVITY TOWARD CURRENT METHODS OF STERILIZATION

This section first establishes whether or not the subject is part of a sterilized couple. Only those women who respond negatively are invited to complete the remainder of the questionnaire. Women's knowledge of sterilization and their friends' prior experience with such procedures are also ascertained.

Most questions focus on subjects' approval of and actual intentions toward surgical sterilization. Women are asked if they would *seriously consider* having their tubes tied after having finished childbearing; if they actually *intend* to eventually undergo sterilization; and, if they are finished childbearing, whether they *plan* to be sterilized within the following *12 months*. Thus, each successive question more closely measures potential behavior.

In order to understand negative responses, subjects who would not *seriously consider* sterilization or are unsure are asked to explain their feelings (see question 34). Eleven possible explanations are provided, including fears of physical and defeminizing aftereffects; partner objections; preference for vasectomy for one's partner; and objections to permanency, surgery, expense, and limiting one's reproductive potential. Women are asked to check all responses that apply to themselves and to double check their primary objection. Furthermore, women who do not *intend* to undergo permanent sterilization are also asked to note their alternative contraceptive courses. The options provided are "other contraceptive methods," "vasectomy for partner," "use of no method," and "preference for tubal sterilization if less expensive." Although the latter is not an alternative course, it was determined in the first survey that some women felt it was their best response to the question. Again, in an attempt to understand why some women may object to sterilization, subjects are asked if they believe sterilization makes women more or less attractive to men. Interestingly, in the prior study significantly more Mexican- than Anglo-American women were concerned about possible negative changes.[9]

In order to ultimately determine if increased acceptability of a new procedure may make a demographic impact in terms of births or pregnancies averted, women who intend to be sterilized are asked how many years they will wait to undergo the procedure after having their last wanted child and how many children they will have at that time. As in the case of other questions in this section, responses are compared with their respective counterparts in section IV.

SECTION IV—RECEPTIVITY TOWARD NON-SURGICAL METHODS OF STERILIZATION

Questions in section IV essentially duplicate those from the previous section. The list of objections provided to women who either will not seriously consider nonsurgical sterilization or are unsure have been appropriately modified (see question 41). Nine of the 12 objections are identical to those in section III. Objections to surgery and to the expense have been removed. Three additional objections have been substituted. These are: "I do not like the fact that there would be *no* chance to undo or reverse the procedure;" "although nonsurgical sterilization would prevent pregnancy in 95 of 100 women, I am afraid that in my case it would fail," and "although nonsurgical sterilization would cost much less than surgical sterilization, it still may be too expensive."

In order to adapt this question to other methods of nonsurgical sterilization, appropriate objections should be substituted for the inappropriate ones. For example, in the case of future methods of nonsurgical sterilization that may be reversible, the item objecting to the absolute permanence of quinacrine or MCA occlusion would be removed. It would be replaced by a more appropriate response, such as, "Although removing the plugs should allow 95 of 100 women to become pregnant again, I am afraid that in my case it would not work."

SUBJECT RECRUITMENT AND DATA ANALYSIS

Methods of subject recruitment and questionnaire administration employed in the prior study proved cost efficient and productive of consistent and reliable data. They are therefore recommended for this study.

All obstetric/gynecologic patients (except those *obviously* long past reproductive age) appearing on randomly selected days in a particular office or clinic, or all women, or a random sample thereof, residing in a village in a developing country, should be asked to anonymously complete the questionnaire. A research assistant should explain the purpose of the study and check the completed questionnaire in the subject's presence for completeness and consistency of response. Although almost all women are asked to participate, analysis should be confined to responses from potential acceptors of nonsurgical sterilization, that is, those women of reproductive age who are neither sterile, already sterilized, nor in a sexual union with a vasectomized male. Using this procedure, a random distribution of respondents will be achieved; nonproductive coding and statistical analysis will be eliminated, and feelings of discrimination (*e.g.*, on the part of deceptively older-looking women) will be avoided. The research assistant, if unsure that a woman is under 50, should assume it.

The questionnaire is easily coded, and study results lend themselves to straightforward statistical analysis. In order to determine if nonsurgical sterilization is significantly more acceptable than surgical procedures, responses to the questions on attitudes and intentions toward nonsurgical methods should be compared with responses to the equivalent questions on surgical procedures. Specifically, the following computations must be made: of those women initially rejecting surgical sterilization, what proportion accept nonsurgical methods, and of those women initially accepting surgical sterilization, what proportion accept and what proportion reject the nonsurgical procedure. The net difference is then computed and analyzed for statistical significance using McNemar's one-tailed Z test for correlated proportions.[3] The same type of analysis is used to determine whether women's perceptions of female attractiveness following surgical sterilization are any different from those following nonsurgical sterilization.

In order to predict the types of women most likely to be affected by development of nonsurgical sterilization, any or all of the dependent variables concerning attitudes and intentions toward both surgical and nonsurgical sterilization should be cross-tabulated with the independent variables contained in section II and with one of the items contained in section III, "friends' experience with tubal sterilization." After the influence of the various sociodemographic and attitudinal variables on intention to be sterilized (both surgically and nonsurgically) are considered, step-wise discriminant function analysis should be used to determine which variables have a significant independent impact on intention to undergo nonsurgical sterilization and on the response change from initially rejecting surgical sterilization to accepting nonsurgical procedures.[11]

In order to determine whether the availability of nonsurgical sterilization would induce women to wait less time after having their last wanted child to be sterilized (and thus avert the possibility of an unwanted pregnancy) or to have fewer children, the appropriate comparisons must be made. McNemar's one-tailed T test for correlated means should be used to determine the significance of possible differences.[3]

USE IN CLINICAL TRIALS

All patients involved in clinical trials should be asked to complete the questions in section V of the questionnaire. Responses will help the clinician or researcher understand women's feelings toward nonsurgical sterilization immediately after they have undergone the procedure. The questions address the women's feelings about the particular method, specifically, perceived advantages, suggestions for possible improvements, perceived detriments, adequacy of the information provided, current well-being, unanswered concerns, treatment by staff, and future recommendations to friends. Analysis of resultant data will provide a quick overview of how the procedure itself and the service delivery system can be improved to increase acceptability.

The description of chemical occlusion provided in section I, or an adaptation thereof, can be given to patients before they undergo the actual procedure. Most questions in section II (those to be eliminated or modified are appropriately marked) should be administered to all patients if the clinician or researcher wants to know which types of women find nonsurgical sterilization most and least acceptable and why. Sections III and IV are not applicable for use in clinical trials.

SUMMARY AND CONCLUSIONS

In summary, the model questionnaire is a very flexible instrument that previously provided consistent and reliable data. It was easily adapted to evaluate the acceptability of nonsurgical sterilization by way of chemical occlusion. With minor modifications involving description of the study procedure and delineation of possible objections to that procedure, the revised questionnaire can be readily adapted to study the acceptability of other forms of nonsurgical sterilization. It is easily administered and coded, and study results lend themselves to straightforward statistical analysis. In addition to its use in evaluating the acceptability of nonsurgical sterilization before its actual introduction, two sections (II and V) are designed for use in clinical trials. If translated with appropriate attention to nuances of meaning within the given language and to overall cultural equivalence, this research instrument, or a simplified version, can be employed as a prototype in developing countries as well as in developed ones. Its use will serve to integrate biomedical and social research, thus helping to reduce costly trial and error.

REFERENCES

1. BURNHAM JC: American medicine's golden age: What happened to it? Science 215:1474–1479, 1982
2. FRIEDSON E: Prepaid group practice and the new demanding patient. Milbank Mem Fund Q 51:473–488, 1973
3. GUILFORD JP: Fundamental Statistics in Psychology and Education, p 188. San Francisco, McGraw-Hill, 1965
4. KELLER A: Contraceptive acceptability research: Utility and limitations. Stud Fam Plann 10:230–237, 1979
5. MARSHALL JF: Fertility regulating methods: Cultural acceptability for potential adopters. In Duncan G, Hilton EJ, Kraeger P et al (eds): Fertility Control Methods: Strategies for Introduction, pp 125–132. New York, Academic Press, 1973
6. MARSHALL JF: Acceptability of fertility regulating methods: Designing technology to fit people. Prevent Med 6:65–73, 1977
7. POLGAR S, MARSHALL JF: The search for culturally acceptable fertility regulating methods. In Marshall JF, Polgar S (eds): Culture, Natality and Family Planning. Chapel Hill, Carolina Population Center, University of North Carolina, Monograph No. 21, 1976

8. SHAIN RN: Acceptability of contraceptive methods and services: A cross-cultural perspective. In Shain RN, Pauerstein CJ (eds): Fertility Control: Biologic and Behavioral Aspects, pp 229–312. Hagerstown, MD, Harper & Row, 1980
9. SHAIN RN: Objections to tubal sterilization: What reversibility can and cannot overcome. Contraception 3:213–225, 1980
10. SHAIN RN: The potential impact of reversibility on selection of tubal sterilization. Contraception 3:227–240, 1980
11. SHAIN RN, DICKSON HD: Tubal sterilization: Characteristics of women most affected by the option of reversibility. Soc Sci Med 16:1067–1077, 1982

Appendix

Questionnaire on a Nonsurgical Method of Sterilization for Women

I. EXPLANATION OF STUDY

This questionnaire is part of a study on sterilization procedures for women, sponsored by [*the name of funding agency or university*]. We are conducting the study because we want to understand women's feelings toward various methods of sterilization. We, therefore, will be asking you questions about sterilization operations that involve surgery and about another sterilization procedure that does not require surgery. Your answers to these questions will help us decide the importance of developing a nonsurgical method of sterilization. Please answer each question as carefully as you possibly can. Every question has an answer that applies to you. However, you may refuse to answer any or all questions. No one will know how you answered this questionnaire because your name is never used. Moreover, the care you receive will in no way be affected by your participation in this study. We greatly appreciate your cooperation in this matter and will be happy to answer any question you may have.

In order to help you answer these questions, we will first explain the meaning of some of the words we use. Birth control refers to anything men and women do to avoid pregnancies. Sterilization refers to any procedure performed on men or women so as to make it impossible for them to have children. There are various ways in which to surgically sterilize women. All of these operations basically involve tying off the tubes (fallopian tubes) which carry the eggs or removing the tubes and the womb (uterus). These types of operations are usually performed in a hospital, normally under general anesthesia. In this questionnaire we will refer to these sterilization operations for women as tubal ligation, or having one's tubes tied. Male sterilization involves a minor operation in which the tubes or cords that carry the sperm cells, or male seed, are cut and tied off. This operation is called a vasectomy and can be performed in a doctor's office under local anesthesia. Today, sterilization operations performed on men and women involve surgery. Although they are considered permanent operations, occasionally they can be successfully reversed through additional surgery.

Research is being conducted to develop various types of sterilization procedures for men and women that do not require surgery. In this questionnaire we are concerned with *one* method of nonsurgical sterilization for women. It would involve inserting a chemical into the mouth of the uterus (womb) through the vagina, followed by another treatment 1 month later. This would cause the tubes to close within 6 to 12 weeks. During this time other contraceptive methods should be used to prevent pregnancy. In this questionnaire, we will refer to this method of nonsurgical sterilization as having one's tubes blocked or closed. Such a procedure could *never* be undone or reversed. We expect that, when first introduced, it will not be as successful as surgical sterilization in preventing pregnancy. We expect it will be successful in 95% of cases, compared with close to 100% for the surgical procedure. Your tubes would be blocked in the doctor's office, without need for anesthesia. There should not be any short- or long-term side-effects, except for some mild cramping pain at the time of treatment. We estimate that this procedure will cost much less than surgical sterilization.

II. GENERAL BACKGROUND QUESTIONS

1. What is your birth date? ________________________

   What is your present age? ________ years.

2. How many years of education have you completed? Circle the highest level (grade) of education you have completed.

   Grade school: 1, 2, 3, 4, 5, 6, 7, 8, 9, 10, 11, 12
   Business or vocational school: 1, 2, 3, 4
   College: 1, 2, 3, 4
   Postgraduate educcation: 1, 2, 3, 4

3. What is your marital status? Check one:

   _____ a. Married, for the first time
   _____ b. Married, for the second or third time
   _____ c. Married, common law
   _____ d. Separated from husband
   _____ e. Widowed
   _____ f. Divorced
   _____ g. Never married

   If you are married: How long have you been married to your present husband? Years _____ Months _____

4. What is your religion? Check one:

   _____ a. Catholic
   _____ b. Protestant
   _____ c. Jewish
   _____ d. Other (specify) _______

5. What ethnic/racial group do you belong to? Check one:

____ a. Mexican-American ____ c. Black
____ b. Anglo ____ d. Other (specify) ______

6. Do you work? Yes ____ No ____

If yes: What kind of work do you do? ______________________

7. Does your husband work or go to school? Yes ____ No ____
I have no husband ____

If you have a husband who works: What does he do? ______________

8. How much income do you and your husband earn (before taxes)? Check one number in both columns (a) and (b):

	(a) *Husband's income* (if you are unsure, please give us your best guess)			(b) *Your income*	
	Yearly	*Weekly*		*Yearly*	*Weekly*
____	1. No husband		____	1. I do not work	
____	2. Husband does not work....		____	2. Under $3,000 ..	Under $58
____	3. Under $5,000 ..	Under $97	____	3. $3000–4,999	$58–96
____	4. $5,000–6,999......	$97–134	____	4. $5,000–6,999......	$97–134
____	5. $7,000–8,999....	$135–173	____	5. $7,000–8,999....	$135–173
____	6. $9,000–10,999...	$174–211	____	6. $9,000–10,999...	$174–211
____	7. $11,000–12,999 .	$212–250	____	7. $11,000–12,999 .	$212–250
____	8. $13,000–14,999 .	$251–288	____	8. $13,000–14,999 .	$251–288
____	9. $15,000–16,999 .	$289–327	____	9. $15,000–16,999 .	$289–327
____	10. $17,000–19,999 .	$328–384	____	10. $17,000–19,999 .	$328–384
____	11. $20,000–24,999 .	$385–481	____	11. $20,000–24,999 .	$385–481
____	12. Over $25,000...	Over $482	____	12. Over $25,000...	Over $482

9. Are you receiving welfare payments? Yes ____ No ____

10. Does any other person help support you? Yes ____ No ____
If yes: Approximately how much does he or she contribute each year?

11. Do you have any children? Yes ____ No ____
If yes: (a) How many do you have?
Number of boys ____ Number of girls ____
(b) How old are they? List their ages:
Boys ________ Girls ________

*12. Are you pregnant now? Yes ____ No ____
If no: Have you ever been pregnant?
Yes ____ No ____ Unsure ____

---

*Eliminate part 1 of this question for use in clinical trials.

*13. Are you trying to become pregnant now? Check one:
Yes _____ No _____ I don't care _____ I'm already pregnant _____

14. Have you ever tried to become pregnant for 2 years or longer and could not? Yes _____ No _____

15. Do you think you can have (are physically able to have) any (more) children? Yes _____ No _____ Unsure _____
If no or unsure: Why do you feel this way? _____________________

16. When you are pregnant or deliver a baby, do you have any serious health problems or have you been told you will have such difficulties with your next pregnancy? Check one: Yes _____ No _____
Unsure _____ Never been pregnant _____

†17. Do you intend to have any (more) children?
Yes _____ No _____ Unsure _____
If yes or unsure: (a) What is the total number you intend to have? _____
(b) What is the oldest (maximum) age you would want to be when you have your last child? _____ years

18. Does your husband (partner) want you to have (more) children?
Yes _____ No _____ Unsure _____ No husband (partner) _____
If yes: What is the total number he wants you to have? _____

19. Have you at any time in your life used a method of birth control or protected yourself in other ways against pregnancy?
Yes _____ No _____

20. Do you now use a method of birth control or protect yourself in other ways against pregnancy? Yes _____ No _____ I'm pregnant _____
Already sterilized (either partner) _____

If yes: (a) Which method do you *now* use?

_____ 1. The Pill
_____ 2. IUD
_____ 3. Diaphragm and jelly
_____ 4. Condom (rubber)
_____ 5. Foam or jelly
_____ 6. Rhythm
_____ 7. Withdrawal (pulling out)
_____ 8. Douche
_____ 9. Breast-feeding
_____ 10. Other (specify) _____________

(b) Do you use it regularly? (Are you protected every time you have sexual relations, or if you now take the Pill, do you always remember to take one each day that you are supposed to?)

_____ 1. Yes, all of the time
_____ 2. Yes, most of the time
_____ 3. Just sometimes
_____ 4. No

If no: At this point in your life, do you engage in sexual relations? Yes
No _____ Sometimes _____

---

*Eliminate for use in clinical trials.
†Modify for use in clinical trials (eliminate intent, refer to wanting more children).

*IF YOU ARE PREGNANT, TRYING TO BECOME PREGNANT, OR IN THE PAST 2 MONTHS HAVE DELIVERED A BABY OR HAD AN ABORTION OR A MISCARRIAGE, ANSWER QUESTION 21. *IF THIS DOES NOT APPLY TO YOU, GO TO QUESTION 22.*

21. Were you using a method of birth control before this pregnancy or before you started trying to become pregnant? Yes ____ No ____

If yes: (a) Which method did you use most recently? Check one or more:

____ 1. The Pill
____ 2. IUD
____ 3. Diaphragm and jelly
____ 4. Condom (rubber)
____ 5. Foam or jelly
____ 6. Rhythm
____ 7. Withdrawal (pulling out)
____ 8. Douche
____ 9. Breast-feeding
____ 10. Other (specify) ____________________

(b) Did you use it regularly? (Were you protected every time you had sexual relations, or if you were taking the Pill, did you always remember to take one each day that you were supposed to?) Check one:

____ 1. Yes, all of the time
____ 2. Yes, most of the time
____ 3. Just sometimes
____ 4. No

22. Are you satisfied with the method of birth control you are now using? Check one: (If you are not using a method of birth control now because you are pregnant, trying to become pregnant, or in the past 2 months have delivered a baby or had an abortion or a miscarriage, please refer to the birth control method you used most recently.) Check one:

____ a. Very satisfied ____ d. Dissatisfied
____ b. Satisfied ____ e. Very dissatisfied
____ c. Unsure ____ f. I don't use any kind of birth control

23. Have you ever stopped using a method of birth control because you were unhappy with it? Check one:
Yes ____ No ____ I have never used a method of birth control ____

If yes: (a) Which method was this? Check one or more:

____ 1. The Pill
____ 2. IUD
____ 3. Diaphragm and jelly

*Modify for use in clinical trials (eliminate reference to current pregnancy and current attempts at conception, referring only to recent delivery or termination).

_____ 4. Condom (rubber)
_____ 5. Foam or jelly
_____ 6. Rhythm
_____ 7. Withdrawal (pulling out)
_____ 8. Douche
_____ 9. Breast-feeding
_____ 10. Other (specify) _____

(b) Why were you unhappy with it? _____
_____

*24. Do you intend to use any method of birth control in the future? Check one:
Yes _____ No _____ Unsure _____ Already sterilized (either partner)

If yes: Which method do you intend to use? Check one:

_____ 1. The Pill
_____ 2. IUD
_____ 3. Diaphragm and jelly
_____ 4. Condom (rubber)
_____ 5. Foam or jelly
_____ 6. Rhythm
_____ 7. Withdrawal (pulling out)
_____ 8. Douche
_____ 9. Breast-feeding
_____ 10. Tubal ligation (have your tubes tied)
_____ 11. Vasectomy for husband (partner)
_____ 12. Other (specify) _____
_____ 13. Unsure

25. Have you ever had (a) an abortion? Yes _____ No _____
(b) a miscarriage? Yes _____ No _____ Unsure _____

26. Did you want to become pregnant this last time (your last pregnancy)? Check one:

_____ a. I have never been pregnant.
_____ b. Yes
_____ c. No, not at that time. I wanted to wait longer.
_____ d. No, I was finished having children.
_____ e. No, I did not want any children.
_____ f. I didn't care.

27. If you had an unwanted pregnancy, would you seriously consider having an abortion? Yes _____ No _____ Unsure _____

III. QUESTIONS ON SURGICAL STERILIZATION

28. Have you or your husband (partner) had an operation that makes it impossible to have children? Yes, I have _____ Yes, my husband (partner) has _____ No _____

*Eliminate for use in clinical trials.

IF NO, GO TO QUESTION 29.

IF YES, COMPLETE QUESTIONS (a), (b), AND (c), AND THEN YOU ARE FINISHED. THANK YOU FOR YOUR COOPERATION.

(a) Did you or your husband (partner) have this operation because of medical problems or because you wanted to stop having children? Check one:
Medical problems ____ To stop having children ____
Both ____

(b) How old was your youngest child when this operation was performed?
Years ____ Months ____

(c) If it were possible, would you want to have this operation reversed so you could have children? Yes ____ No ____

29. Some women get operated on (have their tubes tied) so as not to have more children. Have you heard of this operation before today?
Yes ____ No ____

30. Do you *approve* of women having their tubes tied (tubal ligation) after they have finished having children? Check one:

____ a. Strongly approve
____ b. Approve
____ c. Disapprove
____ d. Strongly disapprove
____ e. Feel it's up to them

31. Have you ever discussed tubal ligation with your husband (partner)?

____ a. Yes, many times
____ b. Yes, only once or twice
____ c. No, never
____ d. No husband (partner)

32. After a woman's tubes are tied, do you think she becomes either more or less attractive to men? Check one:

____ a. No change
____ b. Yes, a little more attractive
____ c. Yes, much more attractive
____ d. Yes, a little less attractive
____ e. Yes, much less attractive
____ f. Unsure

If yes or unsure: In which way? ____________________

____

33. Have any of your female friends or members of your family (women) had their tubes tied? Yes ____ No ____ Unsure ____
If yes: Are they satisfied? Yes ____ No ____ Some yes, some no ____

34. Would you *seriously consider* having your tubes tied after you have finished having children? Check one:
Yes ____ No ____ Unsure ____
If no or unsure: Why do you feel this way? Check (√) all of the reasons that apply to you, and double check (√√) the *one* reason that is most important.

____ 1. I might change my mind and want another baby.
____ 2. I might lose a child and want another baby.
____ 3. I might lose my husband either through divorce or death and then remarry. I might want another baby with my new husband.
For divorced, separated, and widowed women: I might remarrry and want another baby with my new husband.
____ 4. I want to have as many children as I can
____ 5. The operation is too expensive.
____ 6. I do not want to have any surgery I do not absolutely need.
____ 7. I think my husband (partner) should have a vasectomy. (If you check this reason, please explain why) ____________
____
____ 8. I am afraid I will be less of a woman (If you check this reason, please explain why) ____________
____
____ 9. I am afraid of physical problems resulting from this operation. (If you check this reason, please state what you think such problems would be) ____________
____
____ 10. My husband (partner) would object. (If you check this reason, please explain why) ____________
____
____ 11. Other reasons (specify) ____________
____

35. Do you *intend* to have your tubes tied sometime after you have finished having children? Yes ____ No ____ Unsure ____
If no or unsure: Is this because:

____ 1. It is too expensive. If it were free or cost the same as other methods of birth control, I would eventually have my tubes tied.
____ 2. I prefer other methods of birth control.
____ 3. I will not use any method to prevent future pregnancies.
____ 4. My husband (partner) may have a vasectomy instead.

If yes: (a) After you have finished having children, how many months or years will you wait before having your tubes tied?
____ Months or ____ Years
(b) How many children do you think you will have at this time?
____

36. If you are finished having children, do you plan to have your tubes tied within the next *12 months*? Check one:

____ a. I am not (may not be) finished having children
____ b. Yes
____ c. Unsure
____ d. No

37. Some men get operated on (vasectomy) so as not to have more children. Have you heard of this operation before today? Yes ____ No ____

38. Have you ever discussed vasectomy with your husband (partner)? Check one:

____ a. Yes, many times
____ b. Yes, only once or twice
____ c. No, never
____ d. No husband (partner)

IV. QUESTIONS ON NONSURGICAL STERILIZATION

39. Let us suppose that techniques of nonsurgical sterilization were available for women and men. This would mean that a woman or man could have her/his tubes permanently blocked or closed without having to undergo an operation. If such methods were available, would you *approve* of them for women who have finished having children? Check one:

____ a. Strongly approve
____ b. Approve
____ c. Disapprove
____ d. Strongly disapprove
____ e. Feel it's up to them

40. If a woman's tubes were permanently blocked or closed without surgery, do you think she would become either more or less attractive to men? Check one:

____ a. No change
____ b. Yes, a little more attractive
____ c. Yes, much more attractive
____ d. Yes, a little less attractive
____ e. Yes, much less attractive
____ f. Unsure

If yes or unsure: In which way ________________________________
____

41. Would you *seriously consider* having your tubes permanently blocked or closed after you have finished having children if you did not have to have an operation? Check one:
Yes ____ No ____ Unsure ____

If no or unsure: Why do you feel this way? Check (√) all of the reasons that apply to you and double check (√√) the *one* reason that is most important.

_____ 1. I might change my mind and want another baby.
_____ 2. I might lose a child and want another baby.
_____ 3. I might lose my husband either through divorce or death and then remarry. I might want another baby with my new husband.
For divorced, separated and widowed women: I might remarry and want another baby with my new husband.
_____ 4. I do not like the fact that there would be *no* chance to undo or reverse the procedure.
_____ 5. Although nonsurgical sterilization would prevent pregnancy in 95 of 100 women, I am afraid that in my case it would fail.
_____ 6. I want to have as many children as I can.
_____ 7. Although nonsurgical sterilization would cost much less than surgical sterilization, it still may be too expensive.
_____ 8. I think my husband (partner) should have a vasectomy. (If you check this reason, please explain why) ______________
____
_____ 9. I am afraid I will be less of a woman (If you check this reason, please explain why) ______________
____
_____ 10. I am afraid of physical problems resulting from this operation. (If you check this reason, please state what you think such problems would be) ______________
____
_____ 11. My husband (partner) would object. (If you check this reason, please explain why) ______________
____
_____ 12. Other reasons (specify) ______________
____

42. If sterilization for men and women did not require surgery, would you *intend* to have your tubes permanently blocked or closed sometime after you have finished having children? Yes _____ No _____ Unsure _____

If no or unsure: Is this because:

_____ 1. It may be too expensive. If it were free or cost the same as other methods of birth control, I would eventually have my tubes blocked.
_____ 2. I prefer traditional tubal ligation.
_____ 3. I prefer other methods of birth control.
_____ 4. I will not use any kind of method to prevent future pregnancies.
_____ 5. My husband (partner) might have a vasectomy instead.
_____ 6. My husband (partner) might have a nonsurgical vasectomy instead.

If yes: (a) After you have finished having children, how many months or years would you wait before having your tubes blocked or closed if you did not have to have an operation? _____ Months or _____ Years (b) How many children do you think you would have at this time? _____

43. If you are finished having children, would you plan to have your tubes permanently blocked or closed within the next *12 months* if you did not have to have an operation? Check one:

_____ a. I am not (may not be) finished having children
_____ b. Yes
_____ c. Unsure
_____ d. No

V. QUESTIONS ON NONSURGICAL STERILIZATION FOR WOMEN WHO HAVE UNDERGONE THE PROCEDURE

1. Your tubes have just been blocked without surgery. How do you feel about it? Check one:

_____ a. I am pleased
_____ b. I have some regrets
_____ c. I am sorry it was done

If not pleased: Why? _____

2. What were the advantages of the treatment? _____

_____

3. What could have been done to make it even better? _____

_____

_____

4. Do you think anything should be changed about the treatment? Check one:
a. Yes _____ b. No _____ c. Unsure _____
If yes or unsure: What especially bothered you? _____

_____

5. Were you given enough information about the treatment before you decided to have it done? Check one:
a. Yes _____ b. No _____
If no: Please explain _____

_____

6. Is there anything that was not told to you that you wished you had known? Check one: a. Yes _____ b. No _____
If yes: What was it? _____

_____

7. How do you feel now? Check one:

_____ a. I feel well
_____ b. I feel moderately well
_____ c. I feel poorly

8. Is there anything about the treatment that you are now worried about? Check one: a. Yes _____ b. No _____ c. Unsure _____
If yes or unsure: Please explain ______________________________
____

9. How were you treated by the staff? Check one:

_____ a. Very nicely
_____ b. Not nicely but not poorly
_____ c. Poorly

If you were not treated nicely: Please explain ______________________________
____

10. Would you recommend this procedure to friends who are finished having children? Check one: a. Yes _____ b. No _____ c. Unsure _____
If no or unsure: Why not? ______________________________

5

Discussion: Feasibility and Acceptability of Transcervical Sterilization

JOHN J. SCIARRA, MODERATOR

IN DEVELOPING COUNTRIES, WHERE PHYSICIANS ARE SCARCE, HOW FEASIBLE IS SURGICAL REVERSAL, AND HOW IMPORTANT IS REVERSIBILITY AS A CRITERION, IN EVALUATING A TRANSCERVICAL STERILIZATION METHOD FOR PROGRAMS?

There is considerable discussion of reversibility of sterilization procedures, but considering the physician/population ratios and the distribution of physicians in the developing world, a woman seeking reversal would have difficulty finding a gynecologist who is trained to do reversals. A few centers have been established around the world to offer reversal of currently used sterilization methods, but their capacity for reaching large numbers of people is limited. Relative to the number of sterilizations being done, the demand for reversal is very small.

Reversibility becomes important when it is a major advantage of a method, as with the silicone plug or the fimbrial hood. These techniques might have wide appeal and applicability, especially in countries where conventional procedures are often prohibited.

WHAT ARE THE MINIMUM REQUIREMENTS OF A TRANSCERVICAL METHOD, IN TERMS OF EFFICACY, FOR PROGRAMMATIC USE?

Opinions differ on this question. A conservative standard would be a rate of effectiveness fairly close to that achieved with the IUD, perhaps a 2% to 3% failure rate in terms of pregnancy, preferably with one application, or with some way of determining whether or not the closure has been successful.

In considering effectiveness standards, it is important to distinguish between tubal closure rates and pregnancy rates; the actual pregnancy rate may be lower than one would expect, on the basis of the tubal closure rate. With quinacrine, for example, an 85% bilateral tubal closure rate may not seem adequate, whereas the actual pregnancy rates achieved with the method may be low enough to meet program standards.

Panelists: Carl J. Pauerstein, Ralph M. Richart, Rochelle N. Shain, James D. Shelton. *Discussants:* Jan Brundin, Miriam H. Labbok, Robert S. Neuwirth, Malcolm Potts, Rodolfo Quinones, Earle W. Wilson, Lourens J.D. Zaneveld, Gerald I. Zatuchni.

Also, it is critical from a programmatic viewpoint not to consider failure rates for chemical sterilization procedures on the same basis as the rates for conventional surgical sterilization procedures. The generally accepted pregnancy rate for IUDs over a 5-year period is 9/100, and the usual rate for surgical sterilization is less than 0.5%, although in some instances, the rate is higher.

HOW ACCEPTABLE, CULTURALLY AND PROGRAMMATICALLY, IS A METHOD REQUIRING TWO OR EVEN THREE TREATMENTS (AND VISITS TO THE CLINIC) TO ACHIEVE REASONABLE EFFICACY?

A two-treatment procedure is reasonably acceptable, provided that the first visit is not an unpleasant one; however, much depends on the woman's experience during the first visit. The acceptability literature provides information on factors that might seem like frills to the investigator but are important determinators of acceptance, such as availability of child care, not keeping women waiting 6 or 8 hours for a procedure but treating them in perhaps half an hour, provision of good support from the staff, the relative ease with which the service is provided, the distance the woman has to travel to the site of the procedure, and other factors. If at the first visit the experience does not cost a woman a day's absence from her work and it is not humiliating or unduly painful, then she is likely to return for a second treatment. If it is difficult for her, then getting her to return will be difficult. There is an enormous variation in the quality of service provided in different programs around the world, and these factors can create an enormous variation in the success and acceptability of a procedure.

Another significant consideration is the availability of other contraceptive options. Assuming that for much of the population of the developing world, sterilization is unavailable, in terms of the physician/population ratios, then the choice is for the woman to become pregnant again and again using ineffective methods or no methods, or to have a lower pregnancy rate by using the more simply applied and cheaper method, which might be available through less highly trained physicians or paramedical personnel, or which might require several visits to a clinic.

One concept of program strategy is to offer a broad enough range of options, in a kind of family planning cafeteria, with methods varying in price, effectivity, and ease of delivery and permanence, so that almost everyone will like something on the menu.

WHAT PHARMACOLOGIC MEANS ARE AVAILABLE TO RELAX THE TUBAL OSTIA TO ENSURE ADEQUATE INSTILLATION OF AN AGENT?

Swedish investigators are having fairly good success in humans using β_2-adrenergic agents for the relaxation of the intramural part of the oviduct. The relaxation effect lasts for 15 to 20 minutes.

ARE THERE ANY DATA INDICATING THAT PROGESTIN SIGNIFICANTLY INHIBITS TUBAL REPAIR AND THAT IT WOULD INCREASE THE EFFECTIVENESS OF ANY OF THE TRANSCERVICAL METHODS?

There does not seem to be any evidence that progestin would be useful for inhibiting repair. Some investigators have tried unsuccessfully to *accelerate* healing in laboratory animals by hormonal methods.

In a study of patients treated with methyl cyanoacrylate, the data were analyzed for differences in closure rates in patients using Depo-Provera or oral contraceptives versus closure rates in patients using condoms and diaphragms. No statistically significant difference was seen.

One observation may be pertinent: a study of the pregnancy rates of women who are operated on because they have true tubal occlusion and who undergo salpingostomy shows that a large proportion of pregnancies occurring in the first 6 months after the operation are ectopic, whereas nearly all the intrauterine pregnancies cluster in the third 6 months after the operation, with some intrauterine pregnancies in the middle 6 months. One possible, although weak, inference from this is that some type of regeneration has taken place over time; but what kind is not known.

WHAT IS THE INCIDENCE OF ECTOPIC PREGNANCIES WITH CHEMICAL STERILIZATION TECHNIQUES? HAVE ALL THE FAILURES BEEN INTRAUTERINE?

One of the major concerns with the nonsurgical or chemical methods of female sterilization has been failures resulting in intrauterine pregnancies, but, more importantly, perhaps, are those resulting in ectopic tubal pregnancies. A review of the literature of the chemical techniques used at present, as well as of those used in the past, does not reveal any cases of ectopic pregnancy with these methods. The numbers are very small, however, and the follow-up is limited.

DOES HYSTEROSCOPY AID IN IDENTIFYING THE TUBAL OSTIA?

In one center, where investigators are highly skilled in hysteroscopy, they have observed through the hysteroscope that the tubal orifice modifies its shape as pressure is increased and they have found that if the pressure inside the uterus is kept constant, whichever distending medium is used, that identification of the tubal orifices is easy. They use a special uterine insufflator for fluids that keeps the pressure constant at 180 mm Hg. Besides providing easy visualization of the tubal ostia, this approach avoids bleeding in the uterine cavity, even during training sessions lasting 10 or 15 minutes.

In a group of 1284 patients undergoing sterilization by electrocoagulation, the operators failed to identify the tubal orifices in only two patients. One woman had a polyp in the cornual region, and the other patient was in the wrong phase of the cycle. The mucus plugs were easily removed from the tubal orifice through a Storz hysteroscope with a double surgical channel. Most tubes could be catheterized if no more than 1 cm to 1.5 cm of the catheter was introduced into the tube.

However, very few hysteroscopists have the skill and experience to visualize the tubal ostia almost every time. The procedure must be performed during the early proliferative stage of the cycle, and even then there is about a 10% failure to find both tubal ostia. This is an important consideration when hysteroscopy is evaluated for programmatic use.

WHAT EFFECT DOES THE LITERACY OF THE SUBJECTS HAVE IN THEIR ABILITY TO RESPOND TO THE ACCEPTABILITY QUESTIONNAIRE?

Obviously, in areas where literacy is very low, the woman herself does not fill out the questionnaire; an interviewer administers it. It is quite extensive, and a woman must be fairly literate to fill it out. However, with a population such as one in Los Angeles of newly arrived women from Mexico, use of an interviewer works very well and the data seem reliable. The investigators tested it for reliability in a poor Mexican-American clinic in San Antonio. If the woman filled out the questionnaire before she went in to see the physician, she was asked to repeat her answers to certain questions after she had finished her appointment, and the reliability was close to 97%.

IS PATIENT REFERRAL OF FRIENDS FOR PARTICIPATION IN A STUDY PROGRAM A RELIABLE INDEX OF ACCEPTABILITY OF A METHOD UNDER INVESTIGATION?

In various clinical trials over the years, one good measure of acceptability has been whether patients would subsequently refer their friends for treatment. In acceptability studies this is considered a reliable index of acceptability that the individual researcher might use. In one analysis of the results of a study looking at characteristics of women most affected by the attribute of reversibility, one of the variables having a strong impact on selection of sterilization, either a permanent or reversible method, was a friend's prior experience with sterilization. That fact overwhelmed almost all of the other variables.

WHAT NAME IS SUITABLE FOR THE PROCEDURES BEING DISCUSSED?

Chemical transcervical methods of sterilization are hopeful as another "dish on the menu," but providing a proper name for them that will be easily understandable and acceptable to consumers is a problem. These procedures probably should not be called nonsurgical sterilization because people associate sterilization with surgery, so it would sound to people like nonsurgical surgery. Logically, these are contraceptives with a low failure rate and a 100% continuation rate. However, that is difficult to explain to a lay audience, so a new name is needed.

6

Pharmacology of Quinacrine Hydrochloride With Emphasis on its Use as a Tubal Occluding Agent

NORMAN H. DUBIN

TIM H. PARMLEY

MARIA C. DIBLASI

RAMESH B. GHODGAONKAR

MOHAMMED T.M. JIFFRY

DAVID A. BLAKE

THEODORE M. KING

An intensified program for identification of synthetic antimalarial drugs was conducted in Germany during the 1920s. Quinacrine was one of 12,000 synthetic chemicals found to be effective in treating malaria and was widely used prior to World War II. Quinine remained the chief antimalarial drug, however, until the Japanese invasion of the South Pacific cut supplies and expanded US production of quinacrine became imperative, increasing from a prewar level of 1200 lb/year to almost one ton/day.[9] Much of the pharmacologic knowledge about quinacrine was acquired from observations and studies made during that time.[16]

Quinacrine is a bright yellow crystalline powder. The structure of quinacrine hydrochloride is shown in Figure 6-1. The metabolic fate of quinacrine is incompletely understood. In humans, urinary products include the unmetabolized form as well as the O-demethylated derivative, the side-chain–cleaved amine derivative, and an O-demethylated side-chain–cleaved amine.[16] The pharmacokinetics of quinacrine has been studied primarily in regard to ingestion of the drug.[15] Because the mode of administration may alter the absorption of a drug and its distribution, we investigated the pharmacokinetic properties of quinacrine following intrauterine injection. The data are presented later in this chapter.

Besides its use in the management of malaria, quinacrine has been used to

These studies were supported by contracts from the International Fertility Research Program (IFRP) #601 and #603 and AID DSPE/C/0054.

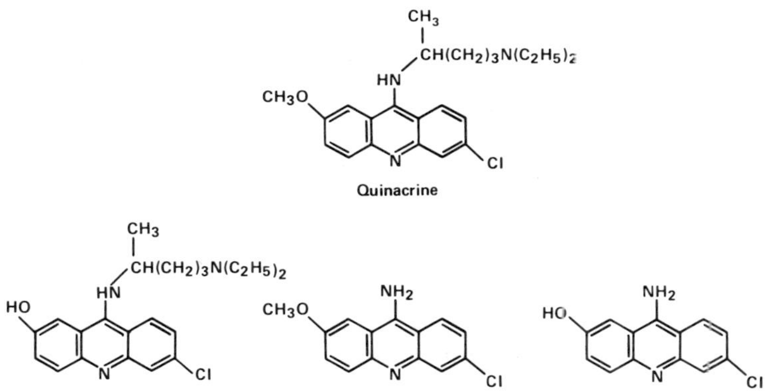

FIG. 6-1. Structure of quinacrine and urinary metabolites. Metabolites (left to right) are O-demethylated, side-chain cleaved, and O-demethyated side-chain cleaved derivative (based on Steck EA: Chemotherapy of Protozoan Disease, vol III, pp 23–172 Walter Reed Army Institute of Research, US Government Printing Office, 1982)

treat tapeworm infection, cutaneous leishmaniasis, and lupus erythematosus and to control neoplastic effusions in the pleural and peritoneal cavities.

Numerous toxic effects of quinacrine have been reported, some of which are listed below:

Skin:
- Lemon-yellow pigmentation
- Dermatitis
- Atrophy of sebaceous and sweat glands

Gastrointestinal tract:
- Nausea
- Vomiting
- Abdominal cramps
- Diarrhea

Cardiovascular system:
- Lowering of blood pressure
- Decreased cardiac output
- Bradycardia

Central nervous system:
- Motor acceleration
- Epileptiform convulsions
- Delusions
- Hallucinations

Other:
- Fever
- Headache

The occurrence of these symptoms depends on dose, length of treatment, mode of delivery, and patient susceptibility. For a more detailed discussion of side-effects, the reader is referred to Goodman and Gilman[9] and an extensive review by Findlay.[7] The toxic effects of quinacrine as a tubal occluding agent are discussed later in this chapter.

QUINACRINE ADMINISTRATION TO MONKEYS

INTRAVASCULAR VERSUS INTRAUTERINE INJECTIONS

Quinacrine was administered to cynomolgus monkeys by means of intravascular or intrauterine injections.[4,5] The cynomolgus monkey was chosen for these studies because its reproductive anatomy is similar to that of the human, and its cervical canal, although more convoluted than that of a woman, can be penetrated by a blunt-end needle.[13] Thus, quinacrine can be deposited directly into the uterine cavity. A solution of quinacrine was used, so that "worst case" exposure to quinacrine could be evaluated. The dose given (30 mg in 1 ml) is approximately two times the dose, on a body weight basis, that would currently be placed in a woman's uterus at any one time (250 mg is the current human dose).

Following intravascular injection of a 1-ml solution of 30 mg quinacrine, 149 ± 42 ng/ml (n = 3) was observed in the plasma at 0.5 hours (Fig. 6-2). The level declined during the next 3½ hours, with an estimated half-life of 2 hours. Less than 1% of the administered drug was found in the urine over

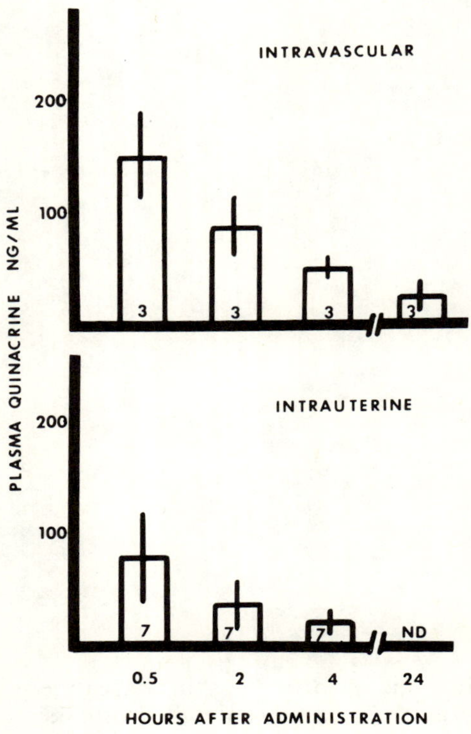

FIG. 6-2. Plasma quinacrine concentrations at various times after intravascular or intrauterine administration of 30 mg quinacrine hydrochloride solution to nonpregnant monkeys. (ND, not detectable; number in bars represents number of observations; Vertical line is ± SEM)

the first 4-hour interval. At 24 hours, the plasma level was 23.5 ± 8.5 ng/ml. Tissues obtained following necropsy at this time were found to have high concentrations of quinacrine. The tissue-plasma ratios are indicated in Table 6-1.

Following intrauterine injections of the 30 mg quinacrine solution, plasma quinacrine levels were 77.1 ± 37.0 ng/ml (n = 7) and declined at a rate similar to that in the group receiving intravascular injections. Thus, quinacrine rapidly enters the circulation when deposited into the uterine cavity. Twenty-four hours after administration, quinacrine was found not only in the uterus and other reproductive organs but also in all organs listed in Table 6-1, except cerebellum and skeletal muscle. It is significant that high concentrations of quinacrine could be detected in the isthmus and ampulla of the oviduct, indicating the possibility of spill into the peritoneal cavity. Many of the tissues from animals that received intrauterine quinacrine and were necropsied 1 week later also contained significant amounts of quinacrine; however, these concentrations were, in general, significantly less than those concentrations found at 24 hours. By 28 days, all tissues had undetectable levels of quinacrine or levels near the limit of detection.

Following both intravascular and intrauterine injection of quinacrine, serum glutamic oxaloacetic transaminase, serum glutamic pyruvic transaminase, and lactic dehydrogenase showed significant elevations compared with these measurements in control monkeys receiving 1 ml physiologic saline by way of the intrauterine route. The elevations were moderate and transient, re-

TABLE 6-1. Tissue-Plasma Ratio of Quinacrine 24 Hours After Intravascular Administration of 30 mg Quinacrine to Cynomolgus Monkeys

TISSUE	RATIO
Lung	1676:1
Adrenal	1345:1
Kidney	1211:1
Pancreas	1041:1
Liver	994:1
Spleen	904:1
Heart	723:1
Bone marrow	445:1
Lymph node	378:1
Myometrium	256:1
Ovary	219:1
Hypothalamus	200:1
Endometrium	184:1
Cerebellum	171:1
Uterine cervix	158:1
Midbrain	138:1
Isthmus (oviduct)	131:1
Ampulla (oviduct)	94:1
Skeletal muscle	68:1

turning to preinjection levels within 48 hours. Histologic examination of tissues listed in Table 6-1 revealed no pathology, except for the reproductive tissue in those animals receiving intrauterine injections of quinacrine.[5]

Following intravascular injection of 30 mg quinacrine, two of three monkeys vomited or retched within 3 minutes of the injection. While nausea has been reported following oral administration of quinacrine in humans, this has implied a direct gastrointestinal effect. Since in these monkeys, the symptoms were seen following intravascular administration, this effect appears to be indirect, possibly acting through the central nervous system. No other toxic effects were observed in these animals that could be attributed to quinacrine administration.

INTRAUTERINE INJECTIONS DURING PREGNANCY

Intrauterine injections of quinacrine were also administered to pregnant monkeys between pregnancy days 34 and 46. Administration of 30 mg quinacrine resulted in plasma concentrations that were at least comparable to those in nonpregnant monkeys receiving intravascular administration of the same dose (Fig. 6-3). This may reflect increased vascularity of the uterus during pregnancy, and more rapid absorption of the drug. Following intrauterine administration of 3 mg of the drug, plasma concentrations were approximately 10-fold less than those in monkeys receiving the 30-mg dose.

One pregnant monkey was found dead in its cage 48 hours after intrauterine administration of 30 mg quinacrine. Autopsy did not reveal the cause of death. While there was no direct or statistical evidence that quinacrine was the cause of death, we were concerned, since we have never had a death in a pregnant monkey following intrauterine injections in our studies involving other drugs.[2,3] Also, the plasma quinacrine concentration at 30 minutes was 445 ng/ml, which was higher than any other 30-minute concentration, including concentrations following intravascular injections in nonpregnant monkeys. It is also significant that we were not able to obtain any urine from this animal, although its bladder was catheterized for the 4-hour postinjection collection period. Thus, impaired clearance of the drug may account in part for high plasma levels.

The effect of quinacrine administration on the fetuses of these pregnant monkeys is discussed in Chapter 7.

INTRAPERITONEAL ADMINISTRATION

A danger of intrauterine administration of drugs is either spill of the drug through the oviducts into the peritoneal cavity or perforation of the uterus with direct application of the drug into this cavity. To determine toxicity in case such an event occurs, the following study was performed.

Under ketamine anesthesia, a needle was inserted through the cervical canal and the uterus was punctured. A 1-ml solution containing 30 mg quinacrine was then applied directly into the peritoneal cavity. Three monkeys were subsequently observed for 3 days and showed no abnormal behavior. Laparotomy performed on day 3 revealed slight adhesion of one tube to the uterus in one monkey, but no other effects were observed.

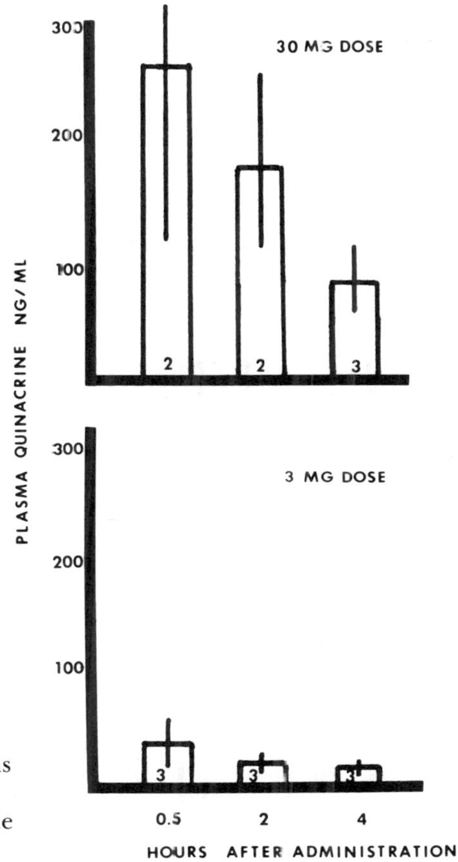

FIG. 6-3. Plasma quinacrine concentrations following intrauterine administration of either 30 or 3 mg quinacrine hydrochloride solution to pregnant monkeys.

A report by Chandra and Malaviya indicated that when high intraperitoneal doses of quinacrine suspension were administered to rhesus monkeys, death occurred within 10 minutes; lower doses caused hyperactivity. The same doses, placed in the uterus of those animals, had no effect.[1]

These studies prompted us to test higher doses of quinacrine in the peritoneal cavity of cynomolgus monkeys. Since pellets are the current form in which the drug is used in women, we elected to use pellets in this study. Three monkeys were studied at one time. Each was immobilized with ketamine and placed under halothane anesthesia. Each received a midabdominal incision and a pellet applicator (supplied by IFRP) was inserted through the incision and pellets were released into the peritoneal cavity. One applicator contained seven pellets (250 mg total dose), one contained 3½ pellets (125 mg), and one contained no pellets (sham control). The animals were then allowed to recover from anesthesia. Periodically, blood was taken from the femoral vein for quinacrine determination. This experimental procedure was repeated on different monkeys on two other occasions, so that each treatment group consisted of three animals.

Of the three monkeys receiving 250 mg quinacrine, two died approximately 2 hours after administration. The third had a seizure, beginning at 2 hours after treatment, which lasted for approximately 1 hour. This animal recovered and appeared to be healthy thereafter. The three monkeys receiving 125 mg quinacrine all survived. One demonstrated slight tremors of the limbs while recovering from anesthesia. All animals receiving intraperitoneal quinacrine pellets, regardless of dose, demonstrated crouching behavior that may have been indicative of abdominal pain. No hyperactivity was observed. The sham monkeys showed more activity than did the treated animals during a 4-hour observation period following treatment.

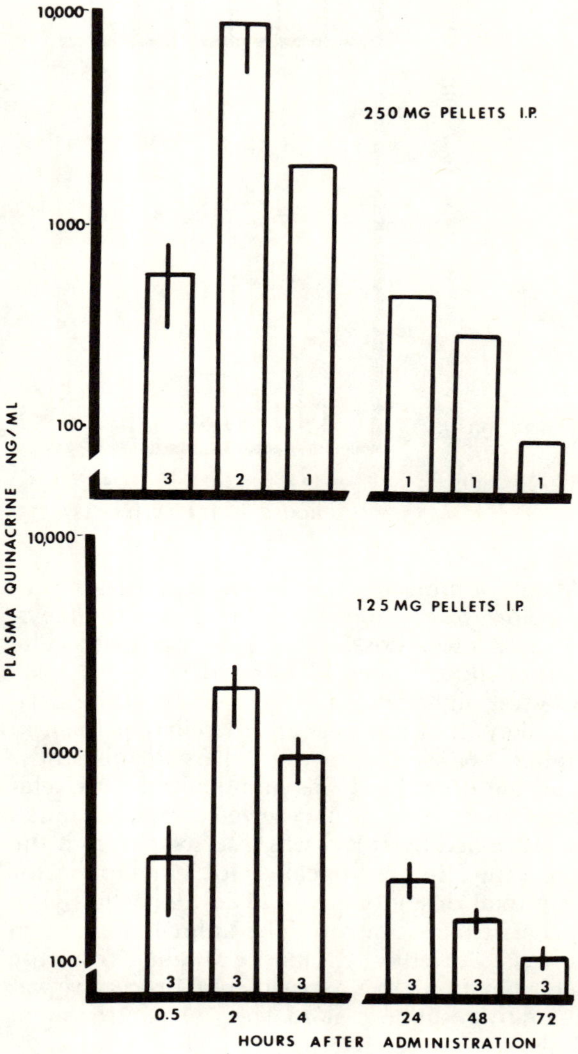

FIG. 6-4. Plasma quinacrine concentration following intraperitoneal administration of 250 or 125 mg quinacrine hydrochloride pellets to nonpregnant monkeys. Note that ordinate is logarithmic.

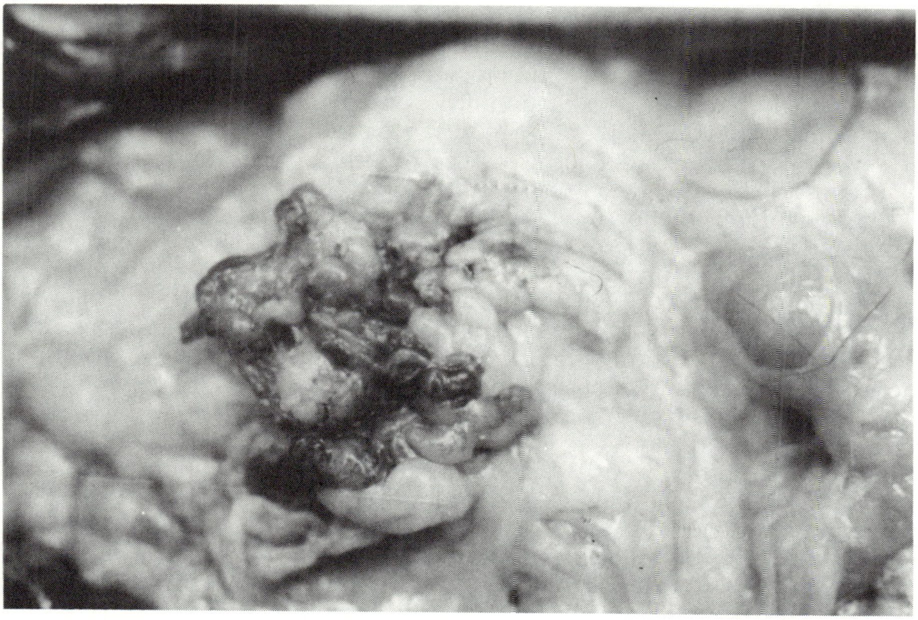

FIG. 6-5. Peritoneal inflammation and adhesions in monkey 3 days following intraperitoneal administration of 125 mg quinacrine pellets.

Plasma quinacrine levels were very high at 30 minutes after treatment (Fig. 6-4). These concentrations increased and we observed the highest levels at 2 hours, the time when the monkeys treated with the high dose died or had convulsions. A blood sample, obtained from one monkey at the time of its death, revealed a quinacrine level of 11,700 ng/ml. In the surviving monkeys treated with quinacrine, plasma concentrations of the drug remained elevated for 3 days after treatment, although they demonstrated a declining trend (see Fig. 6-4).

Surviving animals were autopsied 3 days after treatment. No pellet material could be identified in the peritoneal cavities. One monkey receiving 250 mg quinacrine and another receiving 125 mg quinacrine had an area of inflammation and adhesion directly below the area of incision, corresponding to the area of drug application (Fig. 6-5). Such a reaction could be a source of pain.

COMMENTS

The studies with cynomolgus monkeys indicated three effects that cause concern about the use of quinacrine as a tubal occlusion agent: (1) abdominal pain, (2) central nervous system (CNS) stimulation, and (3) death following administration of the drug.

Some indication of the effect of applying quinacrine directly to the intraperitoneal cavity of humans can be acquired from studies in which quinacrine was used in the control of neoplastic effusions. In one study, 400-mg doses placed directly into the peritoneal cavity caused abdominal pain. The pain is thought to be due to an inflammatory response of the peritoneum to the drug.[8] In another study, instillation of less than 1200 mg resulted in minor toxic symptoms, such as pain or nausea.[14] As the dose exceeded 1200 mg, however, more severe toxic effects were reported, including transient CNS symptoms, such as hallucinatory episodes and "other cerebral difficulties."

The convulsions that occurred in one monkey in our study are of particular significance, because CNS effects were previously reported in people receiving oral quinacrine for treatment of malaria and in women receiving intrauterine quinacrine as a tubal occlusive agent.[17] CNS excitation following treatment of malaria with quinacrine had been noticed and characterized variously as psychic stimulation, motor acceleration, restlessness, insomnia, increased work capacity, and epileptiform convulsions.[9]

A "toxic psychosis" seems to be of two distinct types. In one, there is a sudden increase in motor activity, auditory and visual hallucinations, and delusions. The other type is characterized by gradual clouding of the sensorium, disorientation, amnesia for recent events, and confabulation.[9] That quinacrine, and not the disease, is the source of the symptoms has been demonstrated by the following studies using healthy subjects. In one study, 31 people who had never suffered from malaria were given increasing doses of quinacrine (from 100 mg to 1200 mg daily, orally).[10] Twenty-four reported CNS disturbances of varying degrees. Severe psychic disturbances occurred in 12 subjects, 3 of whom developed frank psychoses, with hallucinations and delusions. Control subjects receiving a placebo reported only mild symptoms, such as insomnia and tension.

In another study, five subjects were given oral doses of quinacrine, ranging from 200 to 1200 mg/day, until plasma levels of the drug exceeded 100 ng/ml.[6] Electroencephalograms were obtained from bipolar fronto-occipital tracings. Frequency of brain waves accelerated when the plasma level of drug exceeded 30 ng/ml. Psychological symptoms, from restlessness to acute panic reaction, occurred concurrent with acceleration in the electroencephalographic patterns.

Following instillation of quinacrine suspension into the uterus, "CNS excitation" was reported in 2% of the patients. However, the symptom has not been reported when pellets are administered.[17]

To date, more than 1000 women have received intrauterine administration of quinacrine, either in solutions or pellets, with no drug-related deaths reported. The studies in cynomolgus monkeys described above, and those in rhesus monkeys, emphasize that the pellet dose that caused death in the cynomolgus monkey was, on a body weight basis, 17 times the dose normally given to women, and the drug was placed directly into the peritoneal cavity.

A 250-mg dose of intraperitoneal quinacrine resulted in the deaths of two of the three monkeys. Assuming an approximate weight of 3 kg for a cynomolgus monkey, this would be about 80 mg/kg. In rats, the maximal tolerable dose is reported to be 250 mg/kg following intraperitoneal administration.[12] A 40-mg dose of quinacrine injected into the rat uterus resulted in a 32% death rate.[11] The mechanism by which death occurs in response to quinacrine is not known, but it appears to be related to the circulating levels of the drug.

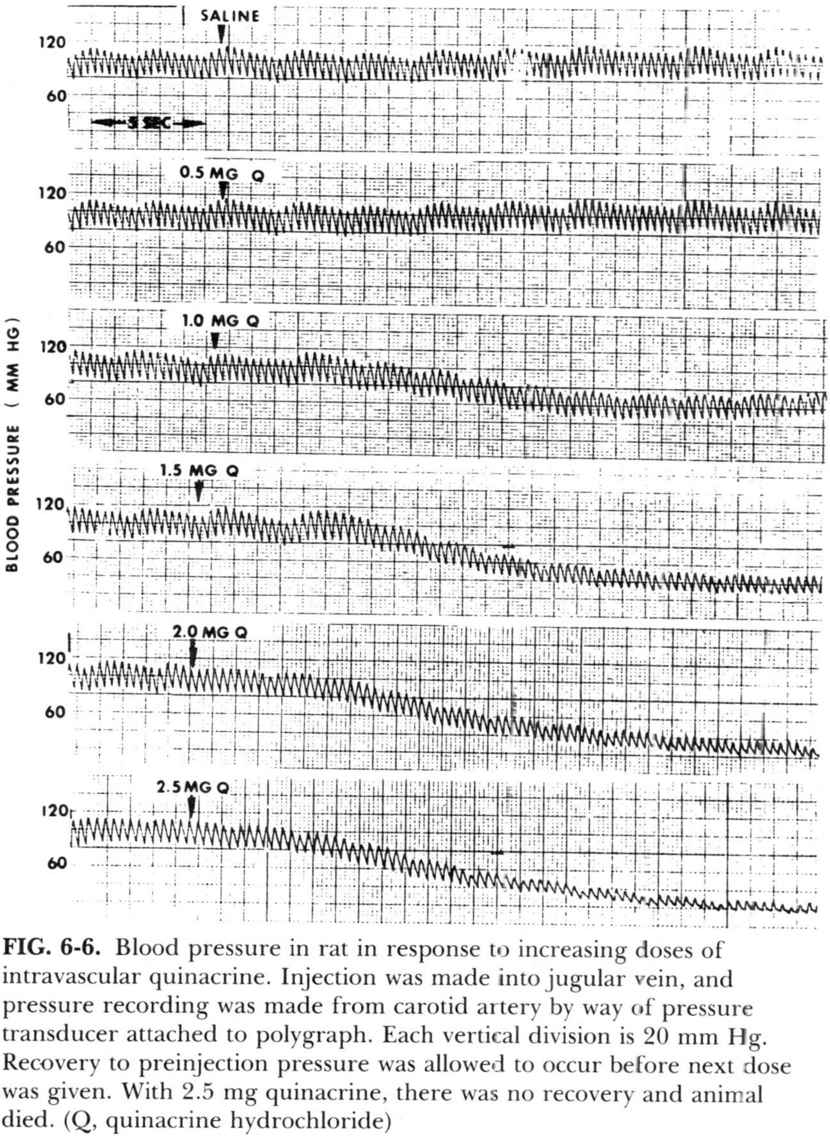

FIG. 6-6. Blood pressure in rat in response to increasing doses of intravascular quinacrine. Injection was made into jugular vein, and pressure recording was made from carotid artery by way of pressure transducer attached to polygraph. Each vertical division is 20 mm Hg. Recovery to preinjection pressure was allowed to occur before next dose was given. With 2.5 mg quinacrine, there was no recovery and animal died. (Q, quinacrine hydrochloride)

We have done preliminary studies in rats demonstrating that intravascular injections of quinacrine, beginning with 1 mg, will cause a decrease in blood pressure from 115/80 mm Hg (systolic/diastolic) to 70/45 mm Hg (Fig. 6-6). This occurs after a lag period of 6 or 7 seconds and is followed by complete recovery after 25 seconds. With increasing doses, there is a greater depression in blood pressure, with prolonged recovery time. Following a dose of 2.5 mg, however, blood pressure dropped to 20/15 mm Hg, there was no recovery, and the animal died. This experiment was replicated in a second animal with the same outcome.

Clearly, there is some risk in the use of quinacrine as a tubal occlusion agent. The importance of these risks relative to the future use of this drug in fertility regulation will be discussed in Chapter 15.

REFERENCES

1. CHANDRA H, MALAVIYA B: Toxic effects of quinacrine hydrochloride in rhesus monkeys. Contraception 24:269, 1981
2. DUBIN NH, BLAKE DA, PARMLEY TH et al: Intrauterine ethanol-induced termination of pregnancy in cynomolgus monkeys (*Macaca fascicularis*). Am J Obstet Gynecol 132:783, 1978
3. DUBIN NH, PARMLEY TH, COX RT et al: Effect of silver nitrate on pregnancy termination in cynomolgus monkeys. Fertil Steril 36:106, 1981
4. DUBIN NH, BLAKE DA, DIBLASI MC et al: Pharmacokinetic studies on quinacrine following intrauterine administration to cynomolgus monkeys. Fertil Steril 38:735, 1982
5. DUBIN NH, STRANDBERG JD, CRAFT CF et al: Effect of intrauterine and intravascular quinacrine administration on histopathology, blood chemistry and hematology in cynomolgus monkeys. Fertil Steril 38:741, 1982
6. ENGEL GL, ROMANO J, FERRIS EB: Effect of quinacrine (Atabrine) on the central nervous system: Clinical and electroencephalographic studies. Arch Neurol Psychiatry 58:337, 1947
7. FINDLAY GM: Recent Advances in Chemotherapy, vol II. Philadelphia, P Blakiston & Son, 1951
8. GELLHORN A, ZAIDENWEBER J, UHMANN J, HIRSCHBERG E: The use of Atabrine (quinacrine) in the control of recurrent neoplastic effusions. Dis Chest 39:165, 1961
9. GOODMAN LS, GILMAN A: The Pharmacologic Basis of Therapeutics, 2nd ed, pp 1167–1173. New York, Macmillan, 1960
10. HOOBLER SW: Psychotic reactions to the ingestion of large doses of quinacrine in normal subjects. Am J Trop Med 27:477, 1947
11. JOSEPH AA, KINCL FA: Toxic and antifertility effects of quinacrine hydrochloride in rats. Am J Obstet Gynecol 119:978, 1974
12. KEELER R, RICHARDSON H, WATSON AJ: Enteromegaly and steatorrhea in the rat following intraperitoneal quinacrine (Atabrine). Lab Invest 15:1253, 1966
13. PARMLEY TH, DUBIN NH, BLAKE DA et al: Hysterosalpingography in cynomolgus monkeys. J Med Primatol (in press)
14. ROCHLIN DA, SMART CR, WAGNER DE et al: The control of recurrent malignant effusions using quinacrine hydrochloride. Surg Gynecol Obstet 118:991, 1964
15. SHANNON JA, EARLE DP, BRODIE BB et al: The pharmacological basis for the rational use of Atabrine in the treatment of malaria. J Pharmacol Exp Ther 81:307, 1944
16. STECK EA: Chemotherapy of Protozoan Disease, vol III, pp 23–172. Walter Reed Army Institute of Research, US Government Printing Office, 1972
17. ZIPPER J, COLE LP, GOLDSMITH A et al: Quinacrine hydrochloride pellets: Preliminary data on a nonsurgical method of female sterilization. Int J Gynaecol Obstet 18:275, 1980

7

Teratologic and Mutagenic Studies With Intrauterine Quinacrine Hydrochloride

DAVID A. BLAKE

NORMAN H. DUBIN

MARIA C. DIBLASI

TIM H. PARMLEY

GAIL STETTEN

THEODORE M. KING

TERATOLOGY

Since 1969, intrauterine quinacrine has been used clinically in various developing countries as a means of effecting tubal closure. The advantage of this procedure is that it is a nonsurgical method of accomplishing sterilization. Because of the possibility that some patients who receive quinacrine might be pregnant at the time of introduction of the drug into the uterus, it is necessary to consider the fetal outcome of such exposure. The following studies were directed toward determining the embryopathic effect and maternal toxicity of an intrauterine injection of quinacrine on pregnant monkeys and rats.

MONKEYS

Methods

Female cynomolgus monkeys were followed for cyclic bleeding and mated during a limited period (3 days) at Hazelton Texas Primate Center, Alice, Texas. If palpation on two occasions revealed that pregnancy had occurred, the monkeys were shipped to Baltimore at approximately 30 days of pregnancy and were placed in individual cages. Pregnancy was confirmed by our personnel by palpation, and treatment was instituted prior to 50 days of pregnancy. We gave a 1-ml intrauterine injection of either 0.9% saline, 3 mg

These studies were supported by contracts from the International Fertility Research Program #601 and #603.

quinacrine HCl, or 30 mg quinacrine HCl (Quinacrine HCl; No. Q 0250FD, F&D lot No. 7-3-2, Sigma Chemical Co., St. Louis, Missouri). While the animal was under ketamine anesthesia, injections were made using a 12-cm 18-gauge blunt-end stainless steel needle inserted through the cervical canal.

Prior to treatment, blood was obtained for blood chemistry and hematology. Blood chemistry determinations included serum glutamic oxalacetic transaminase (SGOT), serum glutamic pyruvic transaminase (SGPT), γ-glutamyl transpeptidase, alkaline phosphatase, lactic dehydrogenase (LDH), cholesterol, triglyceride, total protein, albumin, globulin, blood urea nitrogen, creatinine, direct and total bilirubin, uric acid, glucose, iron, magnesium, sodium, potassium, calcium, phosphorus, and chloride. Hematology analyses included leukocytes, neutrophils, lymphocytes, erythrocytes, hematocrit, and hemoglobin. Food was withdrawn 24 hours prior to treatment. Water was available at all times. Following the treatment, monkeys were returned to their cages and observed daily. Additional blood samples were obtained at 7 and 28 days after treatment for blood chemistry and hematology analyses. On day 28 after treatment, the monkey was repalpated to establish the progress of pregnancy. If pregnancy continued, at approximately 120 days' gestation, the fetus was removed surgically and examined.

Results and Discussion

All monkeys received from the Texas Primate Center appeared in good health, although they appeared thin. Also, after arrival they did not eat for several days, possibly due to the new environment. Pregnancy in all animals was confirmed by palpation. Blood chemistry values prior to treatment were compared with those values obtained from nonpregnant cynomolgus monkeys (obtained from Primate Imports, Port Washington, NY). It was noticed that some values were significantly different. For example, the pregnant group of monkeys had higher SGOT (113.7 ± 20.7 vs. 50.6 ± 3.7 IU/liter, $p < 0.01$), LDH (857 ± 136 vs. 404 ± 34 IU/liter, $p < 0.001$), and γ-glutamyl transferase (42.8 ± 4.7 vs. 26.1 ± 2.0 IU/liter, $p < 0.001$), possibly resulting from the stress of the shipping procedure or from pregnancy.

Following injection of intrauterine physiologic saline, all three animals lost their pregnancies either by spontaneous abortion (*i.e.*, passed fetal tissue; No. 191N and No. 171N) or resorption of the fetus (No. 158N), as indicated by failure of the uterus to grow normally when palpated on day 28 after injection (Table 7-1). This was unexpected, because previous studies indicated that intrauterine physiologic saline injection resulted in a high percentage of normal pregnancies in cynomolgus monkeys (9/13, 70%).[10,11]

All monkeys receiving 3 mg quinacrine resorbed their pregnancies, as indicated by palpation 28 days after injection (see Table 7-1). Following an injection of 30 mg quinacrine one monkey (No. 161N) was found dead in the cage 2 days later. An autopsy disclosed focal peritoneal necrosis and peritonitis, which possibly could have been the result of quinacrine injection but were not believed to be extensive enough to cause death. The possibility that the uterus was perforated and injection made directly into the peritoneal cavity was considered. Because of this possibility, a separate study was instituted to examine the effect of intraperitoneal injection of quinacrine (see Chapter 6). The fetus and placenta showed signs of autolysis indicating that

TABLE 7-1. Summary of Treatment of Each Monkey and Pregnancy Outcome

ANIMAL NUMBER	INJECTION DOSE	PREGNANCY DAY OF INJECTION	OBSERVATION AT 28 DAYS POST INJECTION	FOLLOW-UP
191N	Control	40	Uterus enlarged but hard	Passed tissue 30 days after njection
171N	Control	35	Aborted on day 27	High leukocyte count before and after abortion
158N	Control	45	Not pregnant	
170N	3 mg QHCl	39	Not pregnant	
200N	3 mg QHCl	36	Not pregnant	
180N	3 mg QHCl	46	Not pregnant	
176N	30 mg QHCl	42	Uterus growing but small	Deformed fetus at pregnancy day 115 obtained by hysterectomy
173N	30 mg QHCl	44	Not pregnant	
161N	30 mg QHCl	34	Day 2—mother dead	

QHCl, quinacrine hydrochloride

death of the fetus preceded that of the mother. This was most likely a result of the quinacrine injection.

When palpated on day 28 after injection, the fetus of the third monkey receiving 30 mg quinacrine (No. 176N) was "growing but smaller than expected" as described by the primate technician. The fetus was removed on pregnancy day 115 and examined. It was found to have multiple congenital deformities, including craniorhachischisis, scoliosis, epitheliogenesis imperfecta, atelectasis, ankylosis of the left tarsus, multiple skeletal abnormalities in the digits of paws and feet, and patent foramen ovale. It should be noted that the neural tube completes its closure by day 29 of development in monkeys and since the drug was administered on day 42, it is very unlikely that it could have been the causative factor. Defects such as ankylosis can occur at any stage of development; however, lower limb defects are often associated with neural tube defects in humans and thus there is a reasonable chance that the other defects observed were part of a spontaneous multiple congenital defect syndrome. The incidence of spontaneously occurring grossly observable abnormalities in newborn rhesus monkeys is approximately 1%.[28] Comparable data for cynomolgus monkeys are not available.

Some hematologic changes occurred following treatment. Since there were few animals in any one group, all pretreatment data were pooled, regardless of the treatment group to which the monkeys were assigned. This value was compared with all other data points by a t-test. The only differences that could be attributed to quinacrine were a decline in erythrocytes on day 7 for animals receiving 3 mg ($4120 \pm 100 \times 10^3$ cells/cu mm) or 30 mg ($4575 \pm 195 \times 10^3$ cells/cu mm) compared with the initial value ($5688 \pm 337 \times 10^3$ cells/cu mm). Compared with pretreatment levels, there was a significantly lower hematocrit (22.8 ± 1.2 vs. $36.8 \pm 1.8\%$, $p < 0.001$) and hemogloblin concentration (6.4 ± 0.7 vs. 10.2 ± 0.5 gm/dl, $p < 0.01$) in monkeys 7 days after treatment with 3 mg quinacrine, but levels were normal 28 days after treatment. None of these effects was dose related.

Similar analyses were made with blood chemistries. Total protein was significantly less in monkeys treated with 3 mg quinacrine, compared with pretreatment concentrations (6.4 ± 0.2 vs. 7.3 ± 0.1 gm/dl, $p < 0.01$). By day 28, this value had returned to normal.

There was a slight, but significant ($p < 0.05$) elevation in SGPT at day 7 in monkeys receiving either dose level of quinacrine.

RATS

Methods

Virgin female Sprague–Dawley rats were bred by Charles River Breeding Labs, Wilmington, Massachusetts, or Harlan–Sprague Dawley of Indianapolis, Indiana. In each of the seven treatment groups, approximately 70% of the rats were obtained from Harlan–Sprague Dawley. The day on which a sperm-positive specimen was obtained was designated as day 0 of gestation. The animals were housed in a constant temperature and humidity room and were fed Charles River RMH-1000 formula. Water was provided *ad libitum* from an automatic system. Cages were lined with "Sani-Chips" bedding. The pregnant dams were weighed on arrival at our facility (day 6 of gestation), on the day of treatment, on gestation day 15, and on the day of necropsy (day 19).

Quinacrine hydrochloride (QHCl) was obtained from the same lot used in the study with monkeys. Quinacrine was dissolved in 0.2M sodium phosphate buffer, *p*H 7.4. Because of limited solubility, the highest dose given in the maximum injectable 0.1-ml volume was 4.0 mg. The low dose was 0.4 mg in a 0.1-ml volume.

Laparotomy was performed with the rat under ether anesthesia. The number of visible implantations in each horn was recorded. Intrauterine injections were made with a Hamilton syringe (0.1-ml capacity). In all treatment groups, one horn of each animal served as a control, receiving only the buffer vehicle. Those rats treated early in gestation (day 8) received a single 0.1-ml injection of quinacrine at the cervical end of the uterine horn. The contralateral horn received a single 0.1-ml injection of the buffer. Those rats treated later in gestation (day 12) received the drug in two 0.05-ml injections, one at the cervical end of the horn and the other at the ovarian end. The contralateral horn was treated similarly with buffer. The incision was sutured and the skin was closed with "autoclips." A buffer-sham treatment group had one horn treated with the buffer (0.1 ml) and the contralateral horn subjected to sham injections (insertion of the needle only).

To provide a positive control treatment group, pregnant rats were treated with 4-nitroquinoline-N-oxide (4NQNO; K&K Labs, Plainview, NY) at a dosage of 50 mg/kg by intrauterine injection on day 12 of gestation. The contralateral horn received 0.1 ml of the vehicle dimethyl sulfoxide (DMSO; Fisher Scientific Co, Silver Spring, MD).

All animals were killed by decapitation on day 19 of gestation. The fetuses were delivered by laparatomy/hysterotomy, measured (crown to rump), weighed, and examined for external anomalies. Approximately one of every three fetuses was fixed in Bouin's fluid (Allen's Modification B-15) for visceral examination by Wilson's technique. The remaining fetuses were cleared by glycerin–potassium hydroxide and stained with alizarin red S for skeletal study. Uteri were examined for resorption sites. Ovaries were examined for number of corpora lutea. Each uterine horn with attached ovary was fixed in 10% neutral buffered formalin.

The occurrence of resorptions, fetal death, and skeletal and visceral anomalies in specific treatment groups was examined by χ^2 analysis using the Yates correction.

Results and Discussion

Resorption. QHCl caused dose-related resorptions when given as a direct intrauterine injection on either day 8 or day 12 of gestation (Tables 7-2 and 7-3). Because there was an unequal number of implantations in the treated

ABLE 7-2. Teratogenicity Evaluation of Quinacrine Hydrochloride (QHCl) ollowing Intrauterine Injection on Day 8 in Rats

	TREATMENT*					
	BUFFER	*SHAM*	*BUFFER*	*QHCl 0.4 MG*	*BUFFER*	*QHCl 4 MG*
lumber of uterine orns evaluated	20	20	20	20	20	20
nplantations						
Total number	126	106	108	114	103	137
Mean (± SE)/horn	6.3 ± 0.3	5.3 ± 0.4	5.4 ± 0.4	5.7 ± 0.4	5.2 ± 0.2	6.9 ± 0.5
	($p < 0.05$)				($p < 0.01$)	
esorptions						
Total number	19	14	20	35	19	71
Mean (± SE)/horn	1.0 ± 0.2	0.7 ± 0.2	1.0 ± 1.9	1.8 ± 0.3	1.0 ± 0.2	3.55 ± 0.4
Percent/horn†	15.0 ± 2.4	12.6 ± 3.8	18.4 ± 3.3	31.2 ± 5.3	18.4 ± 3.9	51.8 ± 5.2
			($p < 0.05$)		($p < 0.001$)	
iable fetuses						
Total number	107	92	87	78	84	65
Mean (± SE)/horn	5.4 ± 0.3	4.6 ± 0.4	4.4 ± 0.4	3.9 ± 0.4	4.2 ± 0.3	3.3 ± 0.4
Percent/horn‡	85.0 ± 2.4	87.4 ± 3.8	80.6 = 5.2	68.0 ± 5.2	81.6 ± 3.9	47.6 ± 5.2
					($p < 0.001$)	
alformations Total number of malformed fetuses	6	5	8	6	1	2
Percent malformed/ horn§	6.0 ± 3.3	6.3 ± 2.9	10.3 ± 4.5	5.9 ± 2.8	1.0 ± 1.0	6.0 ± 5.0

*Injections made directly into uteri of anesthetized rats. For each rat, one uterine horn was eated with buffer and the other with buffer plus QHCl. Sham treatment involved insertion of the eedle but no injection.

†Percent resorptions = number of resorptions/number of implantations × 100.

‡Percent viable = number of living/number of implantations × 100.

§Percent malformed = number of fetuses malformed/number viable × 100.

TABLE 7-3. Teratogenicity Evaluation of Quinacrine Hydrochloride (QHCl) Following Intrauterine Injection on Day 12 in Rats

	TREATMENT*							
	BUFFER	*SHAM*	*BUFFER*	*QHCl 0.4 MG*	*BUFFER*	*QHCl 4 MG*	*DMSO*	*4NQNO 1.25 MG*
Number of uterine horns evaluated	19	19	18	18	19	19	19	19
Implantations								
Total number	127	97	87	120	93	125	97	114
Mean (± SE)/horn	6.7 ± 0.3	5.1 ± 0.4	4.8 ± 0.4	6.7 ± 0.3	4.9 ± 0.4	6.6 ± 0.4	5.1 ± 0.5	6.0 ± 0.4
	($p < 0.01$)		($p < 0.01$)		($p < 0.01$)			
Resorptions								
Total number	18	22	18	34	28	86	48	92
Mean (± SE)/horn	1.0 ± 0.2	1.2 ± 0.3	1.0 ± 0.3	1.9 ± 0.4	1.5 ± 0.3	4.5 ± 0.7	2.5 ± 0.5	4.8 ± 0.3
					($p < 0.001$)		($p < 0.001$)	
Percent/horn†	14.9 ± 3.3	22.5 ± 6.0	23.3 ± 6.0	27.0 ± 0.5	27.6 ± 4.4	65.5 ± 8.3	45.0 ± 7.9	85.0 ± 4.9
					($p < 0.001$)		($p < 0.001$)	
Viable fetuses								
Total number	109	75	69	86	64	39	49	22
Mean (± SE)/horn	5.7 ± 0.4	3.9 ± 0.5	3.8 ± 0.5	4.8 ± 0.3	3.4 ± 0.3	2.1 ± 0.5	2.6 ± 0.4	1.2 ± 0.4
	($p < 0.01$)				($p < 0.05$)		($p < 0.05$)	
Percent/horn‡	85.1 ± 3.3	77.5 ± 6.0	76.7 ± 6.0	73.0 ± 5.0	71.3 ± 4.4	34.4 ± 8.3	55.0 ± 7.9	15.0 ± 4.9
					($p < 0.001$)		($p < 0.001$)	
Malformations								
Total number of malformed fetuses	10	7	4	9	2	1	1	4
Percent malformed/horn§	9.9 ± 4.1	6.8 ± 3.3	5.5 ± 3.0	9.1 ± 3.3	2.6 ± 1.8	1.3 ± 1.3	5.3 ± 5.3	10.0 ± 5.8

*Injections made directly into uteri of anesthetized rats. For each rat, one uterine horn was treated with buffer and the other with buffer plus QHCl or sham; except for 4NQNO, which was dissolved in DMSO.

†Percent resorptions = number of resorptions/number of implantations × 100.

‡Percent viable = number of living/number of implantations × 100.

§Percent malformed = number of fetuses malformed/number viable × 100.

DMSO, dimethyl sulfoxide; 4NQNO, 4-nitroquinoline-N-oxide.

and control horns in most treatment groups, it was necessary to analyze these data as absolute values and also after normalizing the data by expressing as a percentage of implantations observed at the time of the treatment. A significant effect was observed in the high-dose groups when calculated either way. Susceptibility to QHCl-induced resorption appeared to be somewhat greater in early pregnancy since on day 8, the low dose (0.4 mg) caused a significant effect, whereas on day 12 this dose was ineffective. The magnitude of the resorption effect caused by the high dose of QHCl (4 mg) was similar on day 8 and day 12, taking into account the differences in control (buffer-induced) resorption rates at these gestational ages; the effect attributable to the drug was approximately 34% and 38% for day 8 and day 12 treatments, respectively. Injection of the buffer vehicle had no significant effect, since the resorption rate was not different between buffer and sham-treated (*i.e.*, insertion of needle without delivery of any liquid) groups at either stage of gestation.

Because 4NQNO is known to be a direct-acting mutagen (as is quinacrine), it was used as a positive control.[19] An intrauterine dose of 1.25 mg given on gestation day 12 had a marked resorption effect (see Table 7-3). DMSO was the vehicle used for 4NQNO, and it also appeared to have a significant resorption effect, although not enough to account for the entire effect observed with DMSO and 4NQNO.

Malformations. A low rate of malformation, less than 10% of viable fetuses, was observed in control (buffer, DMSO, sham) groups (Tables 7-2 and 7-3). There was no observed increase in this overall malformation rate in any of the groups treated with QHCl or 4NQNO.

In order to be certain that a teratogenic effect of a specific type had not been obscured by grouping all malformed fetuses, we also analyzed the results according to separate classification by type of malformation (skeletal, Table 7-4; visceral, Table 7-5). No evidence of treatment-related malformations emerged from this analysis. Some malformations are not listed in these tabulations because they were observed only in control groups, perhaps because of their greater number of fetuses.

The malformation data are presented in a manner appropriate for evaluating the possible occurrence of multiple malformation syndromes in treatment groups in Table 7-6. This analysis also failed to identify a teratogenic effect of either quinacrine or 4NQNO.

This study has demonstrated that intrauterine administration of solutions of QHCl to pregnant rats during the period of embryogenesis results in a marked and dose-related resorption effect. The potency (*i.e.*, dose required to produce a significant effect) of quinacrine for inducing resorptions appeared to be greater in early embryogenesis, whereas the efficacy of the drug (magnitude of effect at a maximal dose) was similar in early and late embryogenesis. There was no evidence of any malformations associated with quinacrine treatment. All viable fetuses were carefully examined for gross evidence of malformations. Skeletal and visceral examinations were performed on two thirds and one third, respectively. Therefore, the drug appears to have no teratogenic (*i.e.*, malformation-inducing) effect. Likewise, the positive control, 4NQNO, did not have a teratogenic effect, although like quinacrine, it did induce resorptions.

TABLE 7-4. Results of Skeletal Examinations: Specific Malformations

TREATMENT	NUMBER OF VIABLE FETUSES EXAMINED	NO STERNABRAE	INCOMPLETE SKULL BONES	METATARSALS NOT OSSIFIED	METACARPALS NOT OSSIFIED	14 PAIRS OF RIBS	ADACTYLE
Control						1 (0.9%)	
Sham	112	7 (6.3%)*	1 (0.9%)				
Buffer	353	25 (7.1%)	4 (1.1%)	2 (0.6%)	1 (0.3%)	1 (0.3%)	
Total	465	32 (6.9%)	5 (1.1%)	2 (0.4%)	1 (0.2%)	2 (0.4%)	
QHCl							
Day 8							
0.4 mg	50	5 (10.0%)	2 (4.0%)	1 (2.0%)	1 (2.0%)	1 (2.0%)	
4.0 mg	44	1 (2.3%)					
Total day 8	94	6 (6.4%)	2 (2.1%)	1 (1.1%)	1 (1.1%)	1 (1.1%)	
Day 12							
0.4 mg	58	4 (6.9%)	1 (1.7%)	1 (1.7%)		1 (1.7%)	
4.0 mg	26	1 (3.9%)					
Total day 12	84	5 (6.0%)	1 (1.2%)	1 (1.2%)		1 (1.2%)	
Total	178	11 (6.2%)	3 (1.7%)	2 (1.1%)	1 (0.6%)	2 (1.1%)	
DMSO control	32	1 (3.1%)	1 (3.1%)	1 (3.1%)			
4NQNO	16	2 (12.5%)	1 (6.3%)	1 (6.3%)	1 (6.3%)		1 (6.3%)

*Numbers in parentheses are the percentage of number examined with abnormality.

TABLE 7-5. Results of Visceral Examinations: Specific Malformations

TREATMENT	NUMBER OF VIABLE FETUSES EXAMINED	CLEFT PALATE	CAVITY IN ADRENAL	MISSING ONE KIDNEY, OVARY, AND UTERINE HORN	HYDRO-NEPHROSIS	ANENCEPHALY
Control						
Sham	55		1 (1.8%)		2 (3.6%)	
Buffer	167					
Total	222		1 (0.5%)		2 (0.9%)	
QHCl						
Day 8						
0.4 mg	28				1 (3.6%)	1 (3.6%)*
4.0 mg	21				2 (9.5%)	
Total day 8	49				3 (6.1%)	1 (2.0%)
Day 12						
0.4 mg	28			1 (3.6%)	2 (7.1%)	
4.0 mg	13					
Total day 12	41			1 (2.4%)	2 (4.9%)	
Total	90			1 (1.1%)	5 (5.6%)	1 (1.1%)
DMSO	17					
4NQNO	6	1 (16.7%)				

*Only fetus from the pregnancy, no corresponding control horn.

(%), percent malformed/number examined.

TABLE 7-6. Results of Skeletal Examinations: All Malformations

TREATMENT	NUMBER OF VIABLE FETUSES EXAMINED	NUMBER OF MALFORMATIONS				
		1 OR MORE	*2 OR MORE*	*3 OR MORE*	*4 OR MORE*	*5 OR MORE*
Control						
Sham	112	9 (8.0%)*	1 (0.9%)			
Buffer	353	29 (8.2%)	7 (2.0%)	2 (0.6%)	1 (0.3%)	
Total	465	38 (8.2%)	8 (1.7%)	2 (0.4%)	1 (0.2%)	
QHCl						
Day 8						
0.4 mg	50	6 (12.0%)	2 (4.0%)	2 (4.0%)	1 (2.0%)	
4.0 mg	44	1 (2.3%)				
Total day 8	94	7 (7.5%)	2 (2.1%)	2 (2.1%)	1 (1.1%)	
Day 12						
0.4 mg	58	6 (10.3%)	1 (1.7%)			
4.0 mg	26	1 (3.9%)				
Total day 12	84	7 (8.3%)	1 (1.2%)			
Total	178	14 (7.9%)	3 (1.7%)	2 (1.1%)	1 (0.6%)	
DMSO	32	1 (3.1%)	1 (3.1%)	1 (3.1%)	1 (3.1%)	1 (3.1%)
4NQNO	16	3 (18.8%)	1 (6.3%)	1 (6.3%)	1 (6.3%)	

*Numbers in parentheses are the percentage of number examined with abnormality.

MUTAGENICITY

BACTERIA

Materials and Methods

The following compounds (obtained from Sigma Chemical Co., St. Louis, MO) were tested in the *Salmonella*/mammalian-microsome mutagenicity assay: acridine, chloroquine diphosphate, primaquine diphosphate, and quinacrine hydrochloride. Five dose levels (1,000 μg, 100μg, 10μg, 1μg, and 0.1μg/plate) were assayed with and without exogenous metabolic activation. Higher doses of chloroquine (10,000μg and 2,500μg/plate) were also tested to achieve the maximum noninhibitory dose. All test compounds except chloroquine diphosphate were dissolved in DMSO (Fisher Scientific, Fair Lawn, NJ). Chloroquine was dissolved in double distilled water and then filter-sterilized using a 0.22μm disposable unit (Millipore Corp, Bedford, MA). All dilutions of test drugs were prepared immediately prior to use. Purified sodium azide (NaN_3) (Fisher Scientific, Fair Lawn, NJ) and 4NQNO (K&K Labs, Plainview, NY) were used as direct-acting mutagens. Benzo(a)pyrene (BP; Aldrich Chemical Co., Milwaukee, WI) and 2-anthramine (Sigma Chemical Co., St. Louis, MO) were used as positive controls requiring metabolic activation.

The *Salmonella typhimurium* strains used (TA 98, TA 100, TA 1535, TA 1537, and TA 1538) were provided by Dr. Bruce N. Ames, University of California, Berkeley. On receipt of the strains, the characteristic markers of each were checked as outlined by Ames and associates.[4] Overnight cultures were prepared from frozen (−70°C) stocks by incubation with 2.5% Oxoid nutrient broth (KC Biologicals, Inc, Lenexa, Kansas) for 16 to 17 hours at 37%C.

Rat liver S9 was used as a source of exogenous metabolic activation. Livers were obtained aseptically from adult male Sprague–Dawley rats, 5 days after intraperitoneal treatment with Aroclor 1254 (Monsanto Chemical Co, St. Louis, MO) at a dosage of 250 mg/kg. The excised tissue was homogenized at 4°C with three volumes of 0.15M KCl using a Brinkmann Polytron. The homogenate was centrifuged at 9000 × g for 15 minutes at 4°C. The supernatant fraction (S9) was stored in a −70°C Revco freezer. Protein content was determined by a modified Lowry procedure.[22] The cofactor mixture contained per milliliter: $MgCl_2$ (8 μmole), KCl (33 μmole), glucose-6-phosphate (5 μmole), NADP (4 μmole), and sodium phosphate, *p*H 7.4 (100 μmole). The S9 was diluted with 0.15M KCl so that when added to the cofactor, the final concentration of S9 protein was 1.0 mg per milliliter of S9-cofactor mix.

The assays were performed as suggested by Ames and associates using Vogel–Bonner Medium E–minimal glucose agar plates.[4] Briefly, 0.1 ml of the overnight broth culture, containing approximately 10^8 organisms, was added to 2 ml molten top agar supplemented with 0.5% NaCl, 15μg histidine, and 22μg biotin. The appropriate dose of test compound, solvent, or positive control in a 0.1 ml volume was then added. For metabolic activation assays, the molten agar received 0.5 ml of the rat liver S9-cofactor mix. This molten agar overlay was vortex-mixed after each addition and then poured over the base plate. Hardened plates were inverted and incubated at 37°C for 48 to 60 hours. Colonies were counted by direct inspection using a colony counter (Fisher Scientific, Fair Lawn, NJ). Results are expressed as the ratio of the number of revertant colonies in the presence of test compound to the average number of revertant colonies in the absence of test compound (spontaneous revertants).

Results and Discussion

The results of *Salmonella* mutagenicity tests with acridine, chloroquine, primaquine, and quinacrine are shown in Table 7-7. Acridine, chloroquine, and primaquine had no detectable mutagenic activity with or without a rat liver metabolizing system. Quinacrine was clearly mutagenic to TA 1537, a frameshift test strain; the mutagenic activity appeared to be slightly enhanced by rat liver activation. Acridine, chloroquine, and primaquine are chemically related to quinacrine, and the latter two compounds are commonly used antimalarial agents. A review of published studies on the mutagenic activity of quinacrine is presented in Table 7-8. These results provide evidence of significant genetic toxicity of quinacrine, particularly in bacterial systems. Quinacrine is known to intercalate in deoxyribonucleic acid, and this property is utilized in many karyotyping laboratories for banding of chromosomes. Mammalian mutagenicity tests did not show a high level of activity, and conflicting results appear in the literature. Our unpublished study of karyotypes of lymphocytes from quinacrine-treated monkeys failed to demonstrate any chromosomal abnormalities (see below).

In summary, quinacrine is a direct-acting frameshift mutagen in bacterial systems. Its genotoxic potential in mammalian cells is equivocal. The lack of

TABLE 7-7. *Salmonella typhimurium* Mutagenicity Tests: Ratio of Revertants With Test Compound to Spontaneous Revertants

COMPOUND	μG/ PLATE	TA98		TA 100		TA 1535		TA 1537		TA 1538	
		NA*	S9†	NA	S9	NA	S9	NA	S9	NA	S9
Acridine	1,000	Toxic	Toxic	Toxic	Toxic	Toxic	Toxic	Toxic	Toxic	Toxic	Toxic
	100	0.38	0.55	0.53	0.69	1.23	0.89	1.26	1.00	1.00	1.14
	10	0.57	0.83	0.92	0.79	1.23	0.89	0.85	1.00	0.71	1.00
	1	0.74	0.83	1.05	0.91	0.82	1.04	1.00	1.00	0.81	0.71
	0.1	0.74	0.62	1.05	0.82	0.86	1.14	0.74	1.00	0.62	1.07
Chloroquine	10,000	0.29	0.48	0.34	0.66	0.52	0.65	Toxic	1.18	Toxic	0.61
	2,500	0.82	0.66	0.96	0.96	1.16	0.59	0.64	1.12	0.78	1.04
	100	0.92	0.83	0.88	0.94	ND	ND	1.50	1.00	0.85	1.00
	10	1.04	0.93	0.85	0.94	ND	ND	0.50	0.67	1.08	1.13
	1	0.88	1.10	1.02	0.91	ND	ND	0.63	0.58	0.92	0.93
	0.1	0.92	0.90	1.00	0.99	ND	ND	1.00	0.75	0.92	1.13
Primaquine	1,000	Toxic	0.40	Toxic	0.41	Toxic	0.68	Toxic	1.18	Toxic	Toxic
	100	1.14	0.86	0.98	1.10	0.64	0.89	1.00	0.73	0.71	1.21
	10	1.14	0.74	0.76	0.88	0.82	0.71	0.67	0.91	1.00	0.86
	1	0.95	0.64	0.76	1.06	1.00	1.29	0.44	0.64	1.29	1.21
	0.1	0.91	0.74	0.66	1.03	1.50	0.71	0.56	0.55	0.64	1.07
Quinacrine	1,000	Toxic	0.86	Toxic	Toxic	Toxic	Toxic	TNTC	Toxic	0.71	1.74
	100	0.83	0.84	0.76	1.07	1.27	0.82	6.48‡	11.42‡	1.29	0.61
	10	0.57	1.06	0.90	0.93	1.23	0.96	0.67	1.00	0.67	1.03
	1	0.38	0.86	0.88	0.87	1.27	0.82	0.67	0.74	0.81	1.03
	0.1	0.38	0.83	0.84	0.83	1.00	0.64	0.67	0.89	0.67	0.97
4NQNO	0.5	13.17‡		17.95‡		ND		ND		23.67‡	
QHCl	100	ND		ND		ND		11.80‡		ND	
NaN_3	1	ND		ND		25.06‡		ND		ND	
BP	5		5.96‡		6.72‡		ND		4.22‡		8.89‡
2-anthramine	2.5		67.50‡		28.60‡		2.21‡		26.21‡		63.29‡
	1.0		ND		ND		6.83‡		ND		ND

*NA, no addition

†S9 = 9000 × g supernatant fraction of rat liver homogenates (Aroclor pretreated).

‡Positive mutagenic response.

ND, not determined; TNTC, too numerous to count.

TABLE 7-8. Mutagenicity Tests With Quinacrine

TEST SYSTEM	DRUG	METHOD	RESULTS	REFERENCE
Bacterial tests				
Salmonella typhimurium C207 (frameshift)	Quinacrine 5μg/plate	Ames test	"Weak mutagen" (no data provided)	3
S. typhimurium TA 1537 (frameshift)	Quinacrine 100μg/plate ± S9	Ames test	control 12; control + S9 12 drug 1000; drug + S9 1000	19
S. typhimurium his G46 TA 1530, 1531, 1532, 1534	Quinacrine diHCl	Ames test	positive in TA 1532 only	28
Bacillus subtilis his$^-$ his B103, B201, B204	Quinacrine HCl crystal or solution spot test	Reversion to his$^+$	Positive with his B103	13
Escherichia coli K-12 strain ND 160 lac$^-$	Quinacrine HCl as positive control 10μg/ml medium	Score lac$^+$ revertants	Positive	9
E. coli B/r strain + deficient repair; trp$^-$	Quinacrine HCl 10μg/ml medium 20μg/ml medium	Drug incorporated in postirradiation medium score str^r mutants, score trp$^+$ mutants	Positive enhancement of U-V induced str^r mutational yield in strains with intact repair similar results with trp$^+$ yield	8
S. typhimurium TA 1535, 1537, 98, 100 ± S9	Quinacrine diHCl 4 conc. but amts not listed	Ames test	Positive, but not listed which strain, concentration, etc.	15
S. typhimurium gal E 503	Quinacrine diHCl	Screen for mutagens that cause deletions	Incapable of generating such deletions	2
S. typhimurium G46 mouse host BP substitution	Quinacrine	*In vitro* spot test for his$^+$ revertants *In vivo* host mediated assay plate peritoneal fluid	Negative in both tests	20

TABLE 7-8. Mutagenicity Tests With Quinacrine (*Continued*)

TEST SYSTEM	DRUG	METHOD	RESULTS	REFERENCE
S. typhimurium G46 base pair C3076 frameshift	Quinacrine	Spot test with saturated disc	Positive with frameshift Negative with base pair	6
Mammalian (nonhuman) Rat	Quinacrine diHCl 160 mg/kg	Dominant lethal test	Equivocal, too few animals	12
Mouse sperm	Quinacrine diHCl	Score sperm head abnormalities	Negative	15
Mouse polychromatic erythrocytes of bone marrow	Quinacrine diHCl	Micronucleus assay for chromosome breakage	Negative?	15
Mouse bone marrow erythrocytes	Quinacrine diHCl 0.28 mg/kg b wt. 1P	Micronuclei	Positive: increase of micronucleated erythrocytes (up to 65% increase)	17
Mouse bone marrow erythrocytes	Quinacrine diHCl 35, 70, 95, 142 mg/kg	Micronuclei	Negative: disputes reference 17	21
Chinese hamster ovary cells	Quinacrine diHCL 5μg/ml medium	Determining cell survival after preirradiation and postirradiation to drug	Sensitized cells to killing by x-rays; greater effect with preirradiation exposure to drug may inhibit DNA repair	26
Chinese hamster ovary cells	Quinacrine diHCl 0.2μM, 2μM, 20μM	Score chromosome breaks in metaphase Score abnormal anaphases	Frequency of chromosome breakage 3 to 5 times that of control (not considered high)	16

Mouse leukemic cells L 1210	Quinacrine HCl 0.2μg/ml medium	Score ara C^s → ara C^r	Frequency reduced 5- to 16-fold "Antimutagenic"	5
Rat sarcoma cells (Jensen) asparagine	Quinacrine HCl 0.01μg, 0.1μg, 1.0μg, 5.0μg/ml	Score asp^- → asp^+ cells	Ineffective in increasing or decreasing mutation frequency	24
Miscellaneous systems				
Silkworm pupae	Quinacrine HCl 0.25 mg/capita 0.50 mg	Score mutations by specific locus method	0.5-mg dose increased number of mosaic type mutations in females only	23
Saccharomyces cerevisiae	Quinacrine	Auxotrophic → prototrophic revertants drug-saturated disc placed in center of plate, score ring of mutants	Negative with both strains	6
Human cell tests				
Human sternal marrow cells (D-98)	Quinacrine HCl 0.06μg/ml	Score azaguanine resistant mutants	Cultures with drug contained ½–⅓ the mean of mutants found in control cultures	18
Human peripheral leukocytes	Quinacrine HCl 0.3 g for 14 days	Treated for protozoan infection karyotyped three times pretreatment and posttreatment	No abnormalities prior to treatment After treatment modal no. of 48 chromosomes, abnormal marker chromosomes	1

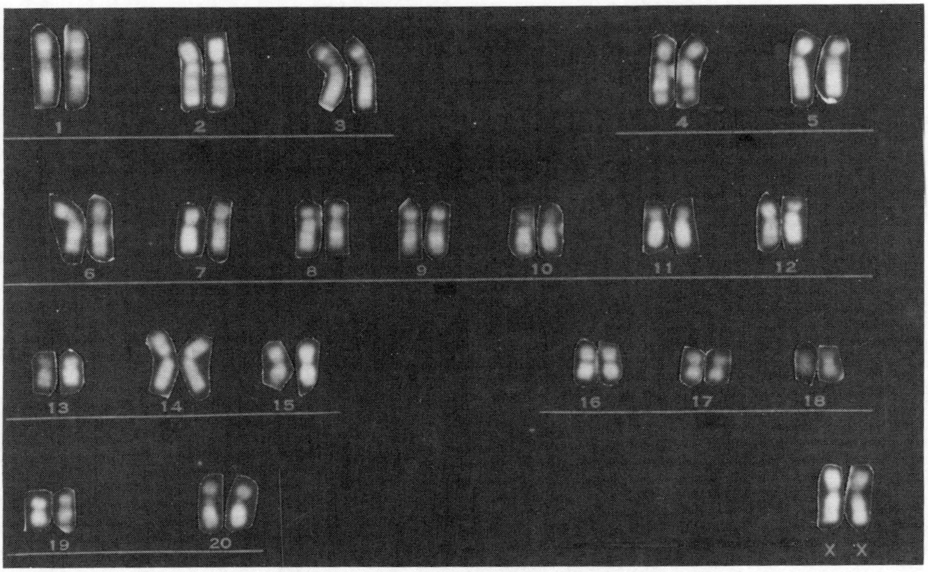

FIG. 7-1. Karyotype of *Macaca fascicularis* arranged according to standard nomenclature.

mutagenic activity (in a bacterial system) for two chemically related antimalarial drugs (chloroquine and primaquine) suggests that the tubal occlusive properties of nonmutagenic analogs of quinacrine may be a productive area for further research.

MONKEY CHROMOSOME ANALYSIS

Peripheral blood samples were taken from a total of 15 monkeys before treatment and at varying times thereafter, ranging from 24 hours to 28 days. Nine received intrauterine quinacrine HCl (30 mg), three received intravenous quinacrine HCl (30 mg), and three received intrauterine saline. Chromosomes were prepared from cultured lymphocytes according to standard human cytogenetic procedures,[25] and slides were prepared for fluorescent banding.[7] For each analysis, 20 banded metaphase spreads were examined and a karyotype was prepared. In every case, the modal chromosome number was found to be 42. No apparent aneuploidy or structural rearrangements were observed for any monkey, regardless of treatment. Chromosome breaks and chromatid gaps were not seen. A typical karyotype for the female cynomolgus monkey is included (Fig. 7-1).

SUMMARY AND CONCLUSIONS

The purpose of these studies was to evaluate the embryopathic potential of quinacrine in the event that the drug is inadvertently administered to a pregnant patient. Such studies in laboratory animals suffer from two major limitations: (1) uncertain suitability as a model for the human and (2) statistical, particularly type II, error (*i.e.*, concluding that no differences due to treatment exist, when in fact they do). Such an error might easily occur in extrapolation of results from a relatively few animal subjects to a much larger population of human patients. We attempted to address these limitations by including two species, the monkey and the rat. We reasoned that although a statistically significant number of rats could be studied, it would be useful to include teratologic testing of a primate species even though the numbers of treated animals would be statistically insignificant. Moreover, although it was difficult to accomplish, we thought it was necessary to use the intrauterine route of treatment in monkeys as well as in rats in order for the study to be relevant to the human circumstance.

The results of the studies in rats clearly demonstrate the embryotoxic potential of quinacrine, manifested as dose-related resorptions. It is important to note, however, that quinacrine treatment did not cause malformations. Thus, strictly speaking, quinacrine is not a teratogen in rats (*i.e* , it does not cause malformed fetuses, although it is quite embryolethal). It is possible, of course, that a much larger study would have demonstrated a low incidence of quinacrine-induced malformations. The sample size (20 pregnant rats per treatment group) was chosen because it is the conventional size for such studies.

Interpretation of the monkey teratologic results is more difficult, primarily because of the small number of animals (three) per treatment group. This is further complicated by the unanticipated result with the control group, where two pregnancies aborted and one resorbed. Our previous experience with intrauterine injections of 0.9% saline in cynomolgus monkeys at this stage of pregnancy suggested a 70% pregnancy continuation rate. However, two of the three control fetuses were aborted (passed tissue) rather than resorbed. This is in contrast to the quinacrine-treated monkeys, in which fetal resorptions occurred but not abortions. Thus, the resorption effect of quinacrine observed in rats also appeared in monkeys. The grossly malformed fetus appeared to be related to factors other than quinacrine, since the type of malformations suggested that they occurred prior to the treatment.

The mutagenicity studies were performed primarily to corroborate what was already published for quinacrine (*i.e.*, it is a direct-acting frameshift mutagen in bacterial systems). As noted in the review of the literature, quinacrine has much less mutagenic activity in eukaryotic cells and no clear mutagenic activity in mammalian systems. It is particularly noteworthy that no chromosomal abnormalities could be detected in the peripheral lymphocytes of cynomolgus monkeys that had received quinacrine by intrauterine or intravenous injection.

Within the limitations of such extrapolations, from these studies quinacrine would appear to have little potential for inducing fetal malformations when administered by intrauterine injection. The embryolethal effect is expected for direct-acting mutagens.

REFERENCES

1. ABE T, MISAWA S, HOSODA S et al: Abnormal (marker) chromosomes in a quinacrine-treated patient with *Isospora* and *Giardia lamblia*. Humangenetik 19:199, 1973
2. ALPER MD, AMES BN: Positive selection of mutants with deletions of the Gal-Chi region of the *Salmonella* chromosome as a screening procedure for mutagens that cause deletions. J Bacteriol 121:259, 1975

3. AMES BN, WHITFIELD HJ: Frameshift mutagenesis in *Salmonella.* Cold Spring Harbor Symposium. Quantitative Biol 31:221, 1966
4. AMES BN, MCCANN J, YAMASAKI E: Methods for detecting carcinogens and mutagens with the *Salmonella*/mammalian-microsome mutagenicity test. Mutat Res 31:347, 1975
5. BACH MK: Reduction in the frequency of mutation to resistance to cytarabine in L1210 murine leukemic cells by treatment with quinacrine hydrochloride. Cancer Res 29:1881, 1969
6. BRUSICK DJ, ZEIGER E: A comparison of chemically induced reversion patterns of *Salmonella typhimurium* and *saccharomyces cerevisiae* mutants, using *in vitro* plate tests. Mutat Res 14:271, 1972
7. CASPERSSON T, LOMAKKA G, TECH L: The 24 fluorescence patterns of the human metaphase chromosomes: Distinguishing characters and variability. Hereditas 67:89, 1971
8. CLARKE CH, SHANKEL DM: Effects of ethidium, quinacrine and hycanthone on survival and mutagenesis of UV-irradiated HCR^+ and HCR^- strains of *E. coli* B/r. Mutat Res 26:473, 1974
9. CLARKE CH, WADE MJ: Evidence that caffeine, 8-methoxypsoralen and steroidal diamines are frameshift mutagens for *E. coli* K-12. Mutat Res 28:123, 1975
10. DUBIN NH, BLAKE DA, PARMLEY TH et al: Intrauterine ethanol-induced termination of pregnancy in cynomolgus monkeys (*Macaca fascicularis*). Am J Obstet Gynecol 132:783, 1978
11. DUBIN NH, PARMLEY TH, COX RT et al: Effect of silver nitrate on pregnancy termination in cynomolgus monkeys. Fertil Steril 36:106, 1981
12. EPSTEIN SS, ARNOLD E, ANDREA J et al: Detection of chemical mutagens by the dominant lethal assay in the mouse. Toxicol Appl Pharmacol 23:288, 1972
13. FELKNEW IC: Mutation induction by the direct treatment of *Bacillus subtilis* deoxyribonucleic acid. Mutat Res 42:175, 1977
14. FERNANDEZ-DONOSO R, LINDSTEN J, NORRBY E: The chromosomes of the cynomolgus monkey (*Macaca fascicularis*). Hereditas 65:269, 1970
15. HEDDLE JA, BRUCE WR: Comparison of tests for mutagenicity or carcinogenicity using assays for sperm abnormalities, formation of micronuclei and mutations in *Salmonella.* Cold Spring Harbor Conference. Cell Proliferation 40:1549, 1977
16. HSU TC, COLLIE CJ, LUSBY AF et al: Cytogenetic assays of chemical clastogens using mammalian cells in culture. Mutat Res 45:233, 1977
17. JESSEN D, RAMEL C, GOETHE R: Induction of micronuclei by frameshift mutagens at the time of nucleus expulsion in mouse erythroblasts. Mutat Res 26:553, 1974
18. JOHNSON HG, BACH MK: Apparent antimutagenic activity of quinacrine hydrochloride in Detroit-98 human sternal marrow cells grown in culture. Cancer Res 29:1367, 1969
19. KUCZUK MH, BENSON PM, HEATH H, HAYES AW: Evaluation of the mutagenic potential of mycotoxins using *Salmonella typhimurium* and *Saccharomyces cerevisiae.* Mutat Res 53:11, 1976
20. LEGATOR MS: The host-mediated assay, a practical procedure for evaluating potential mutagenic agents. In Vogel F, Rohrborn G (eds): Chemical Mutagenesis in Mammals and Man, pp 260–270. New York, Springer-Verlag, 1970
21. MATTER P, SCHMID W: Non-induction of micronuclei by quinacrine. Mutat Res 30:299, 1975
22. MAZEL P: General principles and procedures for drug metabolism *in vitro.* In LaDu HG, Mandel HG, Ways EL (eds): Fundamentals of Drug Metabolism and Drug Disposition, pp 527–545. Baltimore, Williams & Wilkins, 1971
23. MORAKAMI A: Mutagenic activity of quinacrine hydrochloride in the silkworm. Mutat Res 22:295, 1974
24. MORROW J, PRICKETT MS, FRITZ S, VERNICK D, DEEN D: Mutagenesis studies on cultured mammalian cells. The sensitivity of the asparagine-requiring phenotype to several chemical agents. Mutat Res 34:481, 1976
25. SCHWARZACHER HG, WOLF U (eds): Methods in Human Cytogenetics. New York, Springer-Verlag, 1974
26. VOICULETZ N, SMITH KC, KAPLAN HS: Effect of quinacrine on survival and DNA repair in x-irradiated Chinese hamster cells. Cancer Res 34:1033, 1974
27. WASSOM JS, HUFF JE, LOPRIENO N: A review of the genetic toxicology of chlorinated dibenzo-*p*-dioxins. Mutat Res 47:141, 1977/1978
28. WILSON JG: Abnormalities of intrauterine development in nonhuman primates. In Diczfalusy E, Standley CC (eds): Use of Non-Human Primates in Research of Human Reproduction, pp 261–292. WHO Research and Training Centre on Human Reproduction, Stockholm, 1972

8

Histologic Changes Following Intrauterine Administration of Quinacrine Hydrochloride

TIM H. PARMLEY

NORMAN H. DUBIN

J. STRANDBERG

LEONARD E. LAUFE

The histologic changes that occur when quinacrine is placed into the uterus have not been well documented.[1] In addition, the sequential process involved remains unclear.

In this chapter, we will briefly describe a sequence of histopathologic changes taking place in the cornual portion of the fallopian tube subsequent to exposure to quinacrine. This description provides a coherent basis for the two known outcomes of such exposure, tubal closure or tubal patency. Since most of the changes were not observed as part of a prospective timed protocol, the interpretation remains hypothetical.

METHOD

Two pig uteri were examined approximately 2 weeks after the pigs had been treated with quinacrine. In the operation, the uteri had been opened and 125 mg quinacrine was held forcefully against the cornua for 15 to 20 minutes. We also examined the uteri of nine monkeys removed 24 hours (from three monkeys), 7 days (from three monkeys), and 28 days (from three monkeys) after the intrauterine instillation of 30 mg quinacrine in 1 ml sterile water.[1]

HYPOTHESIS

The initial reaction of the tissue lining the endometrial cavity and the cornual portion of the tube is autolysis. In most cases, this damage is superficial. For example, in the cornua, the tube was involved no more deeply than the innermost fibers of muscle surrounding the interstitial tube. Despite gross yellow discoloration of the tube beyond the isthmus in monkeys examined

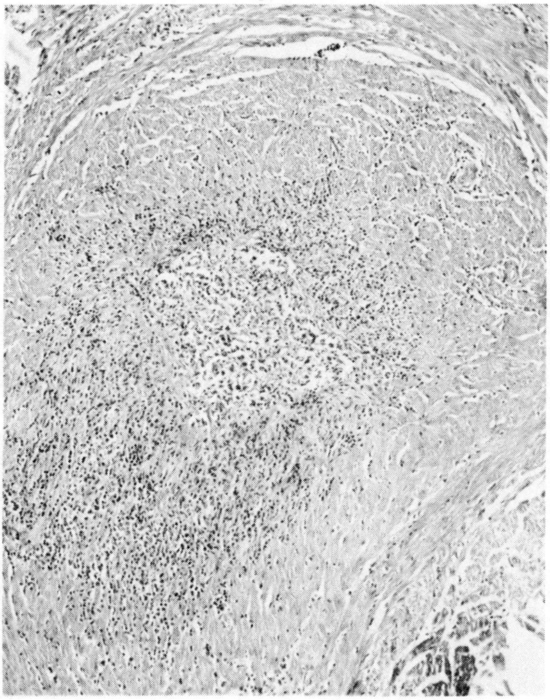

FIG. 8-1. An area of central necrosis, subsequent to autolysis, is being invaded by an inflammatory infiltrate. As yet, there is no proliferative repair. Human tissue.

24 hours after intrauterine quinacrine application, tubal damage did not extend beyond the cornua. On the other hand, in those same monkeys, considerable endometrial damage was found. In most cases, the damage looked superficial with respect to the epithelium, but it extended along this epithelium deep into the glands to the basalis in several spots. In the latter cases, the stroma surrounding the gland might remain relatively intact. There was also one monkey in which there was some endocervical damage, but this damage might have been due to the cervical manipulation required to pass the instillation needle into the uterus.

In several specimens obtained from pigs, however, the damage extended all the way through the myometrium to the serosal surface. It should be noted that the methodology used in these cases was significantly different from that of the rest of the material.

After the initial reaction, the area of autolysis becomes inflamed (Fig. 8-1) and then organized by fibroblastic proliferation and scar (Fig. 8-2). In the cornual portion of the tube, if, as the result of the close apposition of the walls of this narrow portion of the tube, organization occurs in such a manner that the lumen is obliterated, sterilization has been achieved. Occlusion is not always successful, however. If the central or luminal portion of the necrotic area "drops out," presumably because of liquefaction, then this cavity will become reepithelialized before organization occurs (Fig. 8-3). Subsequent or-

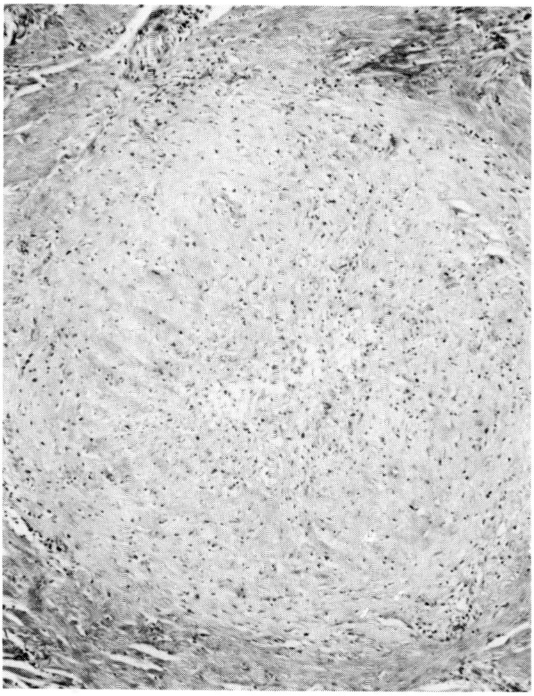

FIG. 8-2 Scar, subsequent to proliferative repair, has almost totally replaced the area of autolysis and necrosis. There is no central epithelium, and the suggestion is that the tubal lumen will be completely scarred across. Human tissue.

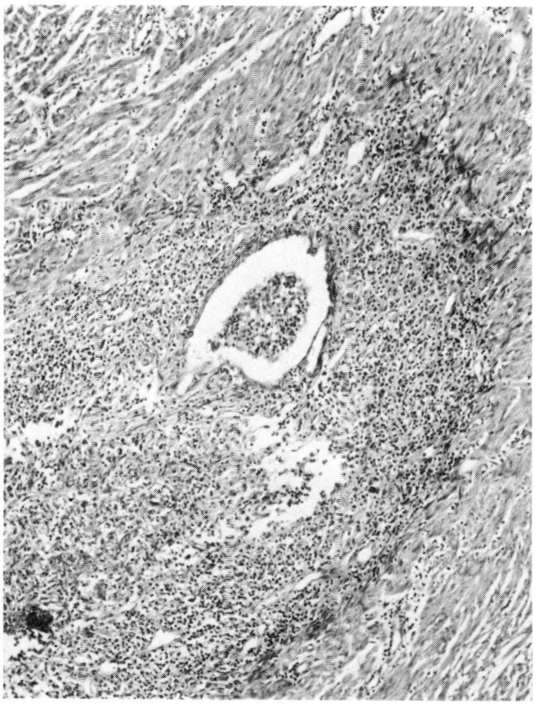

FIG. 8-3. Although a central area of necrosis and inflammation is present, there appears to be a lumen, which already has an epithelial lining. This epithelial lining might be expected to remain even after organization takes place. Human tissue.

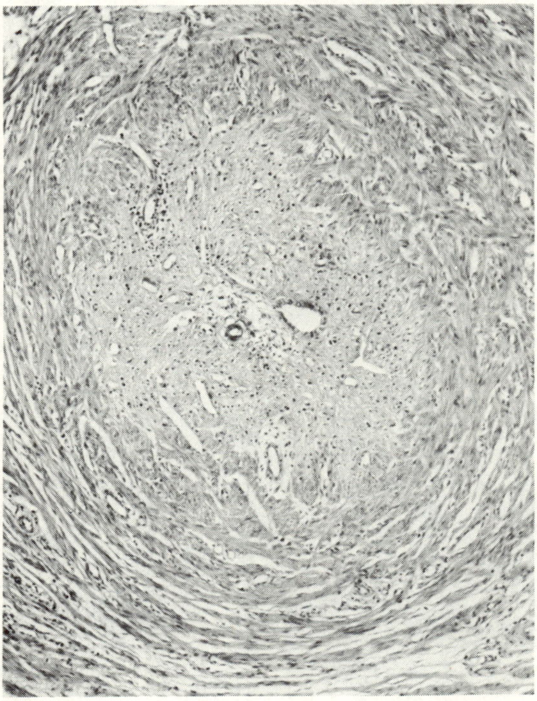

FIG. 8-4. Organization and repair appear to have occurred around two persisting islands of epithelium. Since epithelial surfaces do not adhere, presumably the lumen will not be obliterated in this case. Human tissue.

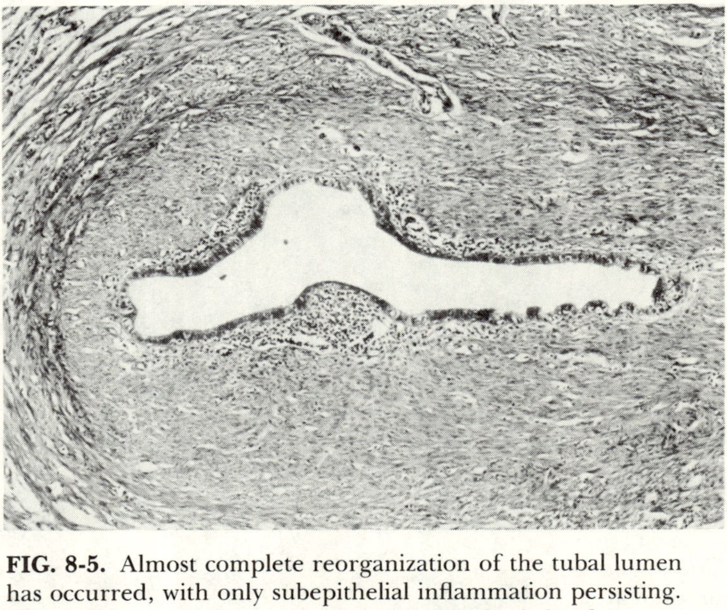

FIG. 8-5. Almost complete reorganization of the tubal lumen has occurred, with only subepithelial inflammation persisting. The flattened tubal epithelium looks metaplastic in places, consistent with its repairing nature. Human tissue.

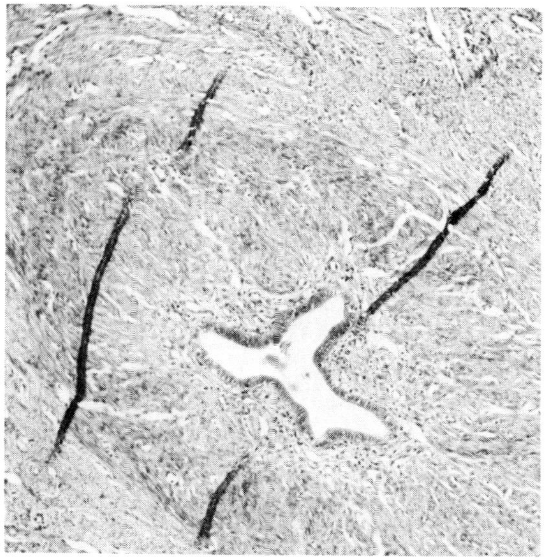

FIG. 8-6. This normal tube has been totally repaired. Human tissue.

ganization does not in this circumstance produce tubal closure (Fig. 8-4) but only the gradual resolution of the inflammatory process (Fig. 8-5) and, eventually, a normal-appearing tube (Fig. 8-6). The frequency with which either outcome occurs is not clear from these data, but it is suggested by clinical efficacy studies reported in Chapters 9, 10, and 12.

In the endometrium of the monkeys examined 1 week and 1 month after the intrauterine of instillation quinacrine, there were two animals in which focal scars were seen. It is not clear that these were related to the quinacrine treatment.

CONCLUSION

Intrauterine administration of quinacrine effectively occludes the central portion of the fallopian tube in a certain proportion of cases. The factors that determine the frequency with which this occurs are still unclear, but intrauterine chemical sterilization with this or a similar agent seems promising.

REFERENCE

1. DUBIN NH, STRANDBERG JD, CRAFT CF et al: Effect of intrauterine and intravascular quinacrine administration on histopathology, blood chemistry and hematology in cynomolgus monkeys. (submitted for publication, 1982)

9

Overview of Clinical Trials With Quinacrine

JAIME ZIPPER

DAVID EDELMAN

LYNDA PAINTER COLE

MIRTA RIVERA

Surgical female sterilization is the most effective method of contraception for women who desire no additional children. In developing countries, the demand for female sterilization usually exceeds the ability of the countries to provide services; therefore, the development of a rapid, effective, and safe nonsurgical method that can be performed by paramedical personnel remains a high priority. In developed countries, such as the United States, a nonsurgical method of sterilization could considerably reduce the high cost of sterilization services, thereby making the method accessible to more women.

For over a decade, Zipper and associates have evaluated the use of the transcervical instillation of quinacrine hydrochloride for effecting permanent sterilization. The results from initial animal studies indicated that quinacrine selectively produced significant morphological changes in the reproductive tract and caused permanent tubal fibrosis and tubal occlusion in the rat.[5] In subsequent clinical trials, various doses, concentrations, and solvents for the quinacrine instillation schedules were evaluated.[6,7] These trials demonstrated that the use of quinacrine was potentially an effective method of permanent sterilization. Other investigators have also found the use of quinacrine to be effective for permanent female sterilization.[1–4]

This chapter presents an overview of the results of three clinical studies conducted to evaluate the safety and efficacy of quinacrine as a method of nonsurgical female sterilization.

MATERIALS AND METHODS

The studies on the safety and effectiveness of quinacrine were conducted at an outpatient clinic in Santiago, Chile. The first study involved 200 patients and evaluated the efficacy of the repeated transcervical instillation of 1500

Partial support for this work was provided by the International Fertility Research Program, with funds from the U.S. Agency for International Development.

mg quinacrine hydrochloride dissolved in 5 ml 2% lidocaine (Xylocaine). All instillation procedures were performed during the proliferative phase of the menstrual cycle. The second instillation was made in the first menstrual cycle following the initial instillation, and the third and last instillation at 6 months after the first. None of the patients used any adjunctive contraceptives. Follow-up visits were scheduled at 6-month intervals after the last instillation.

The second study, in 165 women, evaluated the efficacy of transcervical insertions of 250 mg quinacrine pellets preceded by a single pellet of 20 mg sodium thiopental, a hydroscopic agent used to increase the viscosity of the uterine fluid in an attempt to improve the uterine retention of the quinacrine. The procedure for inserting the quinacrine was essentially the same as is used for inserting an IUD. Insertions were performed only during the proliferative phase of the menstrual cycle. The procedure was repeated 1 month and again 2 months after the first insertion. None of these patients used any adjunctive contraceptives. Clinical follow-up was scheduled at 6-month intervals after the last insertion.

The third study, involving 138 women and also using quinacrine pellets, followed the same protocol as the second but without the sodium thiopental pellets.

For all studies, only those women who requested sterilization for family planning reasons and who did not have a history of psychiatric disorders were selected as subjects. Any woman excluded from the study was either scheduled for a surgical sterilization procedure or provided with another method of contraception. In these studies on the efficacy of quinacrine, the study end point was pregnancy and not tubal patency as demonstrated by hysterosalpingogram.

RESULTS

Mean age and number of live births of women entering the three studies are provided in Table 9-1. Mean age ranged from 31.3 to 33.5 years, and the mean number of live births ranged from 3.7 to 4.7.

Of the women entering the quinacrine solution study, 30% did not complete the three quinacrine instillation schedule, compared with 10.3% in the study of pellets with sodium thiopental and 12.3% in the study of pellets without sodium thiopental (Table 9-2). In part, this was a reflection of a difference in protocol, since in the quinacrine solution study there was a 6-

TABLE 9-1. Age and Live Births for Women Entering Studies of Quinacrine Hydrochloride

	QUINACRINE SOLUTION (N = 200)	QUINACRINE PELLETS WITH SODIUM THIOPENTAL (N = 165)	QUINACRINE PELLETS WITHOUT SODIUM THIOPENTAL (N = 138)
Mean age (years)	31.3	33.4	33.5
Mean number of live births	4.1	4.7	3.7

TABLE 9-2. Reasons Women Did Not Complete Three Administrations of Quinacrine Solution and Quinacrine Pellets

	QUINACRINE SOLUTION (N = 200)		QUINACRINE PELLETS WITH SODIUM THIOPENTAL (N = 165)		QUINACRINE PELLETS WITHOUT SODIUM THIOPENTAL (N = 138)	
	NO.	%	*NO.*	%	*NO.*	%
Reasons for not performing second administration						
Pregnancy	18	9.0	4*	2.4	5†	3.6
Transient psychosis	4	2.0	0	0.0	0	0.0
Ovarian cyst	1	0.5	1	0.6	0	0.0
Cervical synechia	0	0.0	0	0.0	1	0.7
Adnexitis	1	0.5	0	0.0	0	0.0
Amenorrhea	3	1.5	0	0.0	0	0.0
Severe headaches	1	0.5	0	0.0	0	0.0
Nerves	0	0.0	1	0.6	0	0.0
Patient choice	0	0.0	2	1.2	0	0.0
Patient failed to return	4	2.0	2	1.2	3	2.2
Total	32	16.0	10	6.1	9	6.5
Reasons for not performing third administration						
Pregnancy	23	11.5	0	0.0	2	1.4
Cervical synechia	0	0.0	1	0.6	0	0.0
Possible perforation	0	0.0	0	0.0	1	0.7
Cystic mass	0	0.0	0	0.0	1	0.7
Amenorrhea	1	0.5	0	0.0	0	0.0
Metrorrhagia	1	0.5	0	0.0	1	0.7
Intense vaginitis	0	0.0	0	0.0	1	0.7
Allergic skin reaction	0	0.0	1	0.6	0	0.0
Pelvic pain	0	0.0	1	0.6	0	0.0
Headaches	0	0.0	2	1.2	0	0.0
Patient choice	2	1.0	0	0.0	0	0.0
Patient failed to return	1	0.5	2	1.2	2	1.4
Total	28	14.0	7	4.2	8	5.8

*Two women were pregnant at first insertion and one failed to return for second insertion as scheduled.

†Two women were probably pregnant at first insertion and one failed to return for second insertion as scheduled.

month time period between instillation two and instillation three, compared with a 1-month period for both pellet studies. The data show that the unacceptably high pregnancy rate associated with the solution procedure in the time between the first and second instillations appears to have been reduced in the pellet studies. Four of the women who had quinacrine inserted and who were diagnosed as pregnant after the first insertion were thought to have been pregnant at the time of enrollment in the study. Two of these pregnancies were terminated by induced abortion, and two ended in spontaneous abortions.

TABLE 9-3. Gross Life-Table Pregnancy Rates Per 100 Women Completing Three Administrations of Quinacrine Solution and Quinacrine Pellets

	QUINACRINE SOLUTION (N = 131)	QUINACRINE PELLETS WITH SODIUM THIOPENTAL (N = 147)	QUINACRINE PELLETS WITHOUT SODIUM THIOPENTAL (N = 122)
6 month rate	6.5 ± 2.2 (95.2)*	1.4 ± 1.0 (96.6)	3.1 ± 2.2 (42.0)
12 month rate†	9.9 ± 2.7 (88.9)	4.3 ± 1.7 (93.0)	3.1 ± 2.2 (33.9)
24 month rate	13.1 ± 3.3 (49.6)	6.5 ± 2.1 (79.0)	

*Follow-up rate.

†Difference in the cumulative rates over 12 months (Mantel-Cox): quinacrine solution, quinacrine pellets with sodium thiopental, $p < 0.11$; quinacrine solution, quinacrine pellets without sodium thiopental, $p < 0.22$; quinacrine pellets with sodium thiopental, quinacrine pellets without sodium thiopental, $p < 0.70$.

The use of quinacrine pellets appears to have reduced the incidence of transient psychosis, a side-effect that has been observed in studies using intrauterine quinacrine solutions. No women in the pellet studies developed transient psychosis, compared with 2.0% in the solution study. In the pellet study without sodium thiopental, one women, after the second insertion, developed an acute pelvic inflammatory reaction that lasted 48 hours. We suspected that the pellets had perforated into the peritoneal cavity. The woman was treated with penicillin. No additional problems were encountered, and no more treatment was required.

The pellet method of quinacrine insertion appears to be more effective than the solution method (Table 9-3), although the differences in the cumulative rates are not statistically significant ($p > 0.05$). The gross life-table rate per 100 women at 12 months after the third quinacrine administration was 9.9 for the solution method, 4.3 for the pellets with sodium thiopental, and 3.1 for the pellets without sodium thiopental. To date, 16 women who completed the three instillations of quinacrine solution, 10 who completed the pellets with sodium thiopental regimen, and 7 who completed the pellets without sodium thiopental insertions have become pregnant (Table 9-4). Pregnancies have occurred from 2 to 27 months after the third administration; in some women, the tubes were probably never occluded, and in others, recanalization may have occurred. None of the pregnancies was ectopic. Most pregnancies were terminated by induced abortion. Four women carried their pregnancies to term without any apparent ill effects to the mother or fetus.

Other events reported after three administrations of quinacrine are shown in Table 9-4. It is not known whether all of these events are a result of the quinacrine procedure or are merely the usual problems that would be seen in any gynecologic clinic. In addition to the two hysterectomies for chronic pelvic inflammatory disease reported in Table 9-4, two other hysterectomies were performed for genital prolapse, a condition unrelated to the quinacrine procedure.

TABLE 9-4. Events Occurring After Three Administrations of Quinacrine

	QUINACRINE SOLUTION (N = 124)*		QUINACRINE PELLETS WITH SODIUM THIOPENTAL (N = 145)†		QUINACRINE PELLETS WITHOUT SODIUM THIOPENTAL (N = 83)‡	
	NO.	%	*NO.*	%	*NO.*	%
Events§						
Pregnancy	16	12.9	10	6.9	7	8.4
Menstrual						
Amenorrhea	12	9.7	4	2.8	0	0.0
Menorrhagia	8	6.5	2	1.4	0	0.0
Dysmenorrhea	0	0.0	1	0.7	0	0.0
Pelvic						
Pelvic inflammatory disease	4	3.2	3‖	2.1	0	0.0
Endometritis	1	0.8	7	4.8	1	0.3
Leukorrhea	3	2.4	1	0.7	0	0.0
Urinary tract infection	3	2.4	3	2.2	3	3.6
Ovarian cyst	2	1.6	4	2.8	0	0.0
Adnexal mass	0	0.0	1	0.7	0	0.0
Uterine synechia	2	1.6	3	2.1	2	2.4
Myoma	0	0.0	4	2.8	0	0.0
Transient complaints						
Pelvic/abdominal pain	7	5.6	2	1.4	2	2.4
Headaches	3	2.4	6	4.1	0	0.0
Dispareunia	1	0.8	1	0.7	0	0.0
Total women with one or more events	50	40.3	40	27.6	16	19.3

*Of the 140 patients completing three instillations of quinacrine solution, 124 returned for one or more follow-ups.

†Of the 148 patients completing three insertions of quinacrine pellets with sodium thiopental, 145 returned for one or more follow-ups.

‡Of the 122 patients completing three insertions of quinacrine pellets without sodium thiopental, 83 returned for one or more follow-ups.

§Multiple events may be reported for each woman.

‖Two women underwent hysterectomies.

CONCLUSION

Extensive research has been undertaken to develop a simple method of nonsurgical female sterilization. The intrauterine use of quinacrine hydrochloride as a method of nonsurgical sterilization has evolved from instillations of a solution, to the development of pellets used with a potentiating agent, and then to the use of quinacrine pellets alone.

The major adverse effect of quinacrine solution administration was transient psychosis (2.0%); the use of pellets seems to have eliminated the risk of that complication (0.0%), probably because the pellet dissolves relatively slowly

(≤10 minutes) within the uterine cavity, reducing the risk of rapid intravascular absorption.

Animal studies were initiated to identify problems occurring if perforation occurs and quinacrine is accidentally placed in the peritoneum. At high doses, several animals died (see Chapter 6).

Excessive peritoneal absorption produced a high blood level of quinacrine, leading to death, and perhaps caused by a central nervous system reaction. High doses of quinacrine when administered intraperitoneally are clearly toxic. Additional animal studies are planned to determine if, by prolonging the *in utero* rate of release of quinacrine, the toxic side-effects may be avoided without affecting the ability of the drug to cause tubal fibrosis.

A comparison of results from various studies conducted by Zipper show that the pellet method of quinacrine delivery is an improvement over the solution method. Sodium thiopental does not seem to be a necessary adjunct to the procedure. However, the procedure still requires three administrations of quinacrine to be effective, thus falling short of the ultimate goal of an effective, blind, one-insertion procedure.

The erratic performance of the quinacrine pellets in occluding the tubes is probably caused by the uneven distribution of the quinacrine to the tubal ostia. Improvements in the delivery of quinacrine are being explored, including the use of an IUD to deliver the quinacrine to the tubal ostia. Another effort will explore the efficacy of a sustained-release pellet system in the hope that extended exposure of the drug will produce a higher rate of tubal closure.

REFERENCES

1. BENOIT A, MELANCON J, GAGNON M: Chemically induced tubal occlusion in the human female using intrauterine instillation of quinacrine. Contraception 12 95, 1975
2. DAVIDSON O, WILKINS L: Chemically induced tubal occlusion in the human female following a simple instillation of quinacrine. Contraception 7:333, 1973
3. ISRANGKUN C, PHAOSAVASDI S, NEUWIRTH R et al: Clinical evaluation of quinacrine hydrochloride for sterilization of the human female. Contraception 14:75, 1976
4. MEHTAJI S, JADWANI J, GOYAL V: Chemical sterilization with quinacrine. In Fourth Transaction of Scientific Papers, p 167. Bombay, India. India Fertility Research Program, September 1977
5. ZIPPER J, MEDEL M, PRAGER R: Alterations in fertility induced by unilateral intrauterine instillation of cytotoxic compounds in rats. Am J Obstet Gynecol 101:971, 1968
6. ZIPPER J, STACHETTI E, MEDEL M: Human fertility control by transvaginal application of quinacrine on the fallopian tube. Fertil Steril 21:581, 1970
7. ZIPPER J, STACHETTI E, MEDEL M: Transvaginal chemical sterilization. Contraception 12:11, 1975

10

Clinical Report: Quinacrine-Fused Pellets

RENE GUZMAN-SERANI

ALFONSO BERNALES

LYNDA PAINTER COLE

In an effort to meet a demand for female sterilization services that far exceeds the current medical care system worldwide, attention has been given to the development of a safe, effective nonsurgical method that can be performed by paramedical personnel.

Zipper and associates have worked in this area for many years and have identified quinacrine hydrochloride as a chemical likely to produce tubal occlusion when placed in the uterus.[2,3,4,5] Zipper's work led to the development of quinacrine hydrochloride pellets, intended to effect a delivery system that would bring the chemical into prolonged contact with the tubal ostia through uterine retention. Results of an early study were encouraging; at 1 year after three insertions of 250 mg quinacrine pellets, the gross life-table pregnancy rate was 3.1 per 100 women.[1]

The efficacy of transcervical insertions of quinacrine pellets to produce tubal occlusion has been further evaluated in a three-center trial. This chapter reports the results from one of the centers.

MATERIALS AND METHODS

Each quinacrine hydrochloride pellet is cylindrical and has a diameter of less than 4 mm. The pellets are compacted to contain 10 mg quinacrine per millimeter of length. Insertion is accomplished by placing the pellets in a plastic tube with a push rod positioned behind them. The insertion procedure is essentially the same as that for inserting an IUD.

From March through December, 1979, 151 women entered the study, giving informed consent at an outpatient clinic at the Universidad Austral de Chile School of Medicine, Valdivia, Chile. Seven pellets containing a total of 250 mg quinacrine hydrochloride were to be inserted at admission and again at 1 month and 2 months after admission. Insertions were performed during the proliferative phase of the menstrual cycle in women who had not recently

Partial support for this work was provided by the International Fertility Research Program, with funds from the U.S. Agency for International Development.

been pregnant (>42 days since last pregnancy terminated). No additional contraceptives were used. Clinical follow-up was scheduled at 6, 12, and 24 months after the third insertion and at any time when complications or complaints occurred. In this study, tubal patency was evaluated by hysterosalpingography performed at least 3 months after the third insertion.

Only those women who requested sterilization for family planning reasons and who did not have a history of medical or psychiatric disorders were selected as subjects. If the patient appeared to be unduly nervous or had any pathologic pelvic condition (except cervicitis), she was excluded from the study and was either scheduled for a surgical sterilization procedure or provided with another method of contraception.

RESULTS

The women entering the study had a mean age of 31.8 years and a mean of 3.3 live births. At admission, 35.1% reported an irregular menstrual cycle. Only two women (1.3%) did not complete the scheduled three insertions of quinacrine pellets. For one woman, chronic pelvic inflammatory disease, which had been missed at admission, was diagnosed before the second insertion; a bilateral salpingectomy was performed. The second woman contracted a viral infectious hepatitis after the first insertion; the hepatitis had a prolonged course, but 6 months later the woman had fully recuperated. Although she is not presently using additional contraception and never received the third quinacrine insertion, she has not become pregnant.

The procedure was deemed safe (Table 10-1); only minor complications and complaints were reported at insertion or between insertions. In most cases, the complications or complaints were of a temporary nature, disappearing within a few hours or a few days after the procedure. Menstrual disturbances associated with the quinacrine procedure were also transient (Table 10-2). Of those women with regular cycles at the time of the first insertions, 35.7% missed one or two cycles in the 3 months it took to complete the procedures; all had returned to menses by the 6-month follow-up visit. Of those with irregular cycles, 37.7% missed one or more cycles, and only one reported amenorrhea at the 6-month follow-up; she was pregnant.

Four-fifths of the women have returned for 24-month follow-up. Table 10-3 shows the quinacrine pellet method to be very effective. The gross life-table pregnancy rate is 4.1 per 100 women at 24 months. Five pregnancies have been reported; they occurred at 4, 15, 18, 19, and 24 months after the third insertion. Three were terminated by an induced abortion procedure, one ended in a spontaneous abortion, and one was carried to term. The term pregnancy occurred 18 months after the third insertion; the infant was born without any problem.

Hysterosalpingographic results for women who completed three insertions of quinacrine pellets are given in Table 10-4. The hysterosalpingograms showed no patency for three women who later became pregnant.

Other than the pregnancies, follow-up problems were reported by eight women (5.4%) in the 24 months since the third insertion. Most problems were minor and transitory, including two cases of menorrhagia, two of head-

TABLE 10-1. Complications/Complaints Associated With Insertion of Quinacrine Pellets

	PELLET INSERTIONS					
	1 (*N* = 151)		*2* (*N* = 150)		*3* (*N* = 149)	
	NO.	*%*	*NO.*	*%*	*NO.*	*%*
Complications						
Psycho/emotional reaction	1	0.7	0	0.0	0	0.0
Vomiting	1	0.7	0	0.0	0	0.0
Infectious hepatitis*†	1	0.7	0	0.0	0	0.0
Pelvic inflammatory disease*†	0	0.0	1	0.7	0	0.0
Trichomonas†	1	0.7	2	1.3	0	0.0
Vaginal discharge	1	0.7	1	0.7	0	0.0
Fever	0	0.0	1	0.7	0	0.0
Vaginal bleeding	1	0.7	2	1.3	0	0.0
Vaginal spotting	0	0.0	2	1.3	0	0.0
Total women with one complication or more	6	4.0	9	6.0	0	0.0
Complaints						
Pelvic/abdominal pain						
At insertion	21	13.9	12	8.0	18	12.0
Postinsertion	25	16.6	19	12.7	1	0.7
Headache	2	1.3	1	0.7	0	0.0
Muscle pain	1	0.7	0	0.0	0	0.0
Total women with one complaint or more	43	28.5	32	21.3	19	12.8

*Resulted in discontinuation of procedure.

†Unrelated to quinacrine.

aches, and one each of reduced menstrual flow, irregular cycles, episodic pelvic pain, and an ovarian cyst.

CONCLUSIONS

The results of this study suggest that the intrauterine insertion of quinacrine pellets can be an effective, safe, nonsurgical sterilization procedure. In general, complications and complaints associated with the insertion were minor and of a transitory nature. Only 4.1% of the women had become pregnant by 2 years after the third insertion.

Three women who showed no tubal patency by hysterosalpingogram later became pregnant. The possibility of recanalization seems more likely than that the hysterosalpingogram failed to determine tubal occlusion.

Although no deaths have been reported in studies conducted in conjunction with the International Fertility Research Program, two have been reported following the intrauterine instillation of quinacrine solution by other investigators.*† The cause of these deaths is unknown but may be related to

*Atabrine hydrochloride. Product information, Winthrop Laboratories, November 1975.

†Chowdhury A: Personal communication, August 1976.

TABLE 10-2. Amenorrhea Associated With Insertion of Quinacrine Pellets by Menstrual Regularity at Admission

	IREGULAR CYCLE LENGTH REPORTED AT ADMISSION (N = 53)		REGULAR CYCLE LENGTH REPORTED AT ADMISSION (N = 98)	
	NO.	%	*NO.*	%
At insertion II	17	32.1	22	22.4
At insertion III	14	26.4	24	24.5
At 6-month follow-up	1*	1.9	0	0.0
Total women reporting amenorrhea at one or more visits	20	37.7	35	35.7

*Pregnant at time of follow-up.

the rapid absorption of quinacrine. It has been reported that high systemic blood levels of quinacrine from rapid absorption may result in arrhythmias, heart block, impaired cardiac output, hypotension, peripheral vasodilation, and depression of the vasomotor and respiratory centers of the central nervous system.* The pellet method probably decreases the absorption rate, thus reducing the blood level of quinacrine. The decreased absorption rate was part of the reason the pellet method was developed.

A problem with all known blind procedures is that more than one application may be necessary. The quinacrine pellet method used in this study

TABLE 10-3. Gross Life-Table Pregnancy Rates for Women Who Completed Three Insertions of Quinacrine Hydrochloride Pellets

	PREGNANCY RATE	FOLLOW-UP RATE
6 months	0.7 ± 0.7	98.0
12 months	0.7 ± 0.7	97.3
24 months	3.8 ± 1.7	82.8

TABLE 10-4. Hysterosalpingographic Results for Women Who Completed Three Insertions of Quinacrine Hydrochloride Pellets

RESULTS	NO. PATIENTS	%
Neither tube patent	121*	81.2
One tube patent	1	0.7
Both tubes patent	0	0.0
HSG not performed	27†	18.1
Total	149	100.0

*Three women became pregnant.
†Two women became pregnant.

*Atabrine hydrochloride. Product information, Winthrop Laboratories, November 1975.

requires three insertions. Surgical sterilization procedures, in addition to the demands on medical personnel and clinic resources, require multiple visits from the women. At least two visits are recommended: the visit for surgery and the follow-up visit 7 to 21 days later. Surgical procedures also require anesthesia.

Alternative delivery systems that may reduce the number of quinacrine administrations are being explored, including the use of an IUD vector for better delivery of the quinacrine to the tubal ostia and the development of a sustained-release system that will provide extended exposure of quinacrine to the epithelium.

REFERENCES

1. ZIPPER J, COLE LP, GOLDSMITH A et al: Quinacrine hydrochloride pellets: Preliminary data on a nonsurgical method of female sterilization. Int J Gynaecol Obstet 18:275, 1980
2. ZIPPER J, MEDEL M, GOLDSMITH A et al: The clinical efficacy of the repeated transcervical instillation of quinacrine for female sterilization. Int J Gynaecol Obstet 14:499, 1976
3. ZIPPER J, MEDEL M, PRAGER R: Alteration in fertility induced by unilateral intrauterine instillation of cytotoxic compounds in rats. Am J Obstet Gynecol 101:971, 1968
4. ZIPPER J, STACHETTI E, MEDEL M: Human fertility control by transvaginal application of quinacrine on the fallopian tube. Fertil Steril 21:581, 1970
5. ZIPPER J, STACHETTI E, MEDEL M: Transvaginal chemical sterilization. Contraception 12:11, 1975

11

Delivery Systems for Applying Quinacrine as a Tubal Closing Agent

ROBERT G. WHEELER

The use of quinacrine hydrochloride as an effective chemical agent for transcervical female sterilization has been established primarily through the pioneering work of Jaime Zipper.[8,10,11,12] Current research is concerned with making the method commercially available through the development of dosage forms that will enhance the acceptance of the method and through toxicology or related studies that will document the safety of quinacrine chemical sterilization (QCS). The general subject of chemical sterilization has been reviewed by Richart.[6]

The ultimate measure of the success of a specific quinacrine dosage form is the number of failures, measured by pregnancy rates, provider acceptance, user acceptance, and incidence of side-effects. More than 12 years of clinical studies of QCS have been spent in developing a clinically effective method and documenting the results. If the regimen consists of depositing 250 mg quinacrine in tablet form in the uterus three times at monthly intervals, about 2 women per 100 will ever become pregnant again. Available data indicate that quinacrine sterilization is permanent, although efforts to reverse the early stages of occlusion with high doses of estrogen have been successful.[4] Other dosage forms under consideration are slurries of quinacrine powder, pastes, sustained-release tablets, gels, fibers, and plugs intended for direct insertion into the uterotubal junction. IUDs have been tested as vectors to deliver the quinacrine proximal to the uterotubal junction and to provide supplementary contraception.

Quick ways to screen these alternative dosage forms are needed to achieve the benefits of an improved delivery system. A theoretical model of quinacrine sterilization supports the belief that the controlled release of quinacrine could prolong the exposure of the uterotubal junction to high concentrations and reduce the risk of serious side-effects as a result of systemic absorption or accidental delivery of the drug into the peritoneal cavity. Modeling, as presented in a preliminary stage in this chapter, can help focus research on activities that will ensure safe and effective use of QCS systems.

REPEATED EXPOSURE TO QUINACRINE CHEMICAL STERILIZATION

As a first approximation, the probability of successful QCS appears to be constant when quinacrine instillations are repeated at intervals. That is, if one instillation has a 50% probability of occluding a tube, the second instil-

TABLE 11-1. Probability of Producing One and Two Tubal Occlusions, Assuming Both Tubes are Initially Open

	NUMBER OF INSTILLATIONS			
TUBES CLOSED	*1ST*	*2ND*	*3RD*	*4TH*
50% Effective				
0	0.25	0.063	0.016	0.004
1	0.50	0.375	0.219	0.117
2	0.25	0.562	0.765	0.879
80% Effective				
0	0.04	0.002	0.001	0.000
1	0.32	0.077	0.016	0.003
2	0.64	0.922	0.984	0.997

lation will have a 50% chance of occluding any tubes not previously occluded. The work of Westrom on infertility resulting from repeated episodes of pelvic inflammatory disease shows the same trend: repeated cases of pelvic inflammatory disease each have a constant probability of occluding the fallopian tube(s) not previously occluded.[9] Gains to be made if a 50% effective dosage form is improved to 80% effectiveness, assuming constant probability of tubal closure, are shown in Table 11-1.

It is apparent that it takes twice the number of instillations of a 50% effective dosage form as are required for an 80% effective dosage form to get the same tubal occlusion rate. In real situations when multiple instillations are used, pregnancies occur between instillations. The number of pregnancies that occur before the regimen is completed depends on the fecundability of the couple, the effectiveness of the QCS dosage form to occlude tubes, and the use or nonuse of supplementary contraceptives. There are probably a few women whose tubes would not be occluded by any number of QCS instillations. None of the advantages of one dosage form or another comes without a price. In this chapter, the characteristics of several dosage forms are described along with the advantages of each.

QUINACRINE SOLUTIONS AND PASTES

In the initial clinical evaluation of quinacrine as a chemical sterilizing agent, the dosage form was a solution or slurry delivered into the uterine cavity through a cannula attached to a syringe.[11] Solutions and pastes provide a continuum of quinacrine concentrations up to a maximum in the paste form of approximately 800 mg/ml. Since an aqueous solution will hold only 29 mg/ml, Zipper and associates resorted to slurries to achieve the 100 to 1000 mg needed to produce tubal occlusion.[11] This mode of delivery is mostly of historical interest now, since it has been superseded with the solid form because of the low efficacy of the slurries and occasional cortical excitation (toxic psychosis) they produced.[12] High intrauterine pressure can be developed inadvertently when slurries are delivered by a syringe with the possibility of accidental intravenous or intraperitoneal delivery. Use of lidocaine with quinacrine slurries was once thought to be beneficial, but the practice is now out of favor because the lidocaine appears to be unnecessary and possibly hazardous.

Various dispersing agents have been used to make quinacrine pastes and to increase the quinacrine-holding capacity of slurries. If any agent normally safe for food and drugs is used as an additive, care should be taken to ensure that it does not react with the quinacrine and decrease its effectiveness. Polyethylene oxide has been an effective binder for tablets and a dispersing agent for slurry dosage forms over a wide range of polyethylene oxide concentrations. Malaviya and coworkers took advantage of the gel transition temperature of 2% aqueous agar solution containing 800 mg quinacrine per milliliter. They instilled the dose at 50°C in the fallopian tubes of monkeys as a liquid that quickly reverted to a gel *in situ* at body temperature. Forming the gel *in situ* slows down quinacrine absorption and dissolution, thus providing a sustained release. Gel-forming additives in the tablet dosage form also cause gel formation *in situ*. Quinacrine powder in a gelatin capsule is a possible alternative to pellets for delivering solid quinacrine.

QUINACRINE TABLETS

Quinacrine tablets first used by Zipper were made with a simple die and plunger set (Fig. 11-1).[10] The quinacrine powder was moistened to cause binding of the powder into a solid tablet, and the tooling was dusted with magnesium stearate as a lubricant. Two tablets 1.25 cm long and weighing 125 mg each were deposited in the uterus through a 4 mm-diameter polyethylene inserter. Quinacrine has been produced in ⅛-inch diameter 35-mg tablets using commercial tableting equipment. Test lots of tablets were made by the University of North Carolina Division of Pharmacy Services from quinacrine hydrochloride obtained from Sigma Chemical Company, St. Louis, Missouri. To produce free-flowing powder, the quinacrine was granulated through a 35-mesh screen. Tablets were produced with flat-faced ⅛-inch diameter punches on a Stokes Model E single-cavity tablet machine. Tablets with nominal dissolution times of 10, 100, and 800 minutes were produced as described by Onay and associates.[5] Cholesterol was the principal additive used to delay dissolution. The proportions of quinacrine in the tablets varied inversely with the dissolution time and were 89%, 79%, and 46%, respectively. An assembly for insertion of the pellets is illustrated in Figure 11-2.

DELIVERY SYSTEMS FOR TABLETS

A simple polyethylene or polypropylene straw and push rod system (Fig. 11-2) has been an entirely satisfactory method for intrauterine insertion of tablets. There should be some frictional resistance between the inserter straw and the push rod to prevent the rod from falling out and spilling the tablets. A rolled tip on the inserted end of the straw has two functions. It guides the straw through the cervix without scraping and holds the tablets within the straw until they are discharged by pulling the straw over the push rod. Four

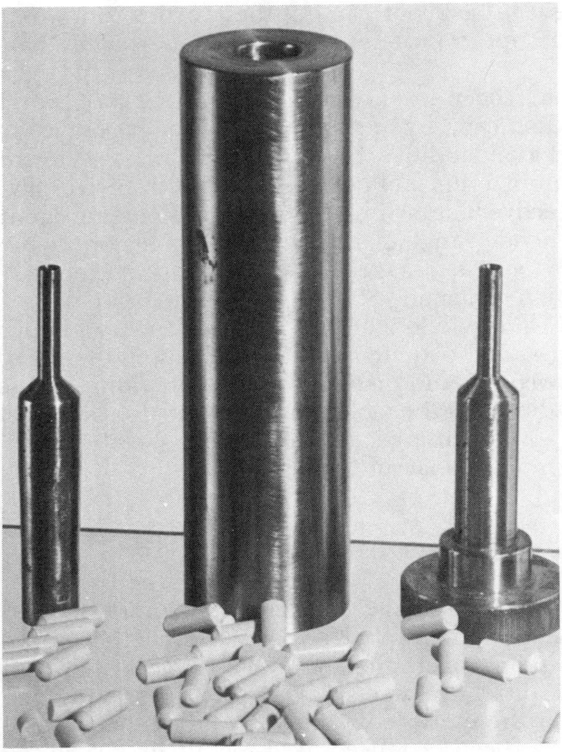

FIG. 11-1. Die and plunger set for fabrication of quinacrine tablets.

diametrically opposed slits in the nosed portion of the straw allow the aperture to expand and pass the tablets. Although curved inserters intended to deliver quinacrine closer to the uterotubal junction have been proposed, there are no published data indicating a curved inserter increases the probability of tubal closure.

The International Fertility Research Program (IFRP) has used a two-step method to ensure the sterility of the quinacrine tablets. The tablets are gamma sterilized in bulk at 2.5 M rad, a dosage that does not denature the quinacrine. The assembled kits are ethylene oxide sterilized. The gamma sterilization step might be avoided if the bioburden of the quinacrine is monitored throughout the production process according to USP guidelines.

UTEROTUBAL PLUGS

The IFRP has cooperated with Dr. R. Quinones in developing a system for placement of small rods of quinacrine directly in the uterotubal isthmus by way of a hysteroscope. A system such as the one illustrated in Figure 11-3 has been tested on specimens from women who have undergone hysterectomy, but no clinical trials have been attempted.

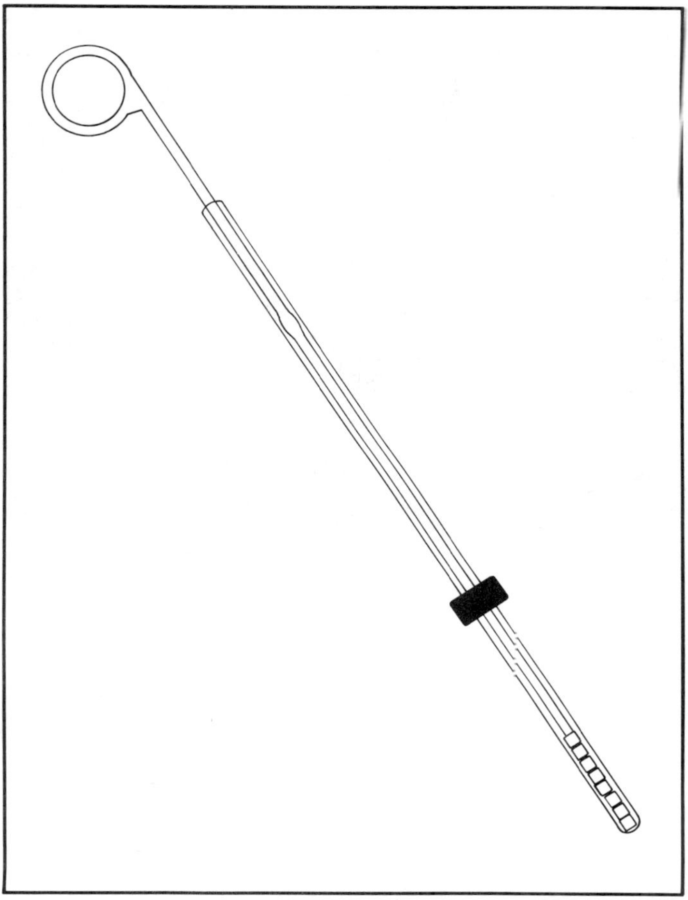

FIG. 11-2. Quinacrine tablet inserter assembly.

QUINACRINE IUDS

A novel combination of family planning methods occurs when an IUD is used as a vector to deliver quinacrine into the uterine cavity and to position the quinacrine close to the uterotubal junctions. (See Chapter 12 for details on this method.) The IUD provides back-up contraception as long as it is retained. Quinacrine itself is spermicidal only at concentrations approaching saturation (20 mg to 30 mg/ml).* The success of quinacrine IUDs as QCS systems depends on obtaining a high probability of tubal closure with one IUD insertion. One insertion of quinacrine pellets when the patient returns

*Chvapil M: Testing the spermicidal effectiveness of quinacrine and potassium sorbate. Personal communication, October 1981.

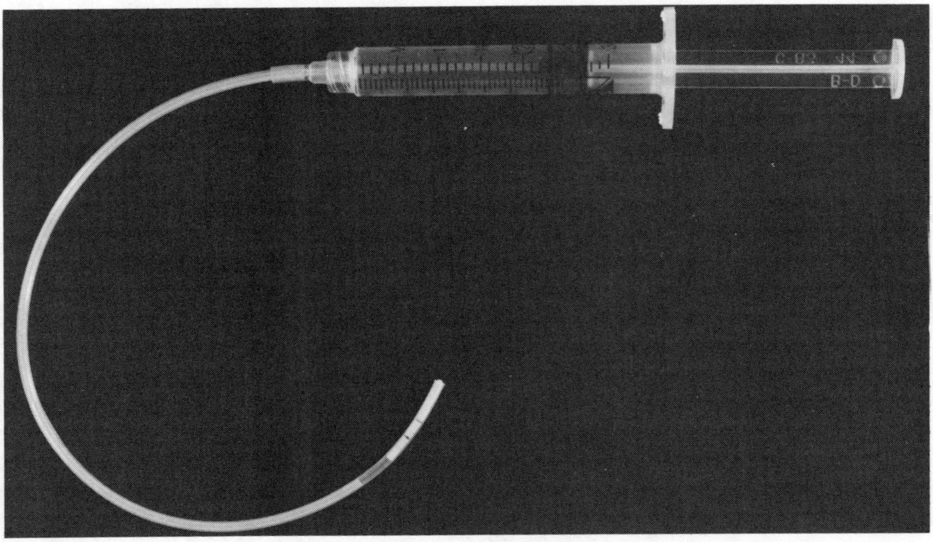

FIG. 11-3. Assembly for direct insertion of quinacrine into the uterotubal junction hysteroscopically.

to have the IUD removed could significantly increase the probability of tubal closure without increasing the amount of medical intervention. Since the IUD displaces a volume that could otherwise be occupied by quinacrine, the amount of quinacrine that can be delivered is less and the amount of cervical dilation is greater for the quinacrine IUD system than for quinacrine tablets.

A THEORETICAL MODEL OF THE QCS SYSTEM

A theoretical model of the QCS system provides a helpful frame of reference for the evaluation of various dosage forms, even though some of the physiological parameters of the model are only estimates. A simple mechanical analog of the system is shown in Figure 11-4. The uterus prior to insertion of the quinacrine tablets is represented in Figure 11-4, *A*. The uterine cavity is expandable as indicated by the spring-loaded piston. Under normal conditions, the amount of fluid flowing into the uterus is less than the water absorption capacity of the uterus, such that the uterine volume remains constant and there is no cervical discharge.

In Figure 11-4, *B*, after the insertion of quinacrine tablets, the water influx exceeds the rate of absorption and causes the uterine cavity volume to increase until there is a discharge of the excess flow out of the cervix. The particulate filter in the mechanical analog ensures that only dissolved quinacrine is absorbed systemically, but the cervical discharge contains both dissolved and particulate quinacrine. A sequence of events might be as follows:

1. Tablets containing 250 mg quinacrine are deposited into the uterus at time zero.

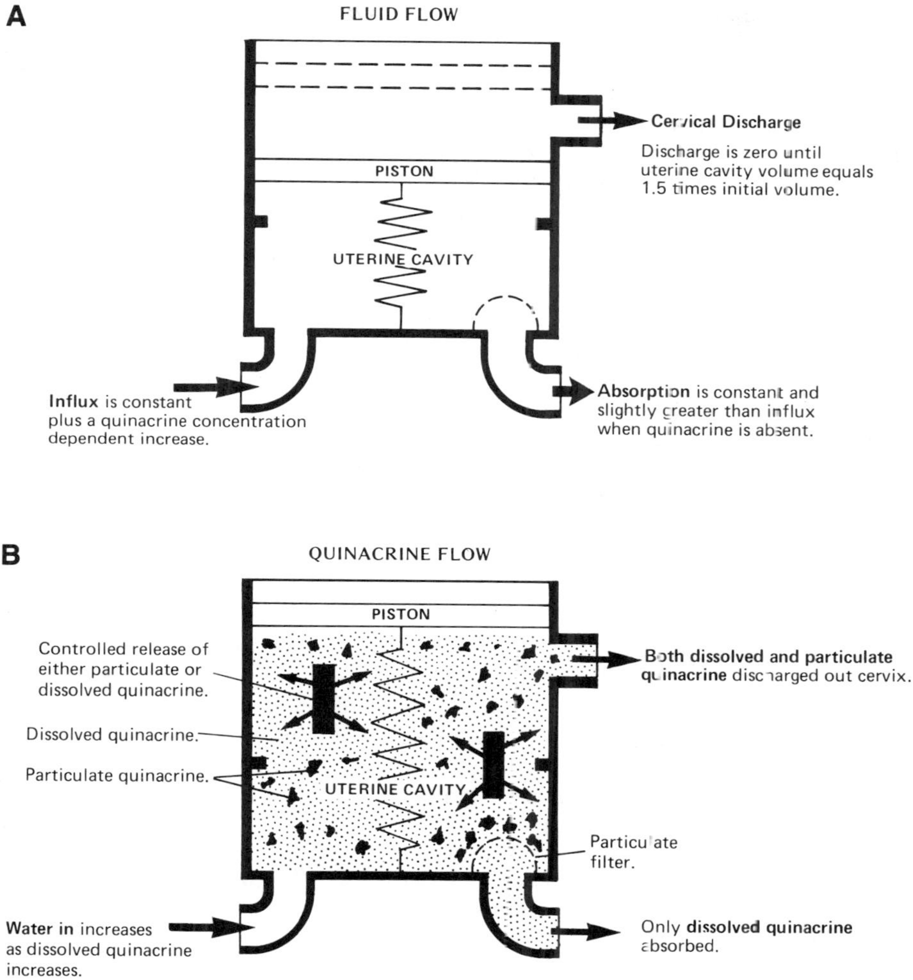

FIG. 11-4. Schematic input-output model of the flow of intrauterine quinacrine. (*A*) Uterus prior to insertion of the quinacrine tablets. (*B*) Uterus after quinacrine insertion.

2. Every minute one half of the weight of quinacrine in tablet form converts to a slurry of particulate quinacrine in the uterine fluids.
3. The particulate quinacrine goes into solution at a rate depending on the concentration of dissolved quinacrine and particle size until the solution becomes saturated at a value of 29 mg quinacrine per milliliter of solution.
4. Quinacrine in solution produces a concentration-dependent osmotic increase of water flow into the uterus until it reaches a maximum value of 1.5 times the nominal preinsertion value of 10 ml/hr.

TABLE 11-2. Predicted Distribution of Quinacrine After Placement of 250 mg Tableted Quinacrine in the Uterine Cavity

AMOUNT OF QUINACRINE PER 250 MG OF TABLETS	FRACTION OF REMAINING QUINACRINE RELEASED PER MINUTE	QUINACRINE ABSORBED SYSTEMICALLY	QUINACRINE DISCHARGED FROM CERVIX	QUINACRINE DISSOLVED IN UTERINE FLUIDS AFTER 30 MINUTES
250	0.5	96	154	16.3
200	0.07	118	82	16.8
125	0.01	112	13	0.94

5. Since the increased water influx is not balanced by an increased water absorption, the excess influx causes the uterus to expand to 1.5 times its nominal volume of 1.0 ml.
6. When the uterine cavity volume reaches 1.5 times its nominal volume, all the excess influx is discharged out the cervix, carrying with it both dissolved and particulate quinacrine.
7. Systemic absorption of quinacrine is linearly dependent on the concentration of quinacrine in the uterine fluids and, in the example represented in Table 11-2, was assumed to be 120 mg/hr at saturation.

Given the above assumptions, the results obtained with 250 mg of tablets having three different quinacrine release rates are presented in Table 11-2. The decrease in the amount of quinacrine available as the release rate decreases represents an estimate of the amount of diluent necessary to delay release. For example, 250 mg of tablets with an 800-minute dissolution time contain only 125 mg quinacrine hydrochloride. The dosage form that releases 0.07 of its contained quinacrine every minute appears to be better than the first example because it is just as effective in maintaining a high concentration of dissolved quinacrine in the uterus. It also has the added safety of using less quinacrine that is released slower. The estimated concentration of dissolved quinacrine in the uterine fluids as a function of time after insertion for the 100-minute dosage form is 16.8 mg at 30 min. Since it takes five to seven tablets to make up 250 mg, there is the option of mixing tablets with different release rates.

Mortality risk may set an upper boundary on systemic absorption. If the risk is to be similar to the risk of mortality from surgical sterilization in the United States, it would be 1:10,000.[2] If the plasma level of quinacrine exceeds a threshold value, there appears to be a small risk of toxic psychosis, a side-effect that carries a mortality risk.[1] Based on early work on the use of quinacrine in the treatment and prevention of malaria, the plasma limits of quinacrine concentration may be around 200 n g/ml.[1] Since psychosis is potentially the most serious known side-effect of QCS, the following is quoted directly:[1]

> Lidz and Kahn (1946) have suggested that mepacrine (quinacrine hydrochloride), without giving rise to actual psychoses, may produce mental impairment as judged by scores on the Kohs-Block test, in which the mental age is assessed by forming standard patterns with coloured cubes, whenever the serum levels are above 18

> μgm per 100 ml. Thus doses of 2.1 gm of mepacrine in seven days were without action in causing impairment of the mental faculties, but 4.5 gm in six days caused a very definite impairment. It would thus seem that mepacrine psychoses are likely to develop only if the plasma or serum levels are allowed to remain at a consistently high level.

To stay below a plasma concentration limit, an upper boundary on the rate of quinacrine release from the dosage form should assume that it has accidentally been delivered into the peritoneal cavity. A guess at this limit is a maximum of 300 mg delivered in 1 hour or less. The product of a low probability of toxic psychosis and a low probability of uterine perforation could make the limit considerably higher unless other effects of interperitoneal quinacrine are controlling.

The estimate of water volume exchange in the uterine cavity is based on the definitive studies of tritiated water volume and exchange in the uterine cavities of rhesus monkeys reported by Shaw and associates.[7] They found the apparent volume of the monkey uterine cavity to be only 0.032 ml and the half-life of the water in the cavity to be 1.17 minutes. This half-life is equivalent to a 24-hour turnover of 19.5 ml. Dubin and co-workers found the half-life of plasma quinacrine to be 2 hours in rhesus monkeys (see Chapter 6). When 1 ml of water saturated with quinacrine (29 mg/ml) was placed in the uterus of the monkeys, a blood plasma measurement 30 minutes after quinacrine instillation fell on the 2-hour half-life decay curve. This failure to observe an initial rise in plasma quinacrine levels indicates an absorption of at least 260 mg/hr. It is probably safe to assume that quinacrine absorption will be equal to the product of water absorption and the concentration of quinacrine in solution. This assumption would give a nominal value of 300 mg/hr when the uterine fluid is saturated with quinacrine.

The rate of quinacrine absorption may correlate with the surface area of the uterine cavity. According to data from Lewis and Zuspan,[3] the surface area of the uterus follows the slightly curvilinear relationship: area = 8.5 $(\text{volume})^{1.115}$ sq cm over the range of 1 to 6 cu cm volume. This relationship was not used in the model, but the work of Lewis and Zuspan was used as a reference to estimate an upper limit of 1.5 ml for the uterine volume.

FUTURE DIRECTIONS

Kessel and Mumford estimate that only one fourth to one third of the potential demand for sterilization in developing countries, excluding China, can be met by surgical sterilization in the 1980s and that quinacrine methods offer the best hope of meeting the demand.[2] Although clinical application of QCS and dosage form development for QCS is in an advanced stage, knowledge of the pharmacology of QCS is less developed. Basic research on the pharmacokinetics of intrauterine quinacrine, uterine fluid exchange, cervical discharge, and time integral of quinacrine concentration effects on tubal occlusion would provide a rational basis for selecting an optimum dosage form. It is likely that clinical QCS will continue to be developed outside the United States where surgical sterilization is physically and financially out of reach of those most in need of sterilization.

REFERENCES

1. FINDLAY GM: Recent Advances in Chemotherapy, 3rd ed, vol VII. Philadelphia, P. Blakiston & Son Co, 1951
2. KESSEL E, MUMFORD SD: Potential demand for voluntary female sterilization in the 1980s: The compelling need for a nonsurgical method. Fertil Steril 37:725–733, 1982
3. LEWIS RB, ZUSPAN F: A method for determining contour volume of the uterine cavity. Contraception 2:249, 1970
4. MALAVIYA B, CHANDRA H, KAR AB: Chemical occlusion of monkey oviducts with quinacrine: Antagonism and reversal with estrogen. Contraception 12:31, 1975
5. ONAY S, OLSEN JL, WHEELER RG: Long-acting quinacrine hydrochloride tablets for female sterilization: An alternative to surgical sterilization (submitted for the Proceedings of the 9th International Symposium of the Sustained Release Society, Ft. Lauderdale, Florida, 1982)
6. RICHART RM: Female sterilization using chemical agents. Research Frontiers in Fertility Regulation, Chicago, Program for Applied Research on Fertility Regulation Vol 1, No. 5, December 1981
7. SHAW ST, AZAR E, MOYER DL: ^3H_2O volume and exchange in uterine cavity of monkeys. Am Physiol 299:1465, 1975
8. Sterilization by occlusion of the fallopian tubes with mucilago phenol: Seven years' clinical observation. Chin J Obstet Gynecol 14:2, April 1979
9. WESTROM L: Incidence prevalence, and trends of acute pelvic inflammatory disease and its consequences in industrialized countries. Am J Obstet Gynecol 138:880, 1980
10. ZIPPER J, COLE LP, GOLDSMITH A et al: Quinacrine hydrochloride pellets: Preliminary data on a nonsurgical method of female sterilization. Int J Gynaecol Obstet 18:275, 1980
11. ZIPPER J, STACHETTI E, MEDEL M: Human fertility control by transvaginal application of quinacrine on the fallopian tube. Fertil Steril 21:581, 1970
12. ZIPPER J, STACHETTI E, MEDEL M: Transvaginal chemical sterilization. Contraception 12:11, 1975

12

Quinacrine IUDs

LEONARD E. LAUFE

ROBERT G. WHEELER

It is 15 years since Corfman reviewed transcervical oviduct occlusion and chronicled the history of the concept.[2] In 1849 a technique was developed to produce tubal occlusion with the application of silver nitrate to the cornua. Many other agents have since been evaluated for their tubal occlusive capabilities, such as zinc, phenol, chloride, sodium morrhuate, salicylic acid, a mixture of gelatin-resorcinol-formaldehyde, and cyanoacrylates.[4] Richart and others at Columbia University have worked extensively with a variety of these drugs and methods, and currently, they are working exclusively with methyl cyanoacrylate.

Zipper, of Santiago, Chile, has worked extensively with quinacrine and his technique has finally evolved into the quinacrine pellet concept discussed in Chapters 9 and 10.

EVOLUTION OF IUD DELIVERY SYSTEMS

As our interest in the further development of the concept of chemical sterilization with quinacrine was pursued, we realized that we must determine the exact pathologic changes induced by quinacrine. In 1980, Bhatt and associates reported on the quinacrine-induced pathologic changes in fallopian tubes.[1] This limited study was accomplished by inserting one application of 250 mg quinacrine pellets into the uterine cavity of 23 women awaiting hysterectomies; therefore, 46 tubes were studied. The changes induced by quinacrine were documented, and in about 50% of the cases an obstructive lesion commensurate with tubal closure was induced.

As a result of this study, a concept was developed to provide a better delivery system of quinacrine to attempt to ensure a more accurate application of the drug to the tubal ostia and to reduce the delivery system to a single event. At that time, studies were initiated using the IUD as a vector for delivering quinacrine. Requirements for these studies were that the par-

The authors wish to express their gratitude to the many collaborators in the IFRP network who have contributed data used in the preparation of this chapter. Appreciation is expressed to the manufacturer of the No-Gravid device and to the contributors in England, Chile, India, and Bangladesh who participated in these studies.

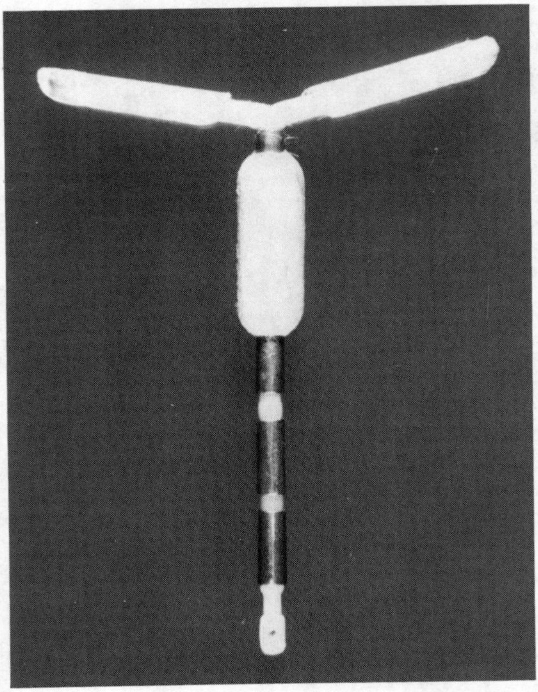

FIG. 12-1. Copper-T 220 with 300 mg quinacrine.

ticipants were awaiting an elective hysterectomy and had no distortion of the uterine body such as myomas and no severe endometrial disturbances. Most of the hysterectomies were in women with prolapse or a premalignant lesion of the cervix. To date, 72 women have been studied. No patient has had any adverse reaction.

In the first five procedures done in Santiago, Chile, a T-vector was inserted, carrying an ethylene vinylacetate (EVA) matrix containing quinacrine. The release rate of the quinacrine from this matrix proved to be extremely limited, and in only one woman could tubal occlusion be demonstrated by hysterosalpingography. Next, a mixture of 80% quinacrine and 20% polyethylene oxide (PEO) was used. PEO is a water-soluble, biocompatible plastic and acts as a binder to hold the quinacrine forms together. The powder mixture was mixed with water to form a very thick paste. The paste was allowed to dry almost completely and was then loaded into a split die and pressed into its final form. The quinacrine/PEO forms were then placed on the arms of the IUD.

The next approach was to add a total dose of 300 mg of the drug to a T-vector, with 75 mg quinacrine at the ends of each of the lateral arms and a central bolus of 150 mg on the stem (Fig. 12-1). The results were erratic, and the central bolus appeared to contribute nothing to the sclerosing effect observed in the tubes. About 50% of the tubes contained a definitive lesion, as with the pellet studies. Results were highly variable. One tube in a given specimen could be totally occluded and the other untouched. The T-vector was next used with the arms upward, as with the original device, but without

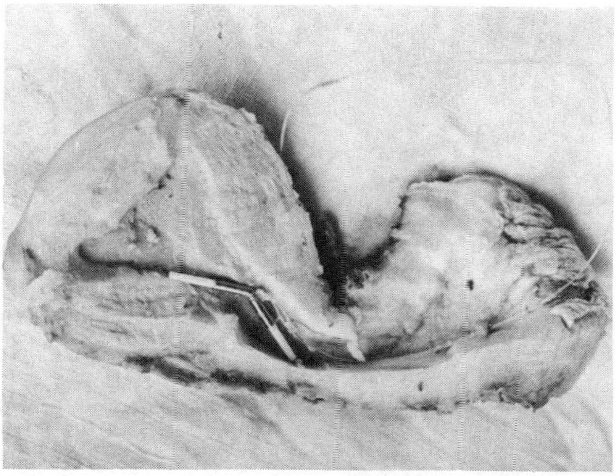

FIG. 12-2. Vaginal hysterectomy specimen with spring device.

the central bolus. In approximately 60% of the tubes, we were able to produce definitive sclerosis.

In the next group, instead of flexing the arms of the IUD upward, we bent them downward by redirecting the mold that applied the quinacrine. This improved the closure rate. In the women treated in this fashion, the tubal closure rate was 75%. Considerable emphasis was placed on proper IUD placement, so that the IUD was reaching the fundus and the arms were properly deployed.

Although the results were improved with the configuration in which a "T" with 75 mg quinacrine on each arm was flexed in a downward posture, examination of specimens with the IUD *in situ* showed that it was not properly deployed in all instances.

An attempt was made to design a vector containing a stainless steel spring in the middle to provide outward flexion of the arms.[3] Devices with this design contained no quinacrine, and we asked contributing physicians to insert them in either fresh hysterectomy specimens or when the patient was on the operating table. These devices proved to be inappropriate, in that either the spring was too weak or it could not be inserted high enough in the fundus to obtain proper deployment of the arms to the tubal ostium (Fig. 12-2).

In the hope of finding a better vector, use of the copper-bearing No-Gravid device made in Verona, Italy, was examined (Fig. 12-3). This device, unlike most IUDs, is made of nylon and is relatively rigid; its arms deploy vigorously toward the tubal ostia. The manufacturer of the No-Gravid provided No-Gravid skeletons. Devices were prepared with 100 mg quinacrine per arm (Fig. 12-4). Twelve hysterectomy specimens have been examined.

During surgery, the devices were left *in situ.* Cornual blocks were taken of each specimen and examined prior to opening the uterus. A uterine fundus containing the device is shown in Figure 12-5. This group of specimens provided the most enlightenment. In all six specimens, the devices were properly deployed and each arm was aimed directly at the tubal ostia. In five uteri, there was bilateral tubal closure throughout the intramural portion of the tubes. In the sixth woman, there was absolutely no effect from the quinacrine,

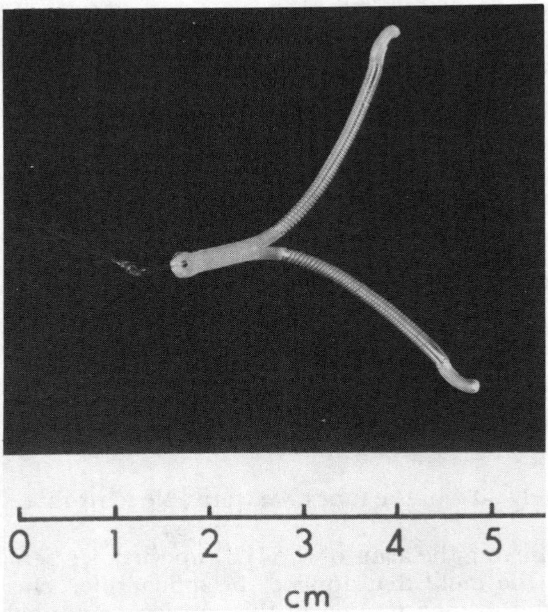

FIG. 12-3. No-Gravid IUD.

and the tubes appeared untouched. The patient had a clinical situation that was unusual. The woman was over 35 years of age and had suffered from extensive menometrorrhagia for the past year. Since a dilation and curettage performed 6 months prior to the IUD insertion revealed no malignancy, she had been treated extensively for 5 consecutive months with high doses of progestational compounds. With this information, we hypothesized that perhaps the extensive use of a progestational compound had made the epithelium resistant to the effect of quinacrine. Another possibility is that her persistent bleeding might have produced rapid dissolution of the quinacrine material and washed it from the uterus.

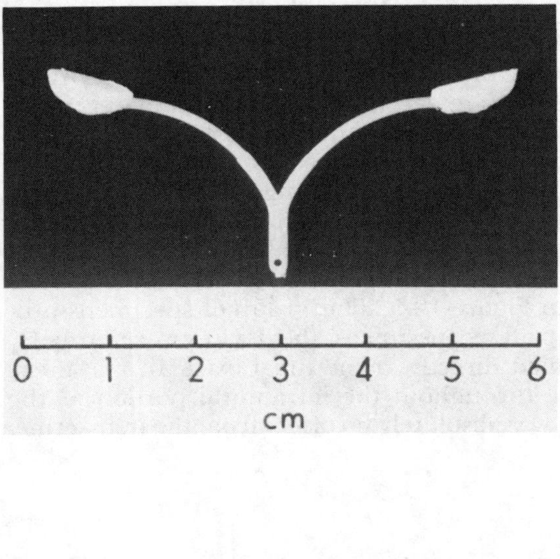

FIG. 12-4. No-Gravid skeleton with 100 mg quinacrine per arm.

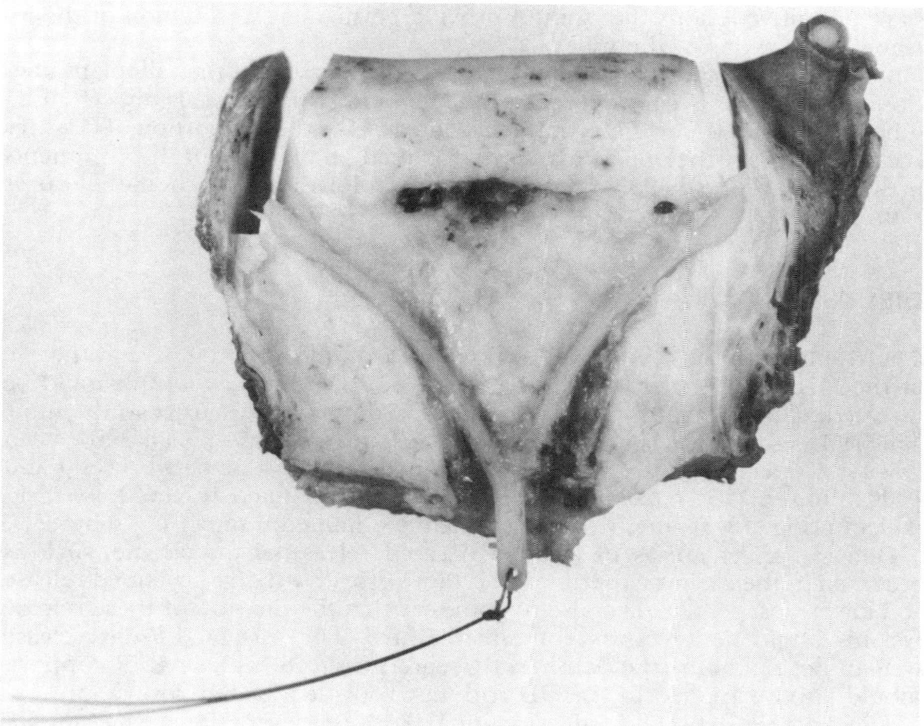

FIG. 12-5. No-Gravid IUD in fixed hysterectomy specimen.

In the early prehysterectomy studies with quinacrine pellets, there was great concern about how the quinacrine acted and whether it operated on the lamina propria in those cases in which the epithelium was intact or had regenerated. One specimen from London, which contained the "T" device, was removed within 10 days of IUD insertion, and we were able to determine that although the epithelium had been damaged it was able to regenerate before sclerosis could occur.

Since the epithelial regeneration of the endometrium and the tubal epithelium is stimulated by estrogen and depressed by progesterone, the next six cases were provided high-dosage progestational therapy 5 days prior to and 5 days following IUD insertion. Megestrol acetate (Megace), 80 mg/day, was used. In these cases ten tubes were found to have definitive large lesions that could only lead to tubal closure. In one tube of one of the specimens, the epithelium was untouched; in one tube of another specimen, there was a mild degree of damage, but whether it would have healed or sclerosed could not be determined.

When these six No-Gravid insertions are added to the first six insertions, definitive tubal lesions are found in 20 of the 24 tubes. If we eliminate the patient with severe dysfunctional bleeding who did not fit the protocol and had received 5 months of intensive progestational therapy, 20 of 22 tubes have definitive lesions that should provide permanent sterilization of the intramural portions of the tubes.

To construct a confidence interval for the proportion of the fallopian tubes closed, each tube is considered an independent experimental unit. If all 24 tubes are included, the 95% confidence interval for the proportion of closures is 0.66 to 0.98. If the one woman is disqualified on the basis of the arguments presented earlier, the 95% confidence interval for the proportion of closures is 0.79 to 1.00.

DISCUSSION

The results with the No-Gravid device appear most encouraging and the use of the IUD as a vector to deliver quinacrine to the tubal ostium should be pursued. Current plans call for variation on quinacrine delivery to the tube. The IUD vector will remain the same. Sustained-release pellets have been developed that leech the quinacrine out over a period of between 800 and 1200 minutes (13 to 20 hours). These have been fixed to the No-Gravid skeleton (Fig. 12-6) and are being studied in a limited number of volunteers.

One can speculate as to whether a rapid release of quinacrine, such as occurred in the earlier experiments, is more effective than a sustained release at a lower dosage. One can also hypothesize that the mixture of these release systems might be necessary for tubal closure. The sustained 7-day release system, developed by the Southern Research Institute with PARFR support, should also be applied to an IUD and may provide a better closure rate.

The original hypothesis of using an IUD as the vector for quinacrine in-

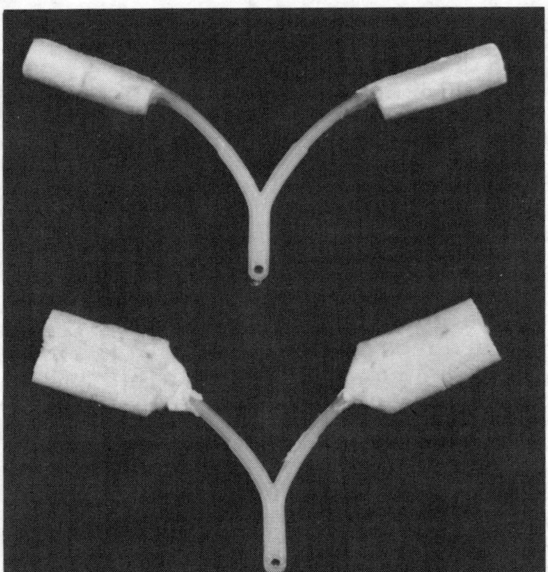

FIG. 12-6. No-Gravid IUD with sustained-release quinacrine pellets.

cluded the idea that the IUD remaining after dissolution of the quinacrine could act as a backup method of contraception. Certainly many variations on this theme are possible. For instance, subsequent to IUD insertion, if the patient wished to have the device removed, a dose of quinacrine pellets could be added at the time of the IUD removal. Patients having the IUD removed could also have a hysterosalpingogram and, if the tubes are patent, could be offered a standard method of surgical sterilization or another quinacrine IUD.

The possibilities are considerable, and we hope that the pursuit of this concept will continue successfully.

REFERENCES

1. BHATT RV, APARICIO A, LAUFE LE et al: Quinacrine induced pathologic changes in the fallopian tube. Fertil Steril 33(6):666–667, 1980
2. CORFMAN PA: Transcervical oviduct occlusion. In Sobrero AJ, Lewit S (eds): Advances in Planned Parenthood. Proceedings of the Third and Fourth Annual Meeting of the American Association of Planned Parenthood Physicians International Congress, Series N138, Vol 1, p 183. Princeton, NJ, Excerpta Medica Foundation, 1967
3. LAUFE LE: Chemical sterilization with an IUD. Contraceptive Delivery Systems 2:343–347, 1981
4. RICHART RM: Female sterilization using chemical agents. In Zatuchni GI (ed): Research Frontiers in Fertility Regulation, vol 1, no 5, December 1981. Chicago, Program for Applied Research on Fertility Regulation

13

Evaluation of Slow-Release Quinacrine Pellets in the Pig

LOURENS J.D. ZANEVELD

ALFREDO GOLDSMITH

A number of studies have established that the uterine instillation of quinacrine in women causes the selective obstruction of the uterotubal junction (UTJ). So far, the procedure has been approximately 90% effective. However, most of the clinical studies performed have employed quinacrine in a suspension or slurry. A number of side-effects have been reported with the use of quinacrine in slurry, including oligomenorrhea, hypomenorrhea, pelvic inflammatory disease, abdominal pain, nervousness, distress, central nervous system excitation, abdominal distention, fever, and chemical vaginitis. Zipper presented evidence that most of these problems can be avoided if the transcervical uterine instillation of the quinacrine is done by a controlled release pellet rather than the injection of fluid. Based on this observation, PARFR contracted the Southern Research Institute to prepare slow-release pellets that liberated quinacrine over a 7-day period (see Chapter 14).

The objective of the present study was to evaluate the efficacy of these slow-release pellets in causing the obstruction of the UTJ and to determine the tissue levels of the quinacrine after it was released from the pellets. The pig was used as the animal model because the pig oviduct is structurally similar to that of the human fallopian tube. Additionally, the pig has two uteri, so one uterus can be used as control and the other uterus as the test.

EXPERIMENTAL PROTOCOL

Pellets were constructed by the Southern Research Institute under the direction of R. L. Dunn (see Chapter 14). Each pellet was tube-shaped and measured 5.0 mm in length and 3.8 mm in diameter. The core of the pellet consisted of 65% quinacrine dihydrochloride in polycaprolactone and was surrounded by a sheath consisting of polycaprolactone. The core contained a central hole that was 0.54 mm in diameter. *In vitro* the pellet had been shown to release

The authors gratefully acknowledge the aid of Dr. R. Richart, Columbia University, New York, in the histologic studies; Dr. N. Dubin and Ms. M. DiBlasi, of Johns Hopkins University, Baltimore, in the quinacrine assays; and Mr. R. L. Dunn, Southern Research Institute, Birmingham, Alabama, in the preparation of the pellets. The project was supported by a contract from the Program for Applied Research on Fertility Regulation.

all the quinacrine in 7 days. Three of the pellets were held together by 4-0 prolene suture that passed through the central hole in the core of the pellets. The average amount of quinacrine in the pellets was 121.0 ± 0.5 mg. Blank (control) pellets were identical to these pellets, except that they did not contain quinacrine.

Ten mature, female pigs of mixed breed were purchased and isolated for 1 month to ensure that they were free of diseases. Before surgery, they were fasted for 12 hours, although water was allowed. The animals were premedicated with atropine (0.05 mg/kg, IM) and xylazine (Rompun) (2.0 mg/kg, IM). The latter is a nonnarcotic drug that produces sedation, analgesia, and muscle relaxation. Anesthesia was induced with thiamylal sodium (2.5%, IV to effect). The animals was intubated with a tracheal tube and maintained on 1.5% to 2.5% halothane with N_2O and O_2 in a 1:2 ratio. During the anesthesia, the animals were monitored electrocardiographically and with an esophageal stethoscope.

With one exception, none of the animals showed any complications during the surgery and recovery was normal. One animal began to show signs of malignant hyperthermia after the administration of halothane, and the anesthesia was immediately discontinued. At a later date, the pig was treated prophylactically with dantrolene (8 mg/kg), 4 hours before induction of the anesthesia. The surgical procedure and postoperative recovery were uneventful.

At the time of surgery, a midline laparotomy was made and the uteri were exposed. The junction between the uterus and the oviduct was isolated, and an incision was made in the uterus, approximately 2 cm long, starting 5 cm from the UTJ. A needle, to which the 4-0 prolene suture with the three pellets was attached, was passed through the incision and threaded through the uterine lumen until it was approximately 0.5 cm from the uterotubal junction. The needle was then pushed through the uterine wall, and the pellets were pulled through the incision into the uterine lumen until the first pellet became situated immediately adjacent to the UTJ, with the other pellets directly adjoining each other. The needle was removed, and the two ends of the suture were tied to each other. The knot was pulled through the incision so that it became situated immediately in front of the last pellet. This prevented the pellets from moving away from the UTJ. The uterine incision was closed with 3-0 Dexon.

The same procedure was repeated on the other uterine horn. One of the uterine horns received the quinacrine pellets and the other received the blank (control) pellets. After the abdomen and skin were closed, the pig was allowed to recover and then was returned to her pen.

The pigs were euthanized after the pellet had been inserted for either 2, 4, 6, 8, or 10 weeks. Two pigs were euthanized at each time period. Immediately on euthanasia, the cervix, uteri, and oviducts were excised. These were divided into several sections to be studied either for histologic changes or for quantitation of quinacrine.

The tissues collected for histology were as follows: 1) the UTJ area, consisting of 5 cm of uterus attached to 2 cm of oviduct; 2) a 3-cm portion of the more cranial uterus, excised 12 cm from the UTJ; 3) a 2-cm portion of the isthmus, excised 9 cm from the UTJ; and 4) a portion of the ovary. These tissues were fixed in phosphate-buffered formaldehyde and shipped to New York, where they were studied by Dr. R. Richart at Columbia University.

For quinacrine quantitation, the following tissues were collected: 1) a 7-cm strip of endometrium, starting 5 cm from the UTJ ("cranial endometrium"); 2) a 7-cm strip of myometrium ("cranial myometrium"), underlying the cranial endometrium; 3) a 7-cm strip of endometrium obtained from the middle of the uterus ("middle endometrium"); 4) a 7-cm strip of myometrium ("middle myometrium"), underlying the middle endometrium; 5) a 7-cm portion of the isthmus, starting 2 cm from the UTJ; 6) a 7-cm portion of the ampulla; 7) a portion of the ovary; and 8) the cervix. Additionally, pieces of the liver, kidney, and the adrenal glands were collected for quinacrine measurements. The tissues were frozen at −20°C and shipped on dry ice to Dr. N. Dubin at Johns Hopkins University.

After the pellets were removed, they were rinsed to cleanse them of blood and sent to R. L. Dunn, at the Southern Research Institute, for quinacrine analyses.

RESULTS

None of the animals showed any side-effects from the surgery or the quinacrine. They continued to gain weight and appeared healthy at the time of euthanasia. At autopsy, none of the animals showed any visible lesions, except that occasional adhesions were present among some of the uterine loops. These occurred with equal frequency on the control and test sides, so they are most likely due to the handling of the uteri during pellet implantation. The incisions in the uteri were completely healed and showed some small scars. In one uterus containing quinacrine pellets, some granulomatous material was detected on the outside wall of the uterus where the incision was made. The suture material was in place in each case and did not cause rupture or strangulation of the uterine wall.

When the uterus was incised, the pellets were found to be still in place, that is, the first one was adjacent to the UTJ. No pellet was visibly altered. In both pigs in which pellets had been implanted for 2 weeks, the endometrium showed yellowish discoloration, starting at the UTJ and extending for 10 cm to 15 cm toward the cervix. None of the pigs with implantations of longer duration showed this, with the exception of one pig with implantations for 4 weeks (No. 801) and one pig implanted for 6 weeks (No. 796). In these animals, some yellowish discoloration was seen at the UTJ. No visible lesions were detected in any of the uteri.

The residual quinacrine in the pellet is shown in Table 13-1. Essentially all of the quinacrine was released from the pellets in all of the animals, even the ones with implantations for only 2 weeks. Therefore, the *in vivo* (uterine) release rate of the pellet is less than 14 days, corroborating the 7-day release rate found *in vitro*.

The tissue levels of quinacrine are shown in Table 13-2. In regard to the test sides, very high levels were present in the cranial endometrium of the animals implanted for 2 weeks. High cranial endometrial levels were also found in one of the 4-week animals (No. 801) and one of the 6-week animals

TABLE 13-1. Residual Quinacrine in Pellets Recovered From Pigs

PIG NO.	WEEKS IMPLANTED WITH PELLETS	QUINACRINE CONTENT OF IMPLANTED PELLETS (MG)	RESIDUAL QUINACRINE IN RECOVERED PELLET AFTER EUTHANASIA (MG)	% OF QUINACRINE RELEASED
797	2	120.8	0.074	99.94
805	2	120.9	0.133	99.89
798	4	120.8	0.037	99.97
801	4	120.9	0.059	99.95
796	6	121.9	0.046	99.96
799	6	120.6	0.042	99.96
802	8	120.8	0.045	99.96
800	8	122.2	0.088	99.93
804	10	120.7	0.040	99.97
803	10	120.7	0.146	99.88

Measurements of quinacrine performed by R. L. Dunn, Southern Research Institute, Birmingham, Alabama.

(No. 796), corresponding to the visual presence of yellowish material (see above). Much less quinacrine was present in the cranial endometria of the other 4- and 6-week implanted animals. Significant amounts were still present in the cranial endometrium of the 10-week implanted pigs. Fairly high amounts of quinacrine could also be found in the cranial myometrium and middle endometrium of the pigs implanted for 2 weeks, the middle endometrium of one of the pigs implanted for 4 weeks (No. 798), and the ampulla and ovary of one of the pigs implanted for 2 weeks (No. 797). Significant amounts of quinacrine were also present in the cervix and isthmus of one of the 2-week implanted pigs, and in the isthmus and middle myometrium of one of the 10-week implanted pigs (No. 804). The ovaries of most pigs tended to possess quinacrine in levels that were often higher than those of the isthmus. In all other cases, tissues showed a concentration of less than 10 ng/100 mg tissue, many of the levels being below detection (< 2.5 ng/100 mg tissue).

The control tracts only showed low levels of quinacrine. Interestingly, the levels tended to be the highest when the corresponding test side was also high in quinacrine (*e.g.*, see the 2-week implanted animals). It was further notable that the ovaries of both the test and control sides possessed approximately the same levels of quinacrine.

Of the nonreproductive organs, only extremely low levels of quinacrine could be detected in the liver and kidney, with the exception of one of the 2-week implanted animals (No. 797). The adrenal gland tended to contain more quinacrine than the liver or kidney, but the levels were only higher than 10 ng/100 mg tissue in the 2-week implanted pigs.

Histologically, all the sections of the oviducts, uteri, and ovaries appeared within normal limits. No evidence of tubal or peritubal changes was noted. One exception was a fragment of granulation tissue in the uterine lumen in pig No. 801, but no further evidence of pathology was found. The UTJs were open in each case, on both the control and the test side.

TABLE 13-2. Tissue Levels of Quinacrine*

PIG NO.	WEEKS PELLETS IMPLANTED	TEST/ CONTROL SIDE	CRANIAL ENDO- METRIUM	CRANIAL MYO- METRIUM	MIDDLE ENDO- METRIUM	MIDDLE MYO- METRIUM	CERVIX	ISTHMUS	AMPULLA	OVARY	ADRENAL GLAND	LIVER	KIDNEY
797	2	Control	X	X	18.3	15.3	21.7	X	X	50.3	18.8	12.1	7.1
		Test	5176.5	394.4	299.3	27.3		22.7	80.5	72.9			
805	2	Control	6.9	5.2	6.1	<2.5	12.0	5.6	9.6	19.6	25.9	<2.5	4.7
		Test	6965.2	33.5	76.9	4.7		29.3	8.9	16.7			
798	4	Control	<2.5	3.5	<2.5	<2.5	4.3	<2.5	X	13.9	<2.5	3.0	<2.5
		Test	156.6	4.7	45.7	3.0		3.4	X	11.1			
801	4	Control	2.8	<2.5	<2.5	<2.5	<2.5	<2.5	X	8.5	9.9	<2.5	<2.5
		Test	1280.4	<2.5	<2.5	<2.5		3.0	X	12.1			
796	6	Control	3.8	9.2	3.1	<2.5	X	2.5	X	8.9	9.4	<2.5	<2.5
		Test	1259.5	3.1	4.4	4.0		3.1	X	8.7			
799	6	Control	<2.5	<2.5	X	<2.5	<2.5	<2.5	<2.5	5.1	3.9	2.5	2.8
		Test	104.6	5.3	<2.5	<2.5		<2.5	<2.5	3.1			
802	8	Control	<2.5	<2.5	3.2	11.0	<2.5	<2.5	X	3.4		<2.5	<2.5
			<2.5	110.6	<2.5	2.6		<2.5	X	2.9	2.8		
800	8	Control	<2.5	<2.5	<2.5	<2.5	<2.5	<2.5	<2.5	<2.5	<2.5	<2.5	<2.5
		Test	4.1	4.1	<2.5	<2.5		<2.5	<2.5	13.6			
804	10	Control	2.9	3.0	3.0	3.2	<2.5	3.0	2.6	3.4	6.5	3.1	2.8
		Test	71.7	9.5	5.3	28.6		12.4	4.4	7.5			
803	10	Control	4.7	5.3	2.5	2.5	2.7	<2.5	3.1	2.7	6.6	3.8	<2.5
		Test	44.6	4.3	4.2	4.0		5.4	2.6	3.1			

*Values are in ng/100 mg tissue. The tissues were analyzed for quinacrine by Dr. N. Dubin and Ms. M. DiBlasi of Johns Hopkins University, Baltimore, Maryland.

X, Not tested.

DISCUSSION

The data show that the slow release of quinacrine over a 7-day period at the UTJ of a pig does not result in the obstruction of the oviductal lumen. This is in direct contrast to the results obtained in women and primates with the quinacrine in slurry or with the 1-day release pellets. Quinacrine solutions were also shown to be active in rats but ineffective in rabbits. These results indicate that the female genital tract of the pig is less receptive to the action and migration of quinacrine than the genital tract of some other species, including the human and nonhuman primate.

Evidence that this hypothesis is correct can be obtained from a study that was performed by researchers by Johns Hopkins University (see Chapters 6 and 7). These investigators injected 30 mg quinacrine into the uteri of cynomolgus macaque monkeys. Tissue levels were measured 24 hours and 7 days after the injection of the quinacrine. Since our quinacrine pellets released their content in 7 days, quinacrine levels in the tissues of the pigs euthanized 2 weeks after insertion of the pellet are comparable to the levels in monkeys observed 7 days after the single instillation of the quinacrine. The endometrial tissue levels were much higher in the pigs than in the monkeys (an average of 3129 ng/100 mg vs. 231 ng/100 mg tissue). By contrast, the levels of quinacrine in the isthmus of the pigs were much lower than those in the monkeys (26 ng/100 mg vs. 1190 ng/100 mg), as were the levels in the ampulla (45 ng/100 mg vs. 1868 ng/100 mg). This can be interpreted to mean that the quinacrine in the pig has a tendency to concentrate in the uterus rather than the UTJ or the oviduct, whereas the quinacrine in the primate concentrates in the oviduct, causing damage to the UTJ.

From a more positive standpoint, the small amount of quinacrine in the nonreproductive organs is very encouraging. In the primate study described above, much higher amounts of quinacrine were found in the adrenal glands, kidney, and liver 7 days after the administration of a solution of 30 mg quinacrine than was found in the pig (respectively, 285, 212, and 120 ng/100 mg vs. 22, 6, and 7 ng/100 mg). Unless species differences exist in this regard, the slow release of quinacrine appears to result in much lower nonreproductive tissue levels of quinacrine than the acute administration of quinacrine and should therefore be less toxic. Since high levels of quinacrine can be released from the slow-release pellets, it can be expected that, in the primate or the woman, the slow release of quinacrine from the pellets should effectively obstruct the UTJ, while causing minimal, if any, side-effects.

14

Controlled Delivery Systems for Quinacrine for Female Sterilization

RICHARD L. DUNN

DONALD R. COWSAR

DANNY H. LEWIS

The transcervical instillation of quinacrine hydrochloride into the fallopian tubes to effect permanent sterilization, as practiced by Zipper and associates, was found to have two limitations: (1) reflux of quinacrine from the uterine cavity to the vagina[6] and (2) leakage of the drug through the ostial opening of the fallopian tubes into the peritoneal cavity.[3] To overcome these problems, investigators sought a system to deliver, at a controlled rate, only the minimum amount of drug needed to induce occlusion of the fallopian tubes.

The quinacrine hydrochloride pellets developed by the International Fertility Research Program were the first attempt to sustain the delivery of quinacrine. The dissolution of the pellets within the uterine cavity reduced the reflux of the drug from the uterus and also reduced the risk of rapid intravascular absorption. As a result, this system decreased both the side-effects and the pregnancy rate associated with the use of quinacrine as an occluding agent. Release of quinacrine from the pellets was sustained for only a few minutes, however, and longer delivery times were desired.

A fibrous polymer delivery system appeared to offer an advantage over other systems in delivering quinacrine to the uterus, because the soft, flexible fibers could be attached to the tips of T- or Y-shaped IUDs and could deliver quinacrine directly to the fallopian tube openings when the IUD was placed in the uterus.

Previous studies showed that a fairly large initial dose of quinacrine was needed for effective occlusion and that a first-order delivery system was desirable in which a relatively large dose of drug is released initially, followed by a gradual decline in amount with time.[1,4] Fibrous polymer delivery systems displaying first-order release kinetics are normally obtained with monolithic fibers, and the drug is dissolved or dispersed within the polymer matrix.[5]

The authors are grateful to the Program for Applied Research on Fertility Regulation (PARFR) for providing support for this research; to Ms. Amelia G. Potter and Ms. Brenda H. Perkins for assistance in the laboratory work; to Dr. Lee R. Beck and Ms. Valerie D. Pope, of the Department of Obstetrics and Gynecology at the University of Alabama in Birmingham, for conducting the studies in rats; and to Dr. Renzo Antonini in São Paulo, Brazil, for conducting the studies in monkeys.

With these considerations in mind, we undertook the studies of fibrous delivery systems, described in the following sections, with the hope of effectively delivering quinacrine to the fallopian tubes at a controlled rate to produce tubal occlusion.

MATERIALS AND METHODS

PREPARATION OF DELIVERY SYSTEMS

Fibers are normally produced by wet-, dry-, or melt-spinning processes. Because melt spinning is the most convenient and the least expensive process, it was used to produce all the fibers in this study. Quinacrine dihydrochloride (Sigma Chemical Company, St. Louis, MO) and quinacrine, prepared as the free base by precipitation of the salt from aqueous solutions with sodium hydroxide, were incorporated into nonbiodegradable polymers (polyethylene and polypropylene) and biodegradable polymers (poly[DL-lactide] and polycaprolactone). These drug/polymer mixtures were then extruded into monolithic fibers with a laboratory melt rheometer.

Coaxial fibers, in which a drug/polymer core was surrounded by a drug-free rate-controlling polymeric sheath material, were prepared by drawing the highly loaded monolithic fibers through a syringe needle that contained solutions of the sheath material in an appropriate solvent. The solvent was evaporated, and the procedure was repeated several times to obtain the desired sheath thicknesses.

Large monolithic rods (>3 mm in diameter), containing high levels of quinacrine dihydrochloride in polycaprolactone, were prepared on a melt rheometer by the same procedure that was used to prepare the smaller fibers. The monolithic rods were then coated with a drug-free sheath of polymer, as described for the fibers, to give coaxial rods.

DETERMINATIONS OF *IN VITRO* RELEASE RATES

The *in vitro* release rates of the quinacrine-loaded fibers were initially determined with a receiving fluid (27.5% by weight ethanol and 72.5% by weight water), to provide infinite-sink conditions for both the salt and the relatively water-insoluble free base. Later, *in vitro* release studies were conducted with the 27.5% aqueous ethanol, distilled water, and acidified saline solution. Aliquots of the receiving fluid were removed periodically and analyzed for quinacrine or quinacrine hydrochloride by ultraviolet (UV) spectroscopy. Appropriate Beer's law plots of absorbance versus drug concentrations were prepared to quantify the mass of drug released from the fiber samples.

DETERMINATION OF *IN VIVO* RELEASE RATES

The first *in vivo* release studies were conducted by implanting 1-cm sections of the best candidate monolithic fibers in the uteri of sexually mature female Charles River rats and recovering the sections after specified periods of exposure. The individual fiber sections were secured to a 7-0 silk suture that was attached to a glass bead and then implanted in rats (under general anesthesia) by puncturing the uterine horn with a 19-gauge needle and inserting the quinacrine-loaded fiber into the uterus by way of the puncture hole. The bead remained free in the peritoneal cavity and prevented the fiber from being expelled from the uterus. Three rats were sacrificed at 2-hour intervals for the first 12 hours after treatment. Additional animals were sacrificed at 1, 2, 4, 8, and 16 days. The fibers were retrieved, cut into small fragments, and extracted with acidified saline solution. The quantity of residual drug extracted from the fibers was determined by UV spectroscopy. In addition, a blood sample from each of the sacrificed rats was assayed by spectrofluorometry for concentration of quinacrine to establish the clearance rate of the drug.[2]

A second series of *in vivo* tests was conducted in *Cebus* monkeys by Antonini in São Paulo, Brazil. Polycaprolactone coaxial fibers loaded with quinacrine were inserted into the uteri of ten *Cebus* monkeys, and two monkeys each were sacrificed at 1, 2, 3, 4, and 5 weeks following treatment. The medicated fibers were removed and analyzed for residual quinacrine dihydrochloride.

RESULTS AND DISCUSSION OF FIBER STUDIES

MONOLITHIC FIBERS

Monolithic fibers were prepared with levels up to 50% by weight of quinacrine and quinacrine hydrochloride in polyethylene and polycaprolactone, with the other polymers giving much lower loadings. In general, fibers containing quinacrine as the free base were of good quality and uniformity; those spun with the dihydrochloride were uniform but of poor quality, owing to the heterogeneous polymer mixture created by the nonmelting of the salt. The fibers containing the free base could be drawn and oriented to give mechanical properties approaching those of normal textile yarns; however, the dihydrochloride fibers were fragile and no drawing or mechanical properties could be obtained. The results of the spinning trials showed that quinacrine as the free base gave better fibers than the salt and that polycaprolactone was the best matrix polymer.

The fraction of the total drug released from the various polymers, when plotted versus time in hours, showed that the rate of release from the monolithic fibers was first order, as expected, and dependent on the polymer matrix, the quinacrine composition, and the loading. Polycaprolactone and polyethylene gave the fastest release rates, with release from polypropylene being very slow. In the first two polymers at the 50% loading, quinacrine dihydrochloride was released at a faster rate than the free base, although this effect was reversed at low loadings.

These results indicate that at the high loadings of quinacrine, dissolution of the quinacrine from the polymer matrix is the rate-controlling step. Because the salt is more water soluble, and is dispersed throughout the fiber as discrete particles, it dissolves faster and creates pores for the penetration of water into the fiber, where the water dissolves more salt. At the lower drug loadings, diffusion of the drug through the polymer membrane is the rate-controlling step and quinacrine as the free base is more permeable than the

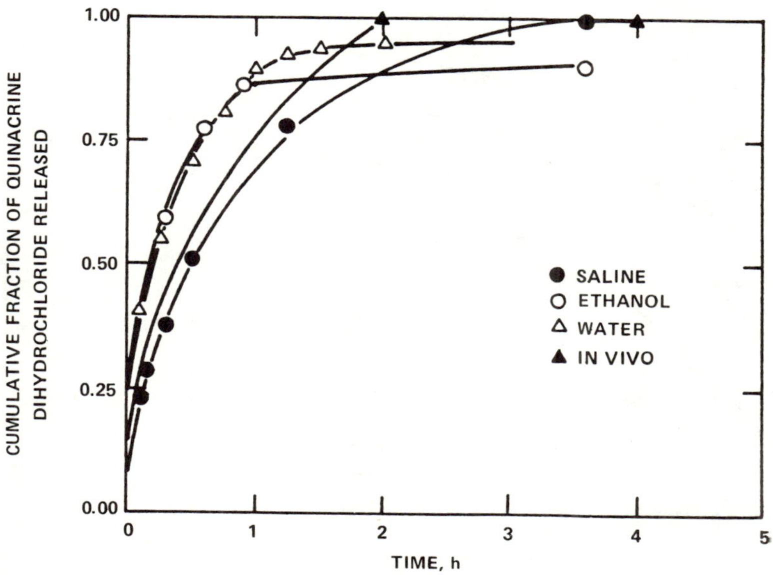

FIG. 14-1. Correlation of *in vitro* and *in vivo* release rates of quinacrine dihydrochloride.

dihydrochloride salt. No major differences in the release rates of either form of quinacrine were observed in the three receiving fluids evaluated.

Because the polycaprolactone monolithic fibers had the best mechanical properties and release rates, samples of these fibers containing quinacrine or quinacrine dihydrochloride (50% by weight) were inserted into the uteri of rats, as described earlier. The cumulative fraction of drug released from each fiber was plotted versus time in hours. These release profiles, given in Figures 14-1 and 14-2, show a good correlation between *in vitro* and *in vivo* release rates for the salt. The data for the *in vivo* release of the free base were scattered, owing to several factors, including fiber nonuniformity, location within the uterus, and incomplete recovery of fiber samples; however, comparison with the *in vitro* release rates showed the same trend. These results confirmed that the *in vitro* model was a suitable system for predicting release rates of quinacrine-loaded fibers.

The amount of quinacrine absorbed into the body was also determined, and Figures 14-3 and 14-4 show the correlation of *in vivo* release with drug levels in the blood of the rats. Although the concentration of quinacrine in the blood was quite low, the levels correlated with the maximum release of quinacrine and its salt.

COAXIAL FIBERS

The release data for the highly loaded monolithic fibers indicated that the delivery of quinacrine and its salt from these systems was too rapid. To in-

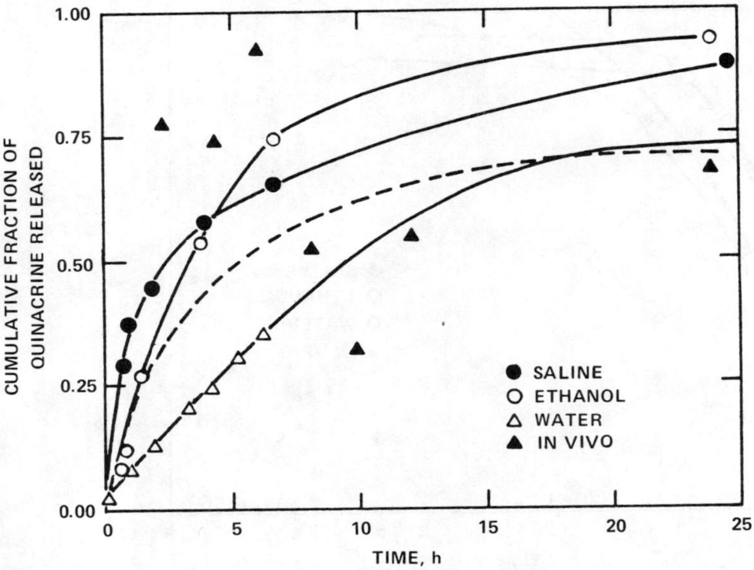

FIG. 14-2. Correlation of *in vitro* and *in vivo* release rates of quinacrine.

crease the duration of drug release of the fibers, quinacrine-loaded coaxial (sheath-core) fibers were prepared with an Estane 5714 or a polycaprolactone sheath and a core matrix of quinacrine or quinacrine dihydrochloride (50% by weight) and polycaprolactone (50% by weight).

The *in vitro* release of samples of these fibers sealed on each end was determined in acidified saline solution. With both fibrous systems, the free

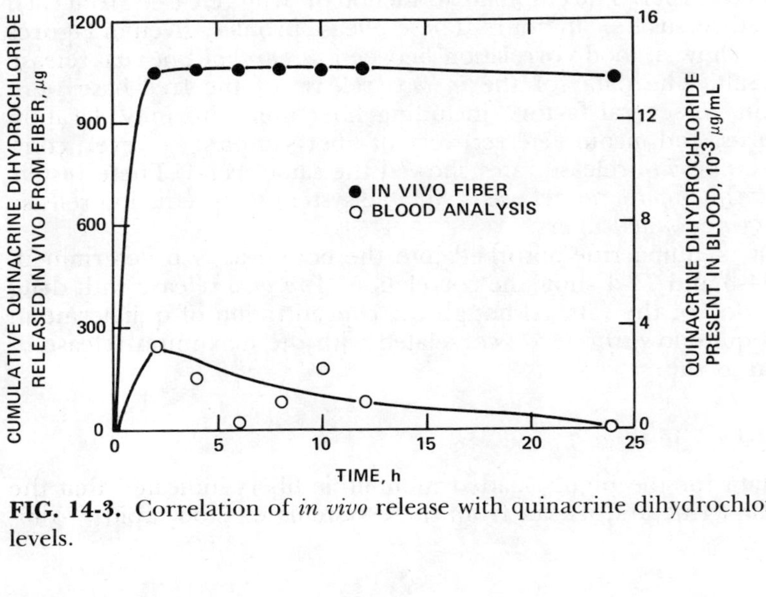

FIG. 14-3. Correlation of *in vivo* release with quinacrine dihydrochloride blood levels.

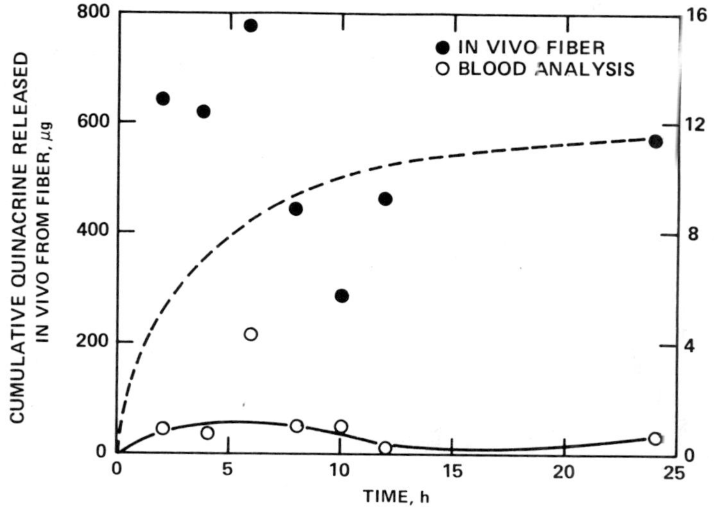

FIG. 14-4. Correlation of *in vivo* release with quinacrine blood levels.

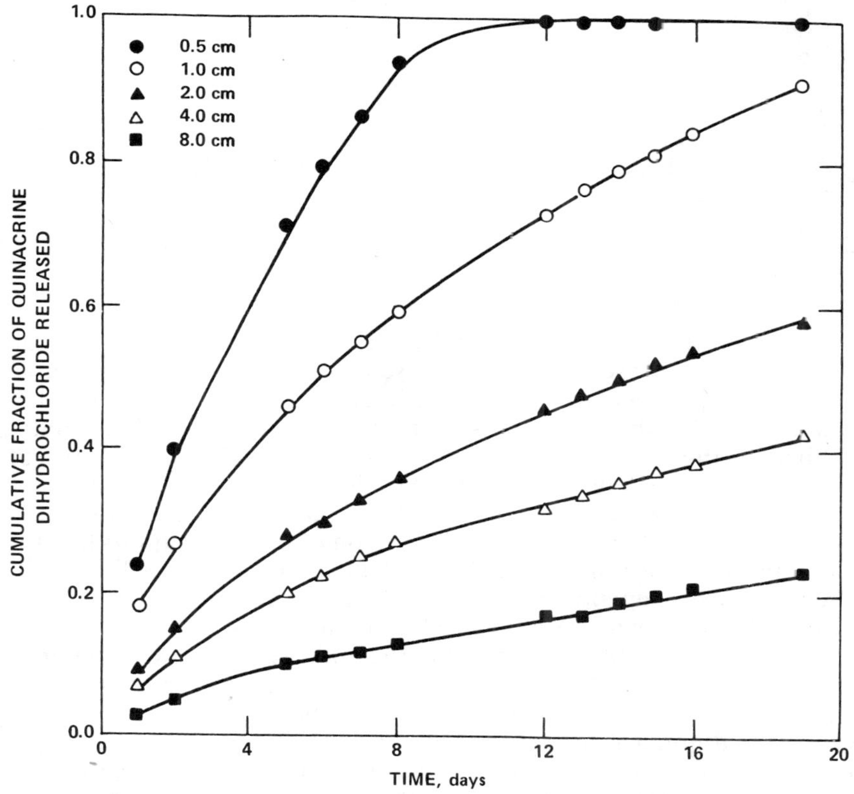

FIG. 14-5. Cumulative *in vitro* release of quinacrine dihydrochloride from various lengths of unsealed coaxial fibers with polycaprolactone sheath.

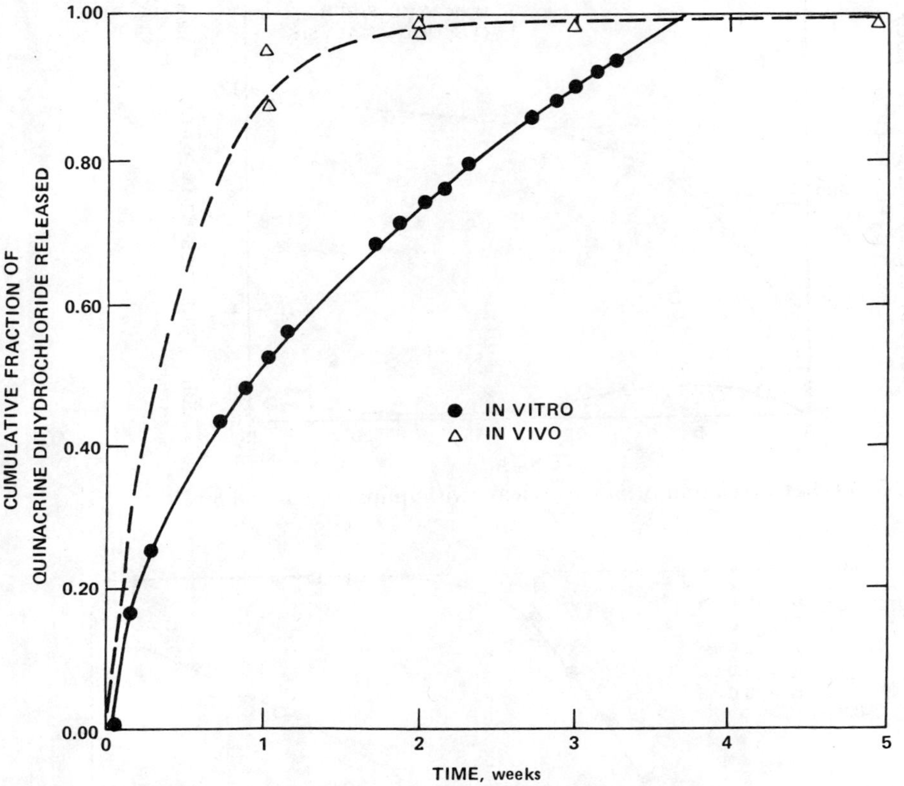

FIG. 14-6. Correlation of *in vitro* and *in vivo* release rates of quinacrine dihydrochloride from coaxial fibers.

base gave the expected decrease in initial burst, but the fiber loaded with the salt gave almost no release at all. These results also indicated that a simple cutting of the coaxial fibers to various lengths should give a controlled delivery of quinacrine dihydrochloride at a rate dependent on the fiber length, because fibers of the same size, when cut to different lengths, have different ratios of unsealed to sealed surfaces. As the salt dissolves from only the unsealed portions, the release rates should correspond. In Figure 14-5, the cumulative fraction of drug released as a function of time for various lengths of unsealed polycaprolactone coaxial fibers shows that the rate and duration of release are indeed dependent on the length of the fiber.

Because of these *in vitro* results, small sections (1 cm in length) of the polycaprolactone coaxial fibers unsealed at the ends were placed in the uteri of *Cebus* monkeys. Although the fibers had a high expulsion rate from the uterus, samples retrieved after the monkeys had been sacrificed were analyzed for residual quinacrine and the rate of *in vivo* release was compared with that determined *in vitro*. The close correlation between the two, with the *in vivo* release being somewhat faster than that predicted by the *in vitro* data, is shown in Figure 14-6.

COAXIAL RODS

Because of the high expulsion rate of the quinacrine fibers in primates and the low quantities of drug available, it was necessary to change the shape of the fibrous quinacrine system for futher evaluations in pigs. In these new studies, a 7-day delivery system with an increased dosage was desired. Therefore, the diameter of the coaxial quinacrine fibers was increased to the size of rods.

The coaxial rods were cut to various lengths, and the release rates were determined in saline solution. These data, and calculations based on the required amount of quinacrine dihydrochloride to be delivered, indicated that the 5-mm length of coaxial rod was the most promising. However, the duration of release from a rod this length was greater than the desired 7 days. To limit the duration of release, two approaches were tried.

The first approach was to drill a hole lengthwise through the core of each 5-mm rod. The hole would create more uncoated surface area and increase the release rate with corresponding decrease in time of release. Although the larger holes gave faster release rates, the duration was only decreased to 11 days.

The second approach was to increase the drug loading of the core of the coaxial rod. The increased drug content would produce a more porous matrix as the quinacrine salt was dissolving and would increase the rate of dissolution of salt from within the coaxial rod. *In vitro* release data on the 65% loaded rod showed a decrease in release of quinacrine to about 9 days.

A combination of the two approaches gave the desired delivery system. The optimum coaxial rod was 3.7 mm in diameter and 5.0 mm in length, with a center hole diameter of 0.6 mm. The rod contained a core of 65% quinacrine dihydrochloride in polycaprolactone, and the sheath was a drug-free layer of polycaprolactone. The *in vitro* release of this system, as given in Figure 14-7, shows an approximately zero-order release of quinacrine dihydrochloride for about 7 days.

Ten devices for controlled delivery of quinacrine dihydrochloride were prepared for use in fallopian-tube occlusion studies with pigs. Each device contained five of the optimum quinacrine coaxial rods, held together with a polypropylene monofilament suture running through the hole of each rod. Ten additional devices, each containing three of the optimum rods, were prepared in the same manner. Each device was sealed in plastic bags and sterilized with ethylene oxide, which had been shown to have no effect on release rates. The devices were then implanted in pigs near the uterotubal junction by Zaneveld (see Chapter 13). The rods were recovered at prescribed times and analyzed for residual quinacrine. These analyses showed that essentially all of the quinacrine had been released within 7 days, as predicted by the *in vitro* release data.

CONCLUSION

The results from this study show that modified monolithic delivery systems can be prepared from quinacrine or quinacrine dihydrochloride with poly-

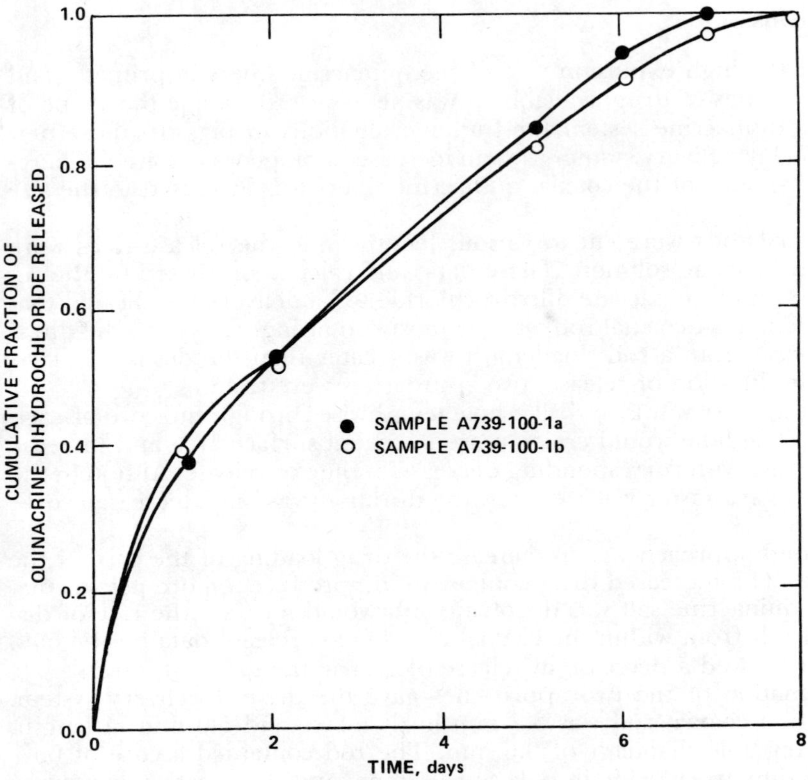

FIG. 14-7. *In vitro* release of quinacrine dihydrochloride from 7-day pellets with polycaprolactone sheath, 65:35 quinacrine dihydrochloride/polycaprolactone core.

caprolactone, a totally biodegradable polymer. These systems, in the form of coaxial fibers or rods, can be designed to give almost zero-order release of quinacrine dihydrochloride for various times, ranging from several days to several weeks. Although the fibers are limited in the quantity of drug they deliver, owing to size and flexibility, both systems provide an effective method of delivering quinacrine at a controlled rate to the fallopian tubes.

REFERENCES

1. BAKER RW, LONSDALE HK: Controlled release: Mechanisms and rates. In Tanquary AC, Lacey RE (eds): Controlled Release of Biologically Active Agents, pp 15–71. New York, Plenum Press, 1974
2. BRODIE BB, UNDENFRIEND S, DILL W et al: The estimation of basic organic compounds in biological materials. J Biol Chem 168:311–318, 1947
3. CHANDRA H, MALAVIYA B, KAR AB: Chemical occlusion of rhesus monkey oviducts with quinacrine. Indian J Exp Biol 12:447–448, 1974

4. COWSAR DR: Introduction to controlled release. In Tanquary AC, Lacey RE (eds): Controlled Release of Biologically Active Agents, pp 1–14. New York, Plenum Press, 1974
5. DUNN RL, LEWIS DH, BECK LR: Fibrous polymers for the delivery of contraceptive steroids to the female reproductive tract. In Lewis DH (ed): Controlled Release of Pesticides and Pharmaceuticals, pp 125–146. New York, Plenum Publishing Corporation, 1981
6. MOULDING TS, THOMPSON H: Distribution of liquids introduced into the uterus with a simple "nonocclusive" cannula. Contraception 9:369–377, 1974

15

Quinacrine Hydrochloride: Future Research

THEODORE M. KING

NORMAN H. DUBIN

DAVID A. BLAKE

TIM H. PARMLEY

Without doubt, there is a need and a demand for a chemical method of tubal sterilization. Chemicals of various categories, including caustic, sclerosing, granuloma-producing, and cytotoxic agents and tissue adhesives have been tested in both animal models and humans.[2] The most effective agent appears to be quinacrine, and, depending on the mode of delivery, it can cause bilateral tubal closure rates in excess of 90%. Clinically, quinacrine has been used in several developing countries.

Efforts have been directed toward improving the efficacy of quinacrine by manipulating the mode of delivery. One approach has been a change from its administration as a slurry to a compacted pellet. V- or T-shaped IUD vectors, with quinacrine located at the tips, have been especially designed to ensure delivery of the drug to the cornual region of the uterus near the uterotubal junction.

As efficacy of quinacrine sterilization improves, safety comes to the fore. In evaluating the elusive risk/benefit ratio of a drug treatment, the therapeutic index is an important consideration. The therapeutic index is the relationship between the dose of a drug that produces an undesirable effect, compared with the dose that produces the desired effect. That index represents, in essence, the "margin of safety" of the drug. A low index, that is, one in which the toxic dose is very close to the effective dose, may be acceptable in the treatment of a life-threatening disease. Thus, digitalis, which has a very low therapeutic index, is nevertheless an acceptable agent for the treatment of congestive heart failure.

In regard to quinacrine, there are numerous known toxic effects; yet, these were of minor importance when this agent was used to treat patients with malaria. However, the risk/benefit assessment of a drug for the treatment or prevention of a debilitating disease like malaria may not be the same as when the agent is used for voluntary tubal sterilization. As an agent for chemical sterilization, it must be assessed against the risks of current methods of surgical contraception, as well as against the risks of other methods of contraception, and of pregnancy itself.

Most of our experience with quinacrine toxicity was gained through its widespread use as an antimalarial during World War II. More pertinent, however, is consideration of potential effects that may occur following intrauterine administration of the drug. Solutions of the drug administered into the uterus are known to be quickly absorbed into the blood and distributed throughout the body. This appears not to cause any toxicity as long as the plasma levels do not exceed some critical level.

That some of the more serious toxic effects of quinacrine are related to elevated plasma levels is shown by the following findings:

Accelerations in electroencephalograms and physiological symptoms occurred in quinacrine-treated human subjects when plasma levels of the drug exceeded 30 ng/ml.

In monkey studies, death or convulsions occurred after quinacrine administration, at the time when plasma levels were at peak concentrations.

In rat studies, a decrease in blood pressure occurred immediately after intravenous infusion of quinacrine, with recovery occurring a short time later, unless the decrease was so severe as to result in death (see Chapter 6).

Central nervous system (CNS) excitation syndromes have been reported following intrauterine administration of quinacrine solutions in 2% of treated women.[1] Studies using pellets suggest a lower incidence of this CNS effect.[3] Possibly, the plasma level achieved in women receiving pellets is less than in those women receiving solutions, but this has not been documented. High plasma levels of quinacrine could also result from inadvertent administration of the drug to pregnant women. Increased plasma levels were observed when the same dose of quinacrine was administered to pregnant as compared with nonpregnant monkeys.

Another consideration is that perforation of the uterus is an inevitable complication, if an intrauterine instrument is used for drug delivery. The subsequent administration of the drug directly into the peritoneal cavity might be expected to result in more rapid absorption of the drug into the blood, and hence higher plasma levels and greater likelihood of toxic reaction (see Chapter 6).

A separate issue is that of potential carcinogenicity of the drug. It is known that quinacrine binds to deoxyribonucleic acid (DNA) and that it acts as a frame shift mutagen in bacterial mutagenicity tests (see Chapter 7). However, no association of quinacrine with mutagenicity or cancer has been demonstrated in mammals, and, theoretically, a single exposure would cause less concern than would a long-term exposure. However, such potential hazards must be considered. It is notable that other analogues of quinacrine were found not to be mutagenic in bacterial test systems (see Chapter 7). However, the efficacy of these drugs as tubal occluding agents has not been documented.

By what mechanism quinacrine closes the tube is still not known. It has been suggested that quinacrine action is related to its ability to intercalate with DNA, and its failure to work in some species, such as the rabbit, is related to the concentration of zinc in the tissue, which inhibits binding with DNA. It is possible, however, that the species differences in response to quinacrine may involve anatomical rather than biochemical factors. For instance, it may be that the close apposition of the luminal surfaces of the uterotubal junction of some species may be more conducive to fibrotic connections between surfaces, rather than to reepithelialization (see Chapter 8).

Furthermore, tubal occlusion may not be the sole *modus operandi* in the antifertility property of quinacrine. It is conceivable that quinacrine affects the reproductive tract in some as yet unknown way to impair the function of the tube, endometrium, or uterine environment.

Further research on quinacrine is needed. Such research might include the following:

Development of a timed release system for quinacrine to give a rate of release that would ensure low plasma levels of this agent, even if it is accidentally placed in the peritoneal cavity, while at the same time yielding high efficacy in causing tubal occlusion

Determination of the tubal occlusion efficacy of nonmutagenic drugs chemically related to quinacrine

Continued testing of alternative drugs with potentially better therapeutic indices for their ability to cause tubal occlusion

More precise definition of the process by which quinacrine results in decreased fertility

Determination of the mechanism by which quinacrine causes tubal closure

On development of improved drug and/or delivery systems, institution of clinical trials, so that such a sterilization technique would ultimately become available.

REFERENCES

1. ENGEL GL, ROMANO J, FERRIS EB: Effect of quinacrine (Atabrine) on the central nervous system: Clinical and electroencephalographic studies. Arch Neurol Psychiatry 58:337, 1947
2. RICHART RM: Female sterilization using chemical agents. In Zatuchni GI (ed): Research Frontiers in Fertility Regulation, vol 1, no. 5, December 1981. Chicago, Program for Applied Research on Fertility Regulation
3. ZIPPER J, COLE LP, GOLDSMITH A et al: Quinacrine hydrochloride pellets: Preliminary data on a nonsurgical method of female sterilization. Int J Gynaecol Obstet 18:257, 1980

16

Discussion: Research and Clinical Experience With Quinacrine

ALFREDO GOLDSMITH

LEONARD E. LAUFE

THEODORE M. KING, MODERATORS

ARE THERE ANY HISTOLOGIC CLUES AS TO THE MECHANISM OF ACTION OF QUINACRINE?

The mechanism of action of quinacrine in producing tubal occlusion is unknown, and the only information presently available has been gained from what can be seen at the histologic level. The term *autolysis* has been used, suggesting a self-dissolving mechanism, and some histologic studies have shown damage in which the neutrophils migrated in from the periphery, as in a classic infarct.

In the limited studies described, the electron microscope was not used, and in only a few cases was the time of injury definitely known to be within 24 hours, so as to provide information on the initial result of injury. The studies suggested that the primary damage was to the cytoplasm and cell wall, rather than to the nucleus. In the early lesions, some nuclei looked reasonably intact; the external structure of the cell was gone, and fragments of nuclei were left floating around in a "soup" that contained no cell membranes.

If a cell wall mechanism were involved, however, then in the *in vitro* tests, at least in the tissue culture systems, one would expect a direct cytotoxic effect, but this has not been seen.

Panelists: Rohit V. Bhatt, David A. Blake, Norman H. Dubin, Richard L. Dunn, David Edelman, Rene Guzman-Serani, Tim H. Parmley, Rodolfo Quinones, Robert G. Wheeler, Lourens J. D. Zaneveld, Jaime Zipper. *Discussants:* Jan Brundin, Nicholas Dodd, Douglas Huber, Miriam H. Labbok, Dean L. Moyer, Robert S. Neuwirth, Carl J. Pauerstein, Ralph M. Richart, Gerald I. Zatuchni

DO THE "SKIP" LESIONS SUGGEST THAT THE QUINACRINE DOES NOT ACT DIRECTLY ON THE EPITHELIUM DURING INTRAUTERINE ADMINISTRATION BUT AS A LOCAL VASCULAR TRANSPORT MECHANISM, FINDING ITS WAY THROUGH THE VARIOUS LAYERS OF THE TUBE TO THE EPITHELIUM?

Not much information is available on the "skip" lesions, except that if one looks carefully at the lesions the damage does not really skip. The histologic findings suggest a direct although superficial effect of the drug. In some of the endometria, the affected area runs down the gland, along the epithelium, all the way to the basalis on the epithelial surface, then up the other side of the gland and down into the adjacent gland, leaving a column of stroma untouched in between. There is no evidence that the drug leaves untouched any areas with which it comes in contact.

The only exceptions are sites exposed to a high concentration of the drug. When quinacrine solution is put into the uterus, it runs out the fimbriated ends of the fallopian tubes; however, invariably, the damage is confined to the interstitial portion and no damage is seen in the fimbrial portion of the tube. Also, no damage is seen on the ovarian surface or peritoneum. These are not skip areas, however. Possibly, in the expansion that takes place, as the drug gets through the isthmus and tube, the concentration decreases dramatically and local anatomical factors, not the tissue type or drug effect, have played the significant role.

HAVE ATTEMPTS BEEN MADE TO RADIOLABEL THE QUINACRINE TO DETERMINE IF ITS EFFECT IS A SURFACE PHENOMENON, AND WHETHER THERE IS LOCAL MICROCIRCULATION OR INTRINSIC VASCULAR REGULATION?

Investigations with fluorescence have provided usable pictures, showing a direct diffusion from the surface in contact with the drug into the subepithelial tissue in a decreasing manner, suggesting surface contact and then diffusion. Tritiated studies with related compounds of quinacrine (not quinacrine itself) show the same type of distribution. A large amount of the compound stayed in the endometrial tissues; some diffused into the myometrium; lesser amounts went down into the cervix and the fallopian tubes; and a small amount went into the ovaries.

WILL INCREASING THE LENGTH OF THE QUINACRINE LESION IMPROVE THE OCCLUSION RATE?

No studies to answer this question have been done. In general, the lesion produced by the quinacrine instillation is small, 2 cm or 3 cm in length, in the intramural portion of the tube. As yet, no investigator has serial-sectioned enough quinacrine-treated tubes to say that a more extensive injury would be more effective. The lesion seems invariably to be confined to the portion of the interstitial tube small enough for wall-to-wall apposition to occur, and that determines the length of the lesion. As some investigators have shown, there is considerable variation in the path that the quinacrine takes, and the size of the lesion varies accordingly.

Eight years ago, clinical trials in Mexico with quinacrine instillation were discontinued because a high percentage of the patients were found to have patent tubes; the quinacrine had been kept in the tube for only about 30 seconds, which is obviously not a sufficient duration of exposure to the drug, even with increased concentrations of the quinacrine solution.

One possible means of improving effectiveness is to place a pellet directly into the tube, instead of near it, since the epithelial damage occurs only in the small narrow area near the tubal orifice. The problem is to keep the pellet in the tube and to know the proper duration of time to produce sufficient epithelial damage. Theoretically, because the quinacrine would be in direct contact with the epithelium, it would not have to be left in place very long and the side-effects would be minimized.

A difficulty with this approach is that very few operators have the necessary skill and expertise with the hysteroscope to place the pellets correctly.

DOES QUINACRINE PRODUCE A LESION THAT IS HISTOLOGICALLY UNIQUE?

Quinacrine-induced changes are not characteristic of any of the routine disease states known to occur in the human female, so in looking at a quinacrine lesion, one would certainly suspect that some sort of trauma had occurred, but whether the lesion is unique to quinacrine is not certain; in fact, other agents are known to have similar effects.

Most observations of the quinacrine lesions are more a reflection of a repair process than of any intrinsic initial effect of the drug.

DOES THE METHOD OF QUINACRINE INSTILLATION AFFECT THE RATE OF ABSORPTION?

No data are available on this, but one would expect that with the quinacrine in solution, the rate of absorption might be increased.

HAVE SPECIES DIFFERENCES IN THE EFFECTS OF QUINACRINE BEEN CONFIRMED, AND IF SO, DO THEY PROVIDE ANY CLUES AS TO THE MECHANISM OF ACTION?

Unlike all the other chemical agents that have been used in the fallopian tubes, which seem to have similar effects in all species, quinacrine apparently acts differently in some species than in others, although there is no evidence that any species has an epithelium that is particularly resistant to the effects of quinacrine.

The variability in species response may be related to the nature of the isthmus. What probably happens is that in some species the interstitial portion of the fallopian tube is sufficiently small in diameter that adherence occurs during the healing process and occlusion is effective. If the interstitial portion is large, or the drug delivery system produces a hole so big that reepithelialization takes place before adherence takes place, the drug is ineffective.

This may explain why quinacrine has not worked well in the pig, an animal in which the junction between the endometrial cavity and the tube is relatively large. In pig studies, even when the drug was sutured directly against the cornua and appeared to completely destroy it, some days later the cornua appeared undamaged and healthy.

HAVE ANY STUDIES CONFIRMED THAT ESTROGEN CAN AFFECT RECANALIZATION OF QUINACRINE-INDUCED LESIONS?

There is very little information on the role of estrogen in recanalization; since the effectiveness of quinacrine seems to result from the outcome of a race between estrogen and the proliferation of the fibroblasts, it would be interesting to do studies in women in a natural hypoestrogenic phase—for example, during early lactation or following danazol treatment—thereby possibly minimizing the effect of endogenously produced estrogen.

Zipper has provided the only report of work in this area, but in his studies women were excluded who had had instillations 40 to 50 days postpartum.

HAVE ANY SERIOUS SIDE-EFFECTS OCCURRED WITH THE QUINACRINE IUD, AND CAN THE CLOSURE RATES BE CONSIDERED RELIABLE?

None of the 72 patients who have worn quinacrine IUDs have had any serious adverse effects. The worst event that occurred in these women was a scanty yellow discharge, which usually lasted 4 to 6 hours and was gone by the next day.

The IUD vector seemed at first to be an ingenious solution to one of the main problems with quinacrine and other chemical agents—the complexity of the delivery system. It provided close proximity for diffusion of the drug and dissociated the delivery from the effectivity. It also provided intermediate protection through its IUD mechanism.

In a significant number of fallopian tubes, however, no histologically demonstrable effect is produced by the quinacrine-laden IUD. The presumed closure rate is based on projections from histologic reminiscences, and although the closure rate in monkeys is 80% to 92%, depending on what denominator is used, these figures should not be considered real rates, because in many cases, although a significant amount of tubal damage was produced at first, epithelialization was extraordinarily efficient. The tube seems to be programmed to stay open, and it does so extremely well.

The problem of how to enhance the activity of the quinacrine is an important one. A promising lead that should be pursued is the concept of prolonged progestational therapy following instillation of quinacrine, with the hope of suppressing epithelial proliferation. Investigators are also looking at delayed-release pellets, and various drug mixtures on the IUD, but these studies are only just being initiated.

IS THE HYSTEROSALPINGOGRAM (HSG) JUSTIFIED AS A PART OF THE STERILIZATION PROTOCOL, CONSIDERING THE VARIABLE RESULTS IN PREDICTING TUBAL CLOSURE, THE RISKS WITH THE METHOD, AND THE POSSIBILITY THAT INJECTING THE DYE MIGHT ITSELF OPEN SOME TUBES?

The HSG has been used strictly as a research procedure in quinacrine studies, to provide comparative data between the quinacrine and methyl cyanoacrylate results. The HSG was never intended to be used in a clinical setting.

Whenever the HSG is used, a diagnosis of bilateral occlusion should be made with caution, because some of the changes in the cornual region produced by the quinacrine are small but important, and an accurate interpretation of the HSG requires considerable skill.

DO THE SAME BLOOD LEVELS OCCUR WITH PELLETS AS WITH OTHER DELIVERY VEHICLES?

There are no good plasma level data with the pellets. However, in an early study, lysed blood samples and saliva measurements were obtained from volunteers who received dosages of 250 mg in pellets and the quinacrine levels in the blood were as high as 40 ng/ml; levels in saliva were less consistent and less reliable.

In another study, the kinetic picture of decay or elimination of quinacrine was shown to be multiphased, with a relatively rapid initial phase and then a much slower phase thereafter. In the initial phase, the ratio between tissue and plasma was 5000:1; the body acted as a sponge, and the drug was greatly absorbed.

Even without calculations one can predict that slow entry of the drug into the circulation, with the pellets, will result in much lower plasma levels than will rapid entry, but whether this is compatible with efficacy will have to be determined in models with the blood levels being measured simultaneously with drug release.

WOULD COMBINING A QUICK AND ACUTE INSULT OF THE TUBE WITH A LONG INSULT IMPROVE THE EFFECTIVENESS OF THE QUINACRINE?

Many investigators believe that chronic exposure by means of a prolonged release rate is critical. What seems to be happening is a race between the epithelium reestablishing the lumen and the fibroblasts obliterating the lumen. The epithelial cells must be kept down while the fibroblasts come in. In most responses, the fibroblasts are relatively resistant to most of the chemicals applied to them, whereas the epithelial cells are highly vulnerable. Thus, a toxic chemical with a slow low-level release rate will probably suppress epithelial regeneration while the scar tissue can form and the tubal occlusion will be effective. Without the scar tissue, recanalization is likely to occur.

WHAT IS KNOWN ABOUT THE QUINACRINE DOSE AND DURATION OF EXPOSURE REQUIRED FOR TUBAL OCCLUSION?

The problem related to the quinacrine lesion in the intramural portion is a matter of time and drug concentration. The time required for dissolution of the pellet is about 10 minutes; just what the actual concentration is in the tube is not known, because the amount of material extruded through the cervical os varies in different patients. Studies in rats indicated that time and concentration are important; a slow-release pellet is required, but a suitable concentration to produce damage is not known and the amount of material inside the uterine cavity apparently must be increased. With a pellet that will last 1 hour, the concentration of the small 10-minute pellets would need to be increased to six times the present size and that would be impractical.

It is doubtful that the slow-release approach alone will produce an adequate effect. A pellet will be required that will give a maximum of 30 minutes instead of 10 minutes. Possibly one can duplicate the size of the pellet, so as to have the same concentration in the blood, but the unstable and higher concentration will be in the uterus. It may be useful to combine the quinacrine with another substance, such as tetracycline or perhaps a chelating agent. It would also be desirable to be able to use a single pellet. Investigators are looking at these possibilities.

HAVE TOXICOLOGY TESTS BEEN DONE WITH THE QUINACRINE ANALOGS?

The US Army has done some toxicology studies of the analogs, but very little of the testing has been done in humans, and none has been done with intrauterine administration.

DO QUINACRINE ANALOGS INTERCALATE WITH DNA?

Whether the analogs molecularly insert themselves between DNA strands is not known. If they do, intercalation is probably not done easily; the analogs have far less avidity for tissue and for DNA than quinacrine does.

WAS THE HIGH BACKGROUND LEVEL OF MALFORMATIONS IN THE SHAM GROUP (6% TO 7%) INFLUENCED BY SOME SPECIAL FACTOR, SUCH AS THE STRAIN OF RATS, DIET, SEASONAL VARIATIONS, OR THE DEFINITION USED TO IDENTIFY A MALFORMATION?

Sprague-Dawley rats, which were used in the study presented, have a higher spontaneous malformation rate than do Long-Evans rats, but this factor alone could not account for the high malformation rate. The definitions used could also make a difference in the malformation rate; many of the malformations were not gross or unusual and might be considered by some investigators to be retarded growth rather than malformations. All malformed fetuses were grouped together, regardless of malformation or number of malformations per fetus. Subsequent analysis of the data by malformation and by syndrome, in terms of combinations of malformations, indicated a dose-related effect.

In a similar study by another group, using Long-Evans rats, the background level was much lower, although serious malformations, including meningomyeloceles and ophthalmia, and minor ones, such as loss of the xyphoid process, were found.

WITH A SLOW-RELEASING DOSAGE, MIGHT THE RESORPTION EFFECT BE AVOIDED AND THEREFORE A HIGHER NUMBER OF MALFORMATIONS BE SEEN?

This is an important point. With a dose system such as a bolus or aqueous type, which delivers the quinacrine rapidly, the number of resorptions increases, thereby precluding some of the malformations that might be noted with the quinacrine pellet, where administration is of an intermediate duration and occurs over many hours or maybe over several days.

WHEN QUINACRINE WAS USED AS AN ANTIMALARIAL DRUG, AND WAS TAKEN BY PREGNANT WOMEN, DID IT AFFECT FETAL GROWTH AND DEVELOPMENT?

Investigators have looked for such reports. Some articles on quinacrine that predate the thalidomide episode claim that quinacrine does not produce malformations. However, a critical systematic evaluation of this problem, either retrospective or prospective, has yet to be done.

WHAT BLOOD LEVELS OF QUINACRINE ARE ASSOCIATED WITH CENTRAL NERVOUS SYSTEM EXCITATION, HEART BLOCK, AND OTHER SERIOUS COMPLICATIONS?

Probably the only data in humans come from an early study by Engle and associates, who looked at the effect of quinacrine on electroencephalograms and psychosis-type phenomena in patients who never had malaria. The study showed that blood levels of about 30 ng/ml were associated with accelerations in the electroencephalographic frequencies. Higher quinacrine levels were associated with nervousness and other central nervous system phenomena, and levels of about 1200 ng/ml were associated with psychotic episodes and hallucinations.

In one quinacrine study, the investigators cannulated the jugular vein of two rats for injection of various doses of quinacrine and also cannulated the carotid artery and attached the cannula to a pressure transducer. They found that injected saline had no effect on the blood pressure, nor did 0.5 mg quinacrine injected directly into the blood. However, 1 mg of the drug began to lower the blood pressure within about 6 seconds, and recovery of normal pressure took about 30 seconds. Higher doses produced lower levels of blood pressure and longer recovery times. With 2.5 mg quinacrine, the blood pressure dropped very low and the animals died.

HAVE ANY DEATHS BEEN ATTRIBUTED DIRECTLY TO QUINACRINE USE?

The two deaths mentioned in association with quinacrine instillation were not related to the quinacrine but to other drug effects.

WHAT IS THE DANGER OF ECTOPIC PREGNANCIES IN QUINACRINE-TREATED WOMEN, IF THE TUBES ARE NOT SUFFICIENTLY DAMAGED?

In Chile, the general ratio of normal to ectopic pregnancies is about 250:1, but in the Chilean quinacrine studies no ectopic pregnancies have been seen in almost 250 pregnancies. The reason for this has not been explained.

WHAT TREATMENT WAS GIVEN TO THE CHILEAN PATIENTS EXPERIENCING CNS EFFECTS FOLLOWING QUINACRINE INSTILLATION? DID THESE PATIENTS EXPERIENCE OTHER SIDE-EFFECTS?

Three to 5 minutes following the instillation, several women became overexcited. They were given phenobarbital, and after resting for 1 or 2 hours they were able to leave the clinic and go home, where they continued to take phenobarbital for 2 days. The process was usually over in 12 to 24 hours. One woman was hospitalized for observation, but she, too, recovered after 24 hours. Her blood pressure was normal, but her urine was yellow, presumably as a result of a massive penetration of the quinacrine slurry into the bloodstream. No hematologic studies were performed on any of the women, but none of the women experienced any prolonged complications.

HAS ANY WORK BEEN DONE ON THE EFFECTS ON NEONATES OF THE PASSAGE OF QUINACRINE IN BREAST MILK?

Information on this question is not presently available, but if this method is to be promoted for developing countries, where a majority of women are either pregnant or lactating, and if it is to be promoted as a method preferable during the quiescent phase of the endometrium, the effects of giving this drug to a lactating woman must be evaluated.

IF THE QUINACRINE IUDS BECOME WIDELY AVAILABLE IN DEVELOPING COUNTRIES, OR IN THE DEVELOPED WORLD, WHAT WILL THE CONSEQUENCES BE IF THE QUINACRINE DEVICE IS MISTAKEN FOR A REGULAR IUD AND ACCIDENTALLY INSERTED IN A WOMAN?

This possibility points up the need to find a name for the quinacrine IUD that totally dissociates it from an IUD, which as a reversible method of contraception is significantly different in intent and effect from the quinacrine IUD.

Every complication that one could imagine and perhaps others that have not even been thought of may occur if one uses this approach of delivering quinacrine; someone may perforate a uterus, someone may put an IUD into a pregnant uterus, and so forth. Still other problems come into question; for example, what will happen if the quinacrine IUD is put into a woman who has a uterine body distorted by myomas? Obviously, the drug will not be delivered uniformly to both sides. And other pelvic abnormalities obviously could contraindicate the use of such an approach.

At present, however, investigators are just promulgating this approach as a vector for delivering the drug more effectively to the tubal ostium; they are still trying to evolve the right device with the right dose and the right release rate. They have no intention at this point of beginning clinical trials of the device. Every case presented thus far has been a prehysterectomy case and will continue to be until the investigators feel they have enough experience to begin a very carefully controlled phase I trial.

If investigators do succeed in finding the right vector with the right dose, they may be able to make the IUD itself a biodegradable component of a whole delivery system, so at the end of 1 or 2 years perhaps, it would completely disappear. However, those possibilities are in the future. Meanwhile, it seems obvious that there is a desire and a need for chemical sterilization and this work will continue.

WHAT IS THE MEXICAN EXPERIENCE WITH QUINACRINE?

When clinical trials with quinacrine in Mexico ended about 8 years ago, some 60 patients had been treated with quinacrine suspension. The drug was instilled in two concentrations: (1) 25 mg in 1 ml of saline solution and (2) 50 mg in 1 ml of saline solution. No problems occurred with introducing the quinacrine, but 10% of the attempts failed. Patients were very carefully selected—only women with grossly normal uteri were accepted—and all procedures were performed with the patient in the proliferative phase of her cycle. In the preliminary report, 6 of 15 patients had both tubes occluded, as shown by a hysterosalpingogram (HSG) 3 months after instillation. The HSG was repeated every 3 months for a year.

The first instillations were done on hysterectomized uteri, to be sure that the quinacrine was being properly introduced into the tube. The procedure was then done in five patients who were waiting to be operated on for another reason. The pathology report on the tissues removed from a patient who was operated on 1 month after the instillation showed an inflammatory reaction in the tubal lumen.

Another patient was operated on 1 year after instillation of quinacrine in one tube and electrocoagulation in the other. The electrocoagulated tube was found to be occluded, but the quinacrine-treated tube was completely normal. This indicated to the investigators that they needed to increase the length of time that the chemical agent was in contact with the tubal epithelium. It provides an impetus for investigating the possibility of a tubal block with a slow-releasing system that could be placed into the intramural portion of the tube.

All the patients had side-effects from the quinacrine, but none of them was serious or of the type described by other investigators. The type and severity of side-effects seemed to depend on the amount of quinacrine instilled. For example, those patients in whom a small amount of quinacrine was instilled prior to operation had no damage of the intraperitoneal structures and no problem with toxicity.

WHAT IS THE EXPERIENCE IN INDIA WITH THE QUINACRINE PELLETS?

If chemical sterilization can be made as effective as the surgical methods, women in developing countries as well as in the developed world would be likely to prefer it to surgical sterilization. However, since it is not presently as effective, its use in developing countries requires careful consideration.

At Baroda, India, investigators have introduced quinacrine pellets into about 85 women and have a follow-up of 2 years. The selection criteria were standard: women had to be in the proliferative stage of the cycle and in the reproductive age-group (average age was 31.4 years, parity was 4.1). Two patients conceived after completing the first instillation and dropped out of the program. Seventeen of 85 women complained of mild to moderate discomfort in the lower abdomen. Menstrual irregularities (delayed cycle and extended period) were experienced by 14% of the women, and pregnancy tests were done in women fearing pregnancy. In a majority of the women, normal cycles returned in about 4 months. Thus far, six pregnancies have occurred, none of them ectopic; one pregnancy occurred at 2 months, one occurred at 8 months, and one occurred at 16 months after a third instillation.

The study has shown that the pellets are more convenient to introduce than quinacrine suspension, which came out through the cervix shortly after instillation. The pellets are sustained *in utero* for a longer time. Pain in the first 48 hours could be prevented or reduced by giving analgesic drugs, then beginning the procedure. There is delay in the return of menstruation in about 10% of cases, and the women worry about possible pregnancy.

The Indian investigators have found that their initial experience with the quinacrine pellets is very encouraging, especially because friends of women in the study are inquiring about whether they, too, can have the treatment. Now the investigators are looking forward to the third generation of IUD quinacrine pellets, which promise even better results than have been seen so far. The 85 women who have had the treatment will be followed for longer than 2 years, in the hope of learning whether any further pregnancies will result.

17

Nonsurgical Procedures for Manual Instillation of a Phenol-Atabrine Paste (PAP) for Female Tubal Occlusion

YU-HAU WU

PEI-LI QIAN

SHUEH-PING TIEN

There is increasing scientific and public interest in the potential of nonsurgical methods for female tubal sterilization. If these methods prove both effective and safe, they are bound to meet with wide acceptance throughout the world. With this objective in mind, we have carried out a series of research projects in animals and humans since 1969.

In the preliminary period from 1969 to 1972, we studied the pharmacological actions and reactions of 11 kinds of chemicals on the mucosa of the tubes of animals and humans, *in vivo* and *in vitro*.[1,2,4,5,7,8,9] As a result of our efforts and those of other investigators,[3,6,10,11] we determined that phenol-Atabrine (quinacrine) paste (PAP) showed promise, and we sought a method by which we could instill the compound into the fallopian tubes transcervically.

MATERIALS AND METHODS

The constituents of the "three in one" PAP are phenol (30 g), Atabrine (35 g), and biligraphine (35 g). The phenol destroys the tubal lining by causing necrosis of the mucosa; Atabrine inhibits the regrowth of tubal epithelium and stimulates the tubal submucosal tissues to proliferate into granulation tissues, occluding the tubal lumen; and biligraphine casts a shadow on the roentgenogram to establish that occlusion has occurred and to determine the amount of PAP instilled into the tubal lumen and the extent of tubal damage.

INSTRUMENTS

We used a stainless-steel cannula about 22 cm in length, with a lumen of 2.5 mm in diameter. The instrument could be bent at an angle of about 140° laterally, so as to fit the curvature of the uterine cavity. A heart-shaped plate was attached at the proximal end of the cannula to serve as a guide. A short piece of rubber tubing was fastened at the distal end of the cannula to prevent trauma of the uterine wall (Fig. 17-1).

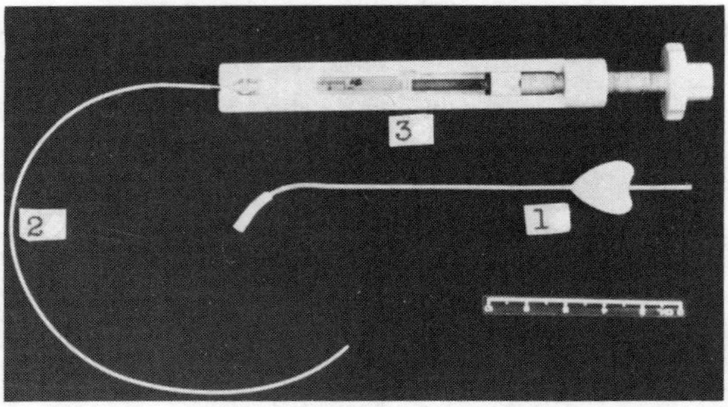

FIG. 17-1. (*1*) Metallic canula. (*2*) Polyethylene tube. (*3*) "Paste driver."

A polyethylene or plastic tube 45 cm in length, with an external diameter of 1.4 mm, an internal diameter of 0.9 mm, and the distal end cut evenly and smoothly, was connected at its proximal end to a 12-gauge needle for instilling PAP into the tubal lumen.

"Paste driver," a specially designed apparatus, was used to push the thick PAP, which would otherwise be difficult to instill into the tube, from a tuberculin syringe into the plastic tube by spiral action.

METHOD

The procedure was carried out in married women, upon their request, and with their husband's consent. It was done in the first half of the woman's menstrual cycle, either 4 months after delivery, during the lactation period, 1 month after early abortion, 4 months after late abortion, or soon after removal of an IUD. Women were not included in the study if they had trichomonal or monilial vaginitis, pelvic inflammatory disease, pelvic cellulitis, pelvic masses, hepatic or renal disease, neuropsychiatric disturbance, or pregnancy.

The manual, nonsurgical procedure was done in the outpatient operation room without the use of anesthesia. The patient was placed in the lithotomy position for cleaning and sterilizing the vulva and vagina. Pelvic examination was done to determine the condition of the cervix and the size, position, and mobility of the uterus and also to rule out any pelvic pathologic conditions. The uterine cavity was sounded to determine its depth, and the curvature, direction, and symmetry of the uterus were ascertained. This preliminary examination was done to locate the uterotubal orifice if possible by means of manual manipulation.

Before its introduction, the cannula was bent to fit in the curvature of the uterine horn, especially at the tubal orifice. The plastic tube was inserted into the cannula until its tip protruded from the opening of the cannula 0.5 cm, the position was marked on it, and the tip of the plastic tube was retracted into the cannula. The cannula with plastic tube was then introduced into the uterine cavity toward the tubal orifice in one of the uterine horns, and the tip of the plastic tube was pushed from the cannula into the tubal orifice; if the tip could not be pushed in farther, the plastic tube, together with the cannula, was drawn back from the uterine mucosa for about 0.5 cm. The plastic tube was then manipulated in different directions in search of the tubal orifice, one more time in each direction, to acquire the feeling of entering the tubal lumen. In a successful entry, the tip of the plastic tube could be inserted 0.5 cm into the tubal orifice without resistance. This sensation of manipulation could be obtained by constant practice.

To test the entry of the plastic tube into the tubal orifice, with the tip of the plastic tube in the tubal lumen, about 20 ml sterilized normal saline was injected, and if the solution did not leak back through the cannula or cervical os, then it was time to inject 0.6 ml to 0.8 ml of 50% sodium saccharide, followed by 5 ml to 10 ml of saline through the plastic tube. Sensations of soreness and bearing down around the anal region, or lower abdominal pain, indicated that sodium saccharide had passed into the abdominal cavity and was stimulating the peritoneum, indirectly proving that the tip of the plastic tube was well inside the tubal lumen.

To instill the PAP, the material was pushed through the plastic tube into the tubal orifice by the spiral action of the "paste driver." A total of 0.42 ml PAP was used, 0.30 ml of which filled the plastic tube while 0.12 ml was pushed into the interstitial portion of the tube. After that amount of PAP was instilled, the cannula and the plastic tube were withdrawn together. The whole procedure was repeated on the opposite side of the tubes.

A plain roentgenogram was taken soon after the procedure. If the result was not satisfactory, the procedure was repeated right away. The linear shadow of PAP in the tube of more than 1 cm was considered success. If possible, the procedure was done under screening, so that direct visualization could be obtained (Figs. 17-2 through 17-5).

The pathologic processes in the tubal lumen were necrosis of the tubal

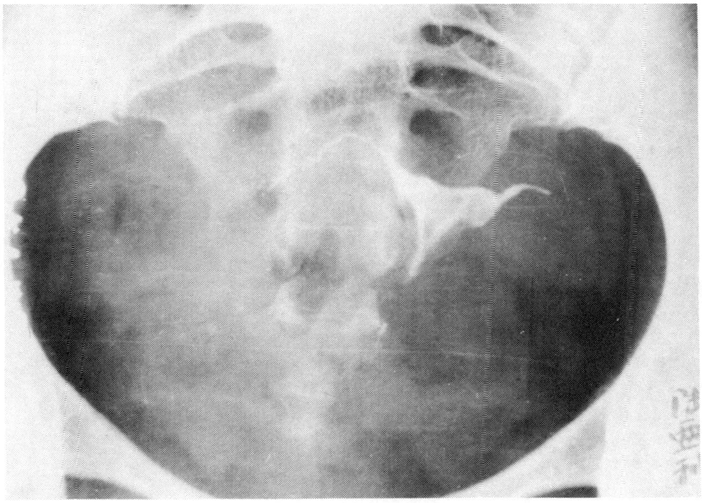

FIG. 17-2 Roentgenogram shows opaque media in uterine cavity and interstitial (left) and isthmic (right) portion of tubes.

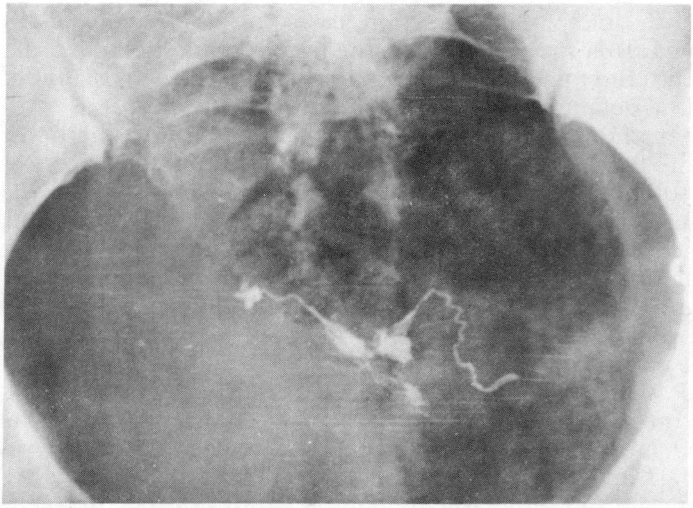

FIG. 17-3. Roentgenogram shows filling of PAP in ampullar portion of tubes.

epithelium (Figs. 17-6 and 17-7), exudation, and sloughing off of the necrotic tubal mucosa. Figures 17-8 and 17-9 show pathologic effects after 5 months. Figure 17-10 shows the female tube 3 months after influx of PAP, with residual chemical granules, proliferation of submucosal granulation tissues, gradual disappearance of foreign body giant cells and inflammatory cells,

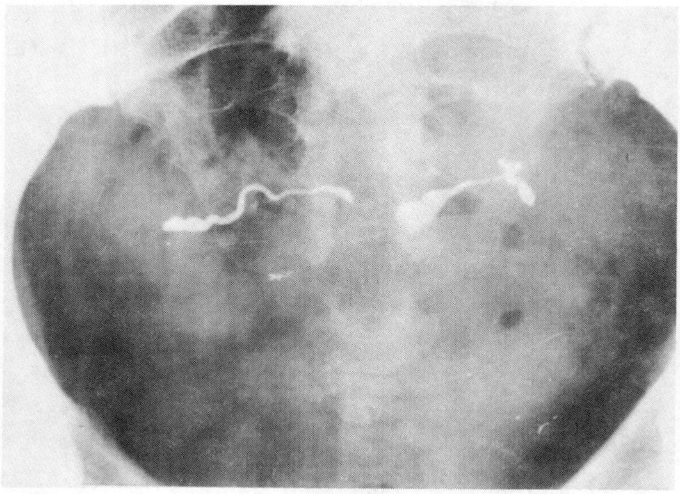

FIG. 17-4. Roentgenogram shows filling of PAP in ampullar portion of tubes (rather thick shadows).

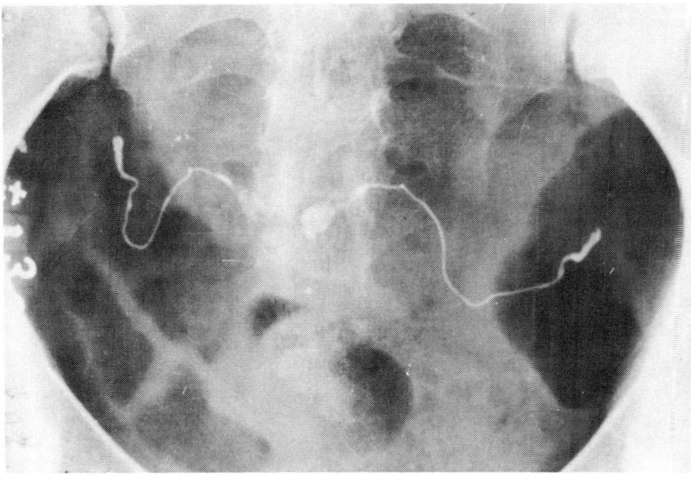

FIG. 17-5. Roentgenogram shows filling of PAP in ampullar portion of tubes (long and thin shadows).

replacement of fibrotic tissues, formation of scar tissue, and, finally, occlusion of the tubal lumen.

RESULTS

Following initiation of the study in 1972, the Shanghai Non-Surgical Cooperative, under Dr. Wu's supervision, performed 1837 PAP instillations into female tubes for occlusion over almost a 4-year period. About ten medical workers from five units of the Cooperative took part in the program after a short period of training. Follow-up of the women was done in two groups (Table 17-1). In the 1837 women undergoing the procedure during a 3-year, 9-month period, radiographic studies revealed that in 129 patients the procedures were considered failures because the linear shadow of PAP was less

FIG. 17-6. Histologic picture of rabbit tube 24 hours after instillation of PAP.

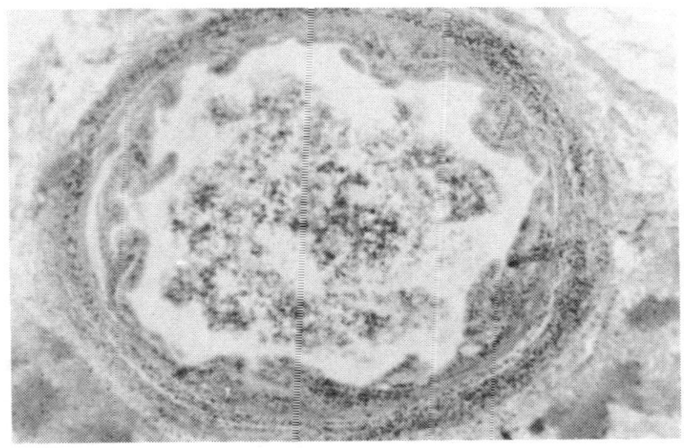

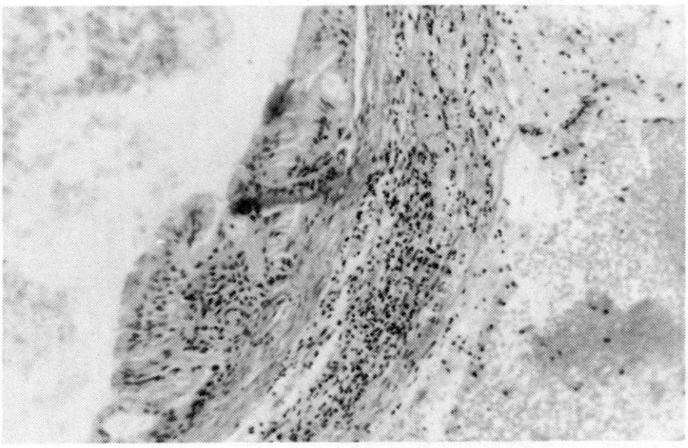

FIG. 17-7. High-power view of rabbit tube in Figure 17-6 shows polymorphonuclear infiltration.

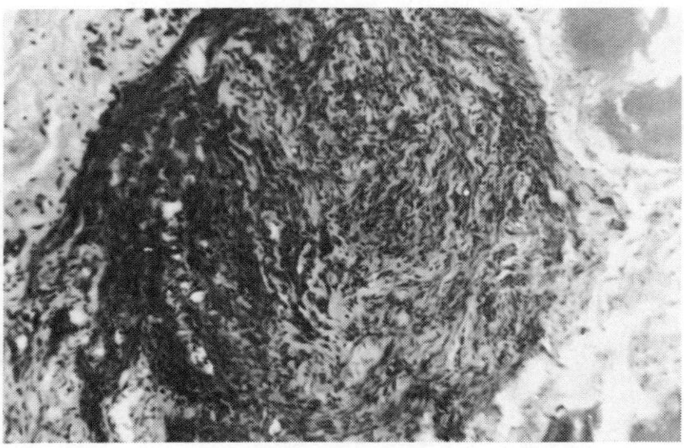

FIG. 17-8. Histologic picture of rabbit tube 5 months after instillation of PAP.

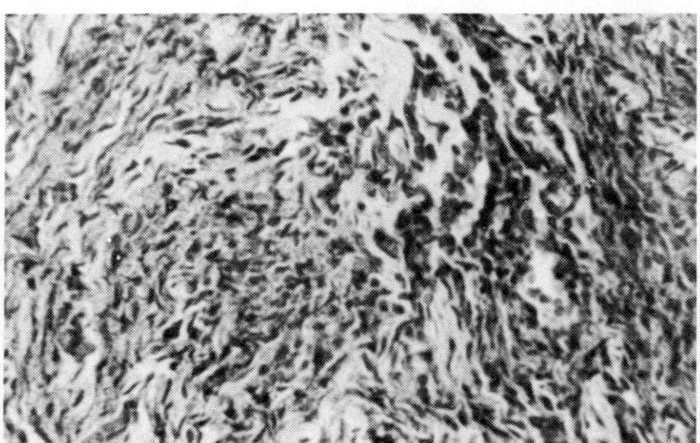

FIG. 17-9. High-power view of rabbit tube in Figure 17-8 shows the tubal lumen completely obliterated.

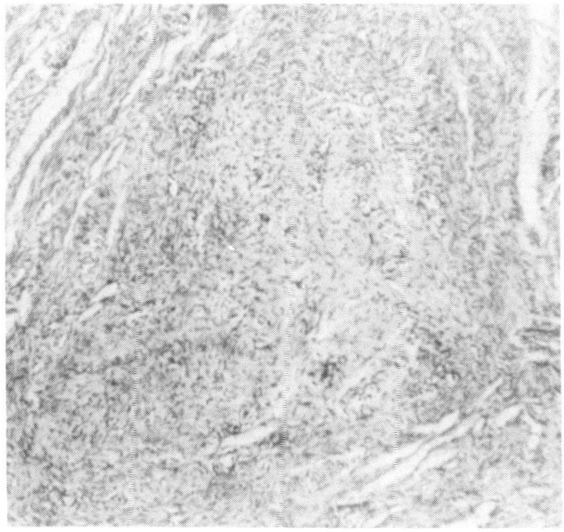

FIG. 17-10. Histologic picture of human female tube 3 months after instillation of PAP shows complete obliteration.

than 1 cm in length (Table 17-1). Therefore, the procedure failure rate was 7.02% (129/1837) and the success rate was 92.98% (1708/1837).

At follow-up, 4 to 7 years after the procedure, only 1637 women were available for study. Of these, 15 women were reported pregnant, thus giving a pregnancy rate of 0.92% (15/1637).

From January to May, 1980, our own staff performed 204 procedures at the Xin Hua Hospital in Shanghai (Table 17-2). Of these procedures, 15 failed, as determined by a radiographic report of less than 1 cm linear shadow of PAP in the tubes. This was a failure rate of 7.35% and a success rate of 92.65%. Of the 189 remaining women with successful procedures, 36 women

TABLE 17-1. Results of PAP Instillations in Women Treated at the Shanghai Non-Surgical Cooperative

RESULT	NO. PATIENTS	(%)
Original study		
Total group	1837	
Successful procedures*	1708	(92.98%)
Failed procedures†	129	(7.02%)
Follow-up at 4 to 7 years		
Total group	1637	
Patient not pregnant	1622	(99.08%)
Pregnancies	15	(0.92%)

*Linear shadow of PAP more than 1 cm in length on roentgenogram.

†Linear shadow of PAP less than 1 cm in length on roentgenogram.

TABLE 17-2. Results of PAP Instillations Performed at Xin Hua Hospital, Shanghai, 1980–1981

TIME FOLLOWING TREATMENT	TOTAL PROCEDURES	SUCCESSFUL PROCEDURES*	FAILED PROCEDURES†	PREGNANCY
January–May 1980	204	189 (92.65%)	15 (7.35%)	
1 year	153	152 (99.35%)		1 (0.65%)

*Linear shadow of PAP more than 1 cm in length on roentgenogram.
†Linear shadow of PAP less than 1 cm in length on roentgenogram.

TABLE 17-3. Length of PAP Shadow as Shown on Plain Film 3 to 5 Weeks Following Instillation

	PAP SHADOW						
	OUTSIDE OF TUBE	*0.5 CM*	*1 CM*	*2 CM*	*3 CM*	*4 CM*	*TOTAL*
Number of tubes	26	27	66	137	222	34	512
Patency on hysterosalpingography	22	4	2	0	0	0	28

TABLE 17-4. Length of Tubal Blockage as Shown by Linear PAP Shadow on Roentgenogram in 15 Women Who Became Pregnant Following PAP Instillations

TYPE OF PREGNANCY	LINEAR PAP SHADOW			
	1 CM	*2 CM*	*4+ CM*	*TOTAL*
Intrauterine	6	4	3	13
Tubal			2	2
Total	6	4	5	15

were lost to follow-up and 153 were followed for 1 year. Only one woman became pregnant and subsequently underwent abortion. Therefore, the pregnancy rate at 1 year was 0.65% (1/153).

In another study, to determine the optimum length of tubal damage, 256 of the 559 patients treated during 1973–1974 were chosen at random for hysterosalpingography 3 to 5 weeks after instillation, and a total of 512 tubes were carefully studied. The comparison of the length of injury and the number of patent tubes, as indicated by hysterosalpingography, is shown in Table 17-3. In the 53 tubes in which the linear PAP shadow was less than 1 cm in length, or was outside the tube, 26 tubes were patent. When the shadow was 1 cm in length, only two patencies were seen, and when the shadow was longer than 2 cm, no patencies were seen. Therefore, we considered a PAP shadow longer than 1 cm to be, in general, an index for a successful instillation. However, as we will show in Table 17-4, the length of the linear PAP shadow does not necessarily correlate with the occurrence of later pregnancy.

Among the 15 women who became pregnant, analysis of the radiographic studies of their tubes indicated that six women had linear PAP shadows longer

TABLE 17-5. Intervals Between the Procedure and Pregnancy

INTERVAL	NO. PATIENTS
3–6 months	4
6–12 months	5
1–2 years	4
2–3 years	2*

*Both ectopic.

than 1 cm, four had shadows longer than 2 cm, and three had shadows longer than 4 cm (Table 17-4). In the two women experiencing ectopic pregnancy, the linear shadow was no more than 4 cm.

The intervals between the procedure and pregnancy are shown in Table 17-5. The two ectopic pregnancies occurred 2 to 3 years following what was described as at least a 4-cm linear PAP shadow.

SIDE-EFFECTS

The side-effects experienced by some patients during the procedure were paleness, sweating, dizziness, nausea, and vomiting. Some felt backache, lower abdominal distention, or a bearing down sensation around the anal region during the first 2 weeks after the procedure, possibly due to congestion, edema, and distention of both tubes. A rare pelvic mass may have resulted from too much PAP injected into the tube, with a leakage through the fimbrial opening into the peritoneal cavity. In these cases, the mass subsided later with treatment. A few patients had loss of appetite or some yellowish or blood-stained vaginal discharge, which usually disappeared in about 10 days.

There were two cases of uterine perforation during the early period of the study. Both perforations happened in the early lactation period, within 4 months after childbirth. One of these women had profuse uterine bleeding, probably due to trauma of uterine mucosa. The women were treated conservatively and recovered without surgery.

TABLE 17-6. Febrile Reactions and Success/Failure Rates Among 1708 Women Following PAP Instillation

	35 G ATABRINE*		NO ATABRINE†		17.5 G ATABRINE	
RESULT	*NO. PATIENTS*	%	*NO. PATIENTS*	%	*NO. PATIENTS*	%
Fever	854	50.0	89	5.6	34	19.65
Success	1698	99.41	1526	96.34	172	99.42
Pregnancy/failure	10	0.59	58	3.66	1	0.58
Total	1708		1584		173	

* 1972–1974.

†1975–1976; paste contains only phenol and radiopaque material.

In 1972–1974, 853 of 1708 patients (50%) experienced fever (38°C to 39°C [100.4°F to 102.2°F]) within 10 days after the instillation of PAP, when 35 g Atabrine was mixed in the paste (Table 17-6). In order to lower the incidence of fever, we removed the Atabrine from the paste during the studies carried out between 1975 and 1976. As a result, the febrile reaction occurred in only 89 of 1584 patients (5.6%). When the sterilization rate of this group was considered, the group in whom Atabrine was used in the paste experienced a failure rate of 0.59%, whereas those without the Atabrine had a failure rate of 3.66%. We then used only half the amount of Atabrine (17.5 g) on 173 women in 1980 for 5 months, and 34 patients developed fever (38°C to 39°C) within 1 week after the instillation (19.65%), a much lower rate than in those patients in whom 35 g Atabrine was used. One pregnancy was encountered, resulting in a pregnancy rate of 0.65%.

DISCUSSION

The secret of successful instillation of PAP into the tubes is to acquire the sensation and skill in introducing the tip of the polyethylene tube into the tubal lumen. The manual techniques can be taught in a short time; in general the technique can be mastered after about 20 trial instillations. A person with more sensitive fingers may need less experience. Of course, this procedure can better be carried out under a screening apparatus for direct visualization.

The constituents of PAP must irritate the tubal lining so as to cause scar formation, thereby occluding the tubal lumen for sterilization. The addition of an opaque medium to the paste for indirect vision is essential, so as to determine the immediate result of the procedure. The PAP must not be too thick or too thin, or it may be difficult to instill or may flow away.

The linear PAP shadow on plain roentgenogram that is longer than 1 cm is regarded as an index of success for tubal occlusion in sterilization.

CONCLUSION

A nonsurgical method by manual instillation of a phenol-Atabrine paste (PAP) into the tubes for occlusion has been evaluated. In a period of 3 years and 9 months in 1972–1976, 1837 procedures were carried out by the Shanghai Non-Surgical Cooperative, composed of five medical units, and the procedures were successful in 1708 cases, giving a rate of 92.98%. In a follow-up study of 1637 immediately successful cases in the 4 to 7-year period, the success rate was 99.08% (in terms of occluded tubes).

The total number of procedures done to date in all of Shanghai between 1972 and 1981 is 9,500, with a successful occlusion rate of 99%.

Among the 200 medical units offering this procedure, a study of 33 such units, located in five provinces, indicates that between 1975 and 1981, 30,000 women have had the procedure, and in those women who have had a follow-up of more than 2 years, a successful occlusion rate of 99% has been obtained. The failures resulted from improper instillation and PAP that was too thick.

The ideal tubal occlusion medium will include a combination of chemicals that will cause fewer side-effects and febrile reactions but will have a high success rate. Although our sterilization procedure is not done under direct vision, the manual technique of inserting the tip of a polyethylene tube into the fallopian tube for instillation of PAP can be learned through proper training.

Our procedure is simple and without severe reaction and it has few complications. So far there is no mortality. The success rate for female sterilization is high, and the results are promising.

REFERENCES

1. CORFMAN PA: Response of the rabbit oviduct to tissue adhesive. Science 148:134, 1965
2. GIAK J, HAHN PE: Quinacrine (Atabrine) mode of action. Science 156:655, 1967
3. GRODE GA, PAVKOV KL, FALB RD: Feasibility study on the use of a tissue adhesive for the nonsurgical blocking of fallopian tubes. Fertil Steril 22:552, 1971
4. SHANGHAI NON-SURGICAL RESEARCH COOPERATIVE: Pharmacological experiments on chemical instillation into fallopian tubes for sterilization. Chin Med J Obstet Gynecol 14(2):87, 1979
5. SHANGHAI NON-SURGICAL RESEARCH COOPERATIVE: Phenol compound paste instillation into female tubes for occlusion in sterilization. Chin Med J Obstet Gynecol 14(2):91, 1979
6. STEVENSON TC, TAYLOR DS: The effect of methylcyanoacrylate adhesive on the human fallopian tube and endometrium. Br J Obstet Gynaecol 79:1028, 1972
7. TSONG-SAN MEDICAL SCHOOL, NO. 2 HOSPITAL, TUBAL OCCLUSION BY CHEMICALS RESEARCH GROUP: Observations on tubal occlusion by introduction of phenol jelly for female sterilization in past 7 years. Chin Med J Obstet Gynecol 14(2):79, 1979
8. ZIPPER J, MEDEL M, PASTENE L et al: Intrauterine instillation of chemical cytotoxic agents for tubal sterilization and treatment of functional metrorrhagias. Int J Fertil 14:280, 1969
9. ZIPPER J, MEDEL M, PRAGER R et al: Alterations in fertility induced by unilateral intrauterine instillation by cytotoxic compounds in rats. Am J Obstet Gynecol 101:971, 1968
10. ZIPPER J, STACHETTI E, MEDEL M et al: Human fertility control by transvaginal application of quinacrine on the fallopian tube. Fertil Steril 21:581, 1970
11. ZIPPER J, STACHETTI E, MEDEL M et al: Transvaginal chemical sterilization. Contraception 12:11, 1975

18

A Study of Phenol-Mucilage–Induced Tubal Occlusion for Sterilization (Analysis of the Results in 4,784 Cases)

HUI-GUO ZHENG

XUE-HUANG CHEN

The use of pharmacologically active agents to induce occlusion of the fallopian tube for sterilization by instrumentation through the uterine cavity was tried in the early part of the 19th century,[5] but it was soon abandoned because of serious complications and the uncertainty of the contraceptive result. It has only been since the 1960s that this method had been restudied by a number of investigators to determine the efficacy of the drugs and to establish the proper techniques for clinical application.[2,3,6,7] With the increasing social demand for fertility regulation and for improvement of the techniques, chemical sterilization has become more and more popular in China, and a number of gynecologists have been very enthusiastic in carrying out this work to accommodate the need of a nationwide project on family planning.

Since 1970, we developed a method using specially prepared phenol-mucilage. This compound was first studied in animals to determine its sclerotic action on the tubal mucosa and was then applied clinically in a large series of cases.

PREPARATION OF PHENOL-MUCILAGE

The phenol-mucilages are prepared by mixing liquid phenol, gum tragacanth, glycerin, and other components in the following proportion:

Phenol-mucilage I

Liquid phenol	35 ml
Gum tragacanth	5 ml
Glycerin	20 ml
Distilled water added up to	100 ml

Phenol-mucilage I was the major preparation used for the first group of sterilization procedures performed between August 1970 and December 1979.

The authors thank Professor Tien-Chi Ho, M.D., for his encouragement and assistance in the preparation of the manuscript; Dr. Shang-Wu Huang, M.B., for reading and explaining the salpingo-roentgenogram; and Mr. Shi-Ye Yao, of the Department of Pharmacy, for initiation and preparation of the pharmacologic agents.

Phenol was the main component because of its corrosive action and sclerotic effect. Gum tragacanth was added for increasing the viscosity to make the mucilage more adherent and thus to prolong contact.

Phenol-mucilage II	
Liquid phenol	35 ml
Gum tragacanth	5 ml
Glycerin	11 ml
Meglucamine iodipamide	35 ml
Distilled water added up to	100 ml

Phenol-mucilage II was used later in the study for simultaneous roentgenography. Meglucamine iodipamide was the contrast medium added for the purpose of visualizing the location and contour of the mucilage in place.

TECHNICAL PROCEDURES

A thin narrow metallic cannula was introduced through the cervical orifice and the uterine cavity to reach the uterine tubal ostia. The tip was conical so that it would fit well into the cornual recess. When the cannula was in place, a polyethylene catheter 1 mm in caliber was passed through to the lumen of the fallopian tube (Fig. 18-1). A test for accuracy of insertion of the catheter was made by injecting 8 ml sterile normal saline to see if there was any leakage

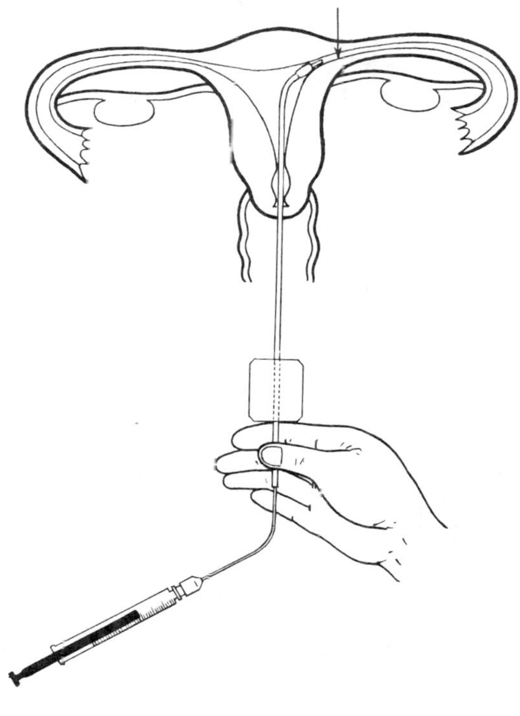

FIG. 18-1. Instillation of phenol-mucilage through the catheter.

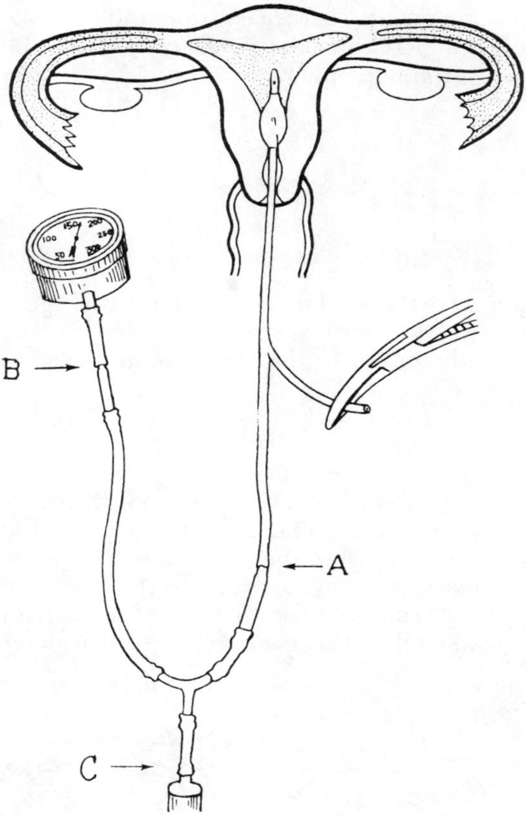

FIG. 18-2. Testing occlusion of fallopian tubes by means of forcing pressure test. (*A*, double-lumen tube; *B*, sphygmomanometer; *C*, syringe for injecting normal saline under pressure).

of it from the uterus. Then 0.10 ml to 0.15 ml mucilage was injected carefully with a small syringe through the catheter. Three months later, complete occlusion of the fallopian tubes was tested by the uterine forcing pressure test, using a double-lumen catheter attached to a pneumonic sphygmomanometer (Fig. 18-2).

CLINICAL MANIFESTATIONS AND RESULTS

From August 1970 to May 1981, 4784 women were studied in our outpatient clinic. They were divided into two groups for comparison:

Group A includes 4336 women treated between August 1970 and December 1979 with phenol-mucilage I. Among them, 2915 were injected from August 1970 to February 1977, with a success rate of 85.32%.[4] Subsequently, another 1421 women were injected in the same way, and the success rate went up to 93.17%. The average success rate was 87.89% (Table 18-1).

During injection, some of the women felt aching and slight lower abdominal distention. In the following days, some felt feverish but actually had no

TABLE 18-1. Result of Occlusion of the Fallopian Tubes With Phenol-Mucilage, as Shown by the Uterine Forced Pressure Test 3 Months After Injection in 4784 Women Treated From August 1970 to May 1981

PHARMACOLOGIC AGENTS	DATES OF INSTILLATION	NO. WOMEN INJECTED	NO. SUCCESSFUL INJECTIONS	% SUCCESSFUL INJECTIONS
Phenol-mucilage I (nonradiopaque)	Aug 1970 to Feb 1977*	2915	2,487	85.32
	Mar 1977 to Dec 1979†	1421	1,324	93.17
Total		4336	3,811	87.89
Phenol-mucilage II (radiopaque)	Jan 1980 to May 1981	488	438	97.77

*Previous cases published in Chin J Obstet Gynecol 14(2):79, 1979.
†Unpublished data.

fever. Forty women developed pelvic inflammation later, but it was well controlled by the use of antibiotics and supportive measures. This complication may be ascribed to contamination by spilling of mucilage into the pelvic cavity. In three lactating women, the uteri were accidentally perforated. All of them healed promptly after surgical repair.

All of the successfully injected women in group A, not including those injected after February 1977, were followed for 5 to 10 years, and 64 women (2.58%) became pregnant, most of them (55) within 6 months to 2 years after injection. A number of the 909 women were rechecked by a hydrotubation test and/or hysterosalpingography for determination of complete tubal occlusion. It was found that the tubes had reopened in 15 patients (1.65%).

Group B included 448 women who were treated between January 1980 and May 1981 with phenol-mucilage II. The procedures were the same as in group A. Roentgenography was done within 1 hour after injection. We noted that the filling shadow varied from 1 cm to 6 cm, with the majority between

TABLE 18-2. Complete Occlusion* of the Fallopian Tubes With Phenol-Mucilage II in Relation to the Status of Filling as Shown in the Roentgenograms

	LENGTH OF OPACITY (CM)							
	1.0–2.0	*2.1–3.0*	*3.1–4.0*	*4.1–5.0*	*5.1–6.0*	*>6.0*	*(2.1– >6.0)*	TOTAL
No. women injected	43	77	104	˙01	68	55	(405)	448
No. successful procedures	37	75	104	100	68	54	(401)	438
Rate of complete occlusion (%)	86.05	97.41	100	99	100	98.18	(99.0)	97.77

*Determined by the uterine forcing pressure test and/or hysterosalpingographic examination 3 months after injection.

3 cm and 5 cm. Women who had a shadow of less than 1 cm underwent reinjection immediately or the next morning.

With such management, 438 of the 448 women (97.77%) experienced successful injection (see Table 18-1). We have found that a good filling of the mucilage to both tubes is important for achieving greater pharmacologic action on the tubal mucosa. With the radiopacity of 2 cm or less, of 43 women, only 37 (86.05%) proved to be successfully injected; whereas in the 405 cases with the opacity longer than 2 cm, 401 women (99.0%) showed evidence of successful injection (Table 18-2).

PATHOLOGIC FINDINGS

Pathologic examinations were done for 157 fallopian tubes of 107 women under the following conditions: tubal ligation after failure of phenol-mucilage injection; tubal ligation after pregnancy; residual pelvic inflammation with the possibility of concomitant associated disease; or some other abdominal lesions requiring laparotomy and the women voluntarily receiving an injection of the mucilage 1 to 2 hours before the operation. With the specimens available for pathologic examination, we found that the tubes had undergone successive changes throughout stage I of tissue damage and inflammation (in the specimens obtained 6 hours to 4 days after injection), stage II of phagocytosis and foreign body granuloma formation (in the specimens of 1 to 6 months), and stage III of fibrous tissue formation (1 or more years). The tubes might have been completely occluded at any stage, but it was by fibrous tissue formation that pertinent tubal occlusion could be obtained. However, recanalization, as denoted by the presence of crypts in the microscopic field, had been seen in some of the specimens. This histopathologic feature of resolution might have resulted in real recanalization if it communicated all the way through. The details were described elsewhere.[1]

DISCUSSION

The phenol-mucilage instillation to the tubal lumen described above may be considered to be a satisfactory method of tubal sterilization. As technical experience increases, the rate of successful injection and sterilization is expected to increase. This technique has been well accepted in our locality, because it is relatively simple, is nonoperative, and can be done in the outpatient clinic.

To avoid complication, cannulation must be done with meticulous care and should be performed at 4 months postpartum, since the uterine wall is more friable then.

This method of cannulation is not done under direct vision, so uterine injury and the possibility that the uterine tubal ostia will be missed exist no matter how experienced the operator is. Therefore, a hysteroscope should be used as an aid in introducing the cannula, and phenol-mucilage II is desirable to aid roentgenography. However, use of the hysteroscope cannot entirely replace the simple method of cannulation, because it is almost impossible for the scope to reach the site so that the cornual recess can be visualized in cases of severe anteflexion or retroflexion of the uterus.

REFERENCES

1. CHEN M-Y, XING L-C, CHEN X-H: Analysis of pathological process in fallopian tubes after injection with mucilage phenol in relation to its sterilization effectiveness. Chin J Obstet Gynecol 14(2):84, 1979
2. CORFMAN PA, TAYLOR HC: An instrument for transcervical treatment of the oviducts and uterine cornua. Obstet Gynecol 27:880, 1966
3. PITKIN RM: Sodium morrhuate for tubal sterilization. Obstet Gynecol 28:680, 1966
4. RESEARCH GROUP OF TUBAL OCCLUSION BY DRUGS, SECOND TEACHING HOSPITAL, ZHONGSHAN MEDICAL COLLEGE: Sterilization by occlusion of the fallopian tubes with mucilage phenol: A seven years' clinical observation. Chin J Obstet Gynecol 14(2):79, 1979
5. RICHART RM: Female sterilization using pharmacologically active agents. In Zatuchni GI, Labbok MH, Sciarra JJ (eds): Research Frontiers in Fertility Regulation, pp 262–269. Hagerstown, MD, Harper & Row, 1980
6. RICHART RM, GUTIERREZ-NAJAR AJ, NEUWIRTH RS: Transvaginal human sterilization: A preliminary report. Am J Obstet Gynecol 111:108, 1971
7. ZIPPER J, MEDEL M, PASTENE L et al: Intrauterine instillation of chemical cytotoxic agents for tubal sterilization and treatment of functional metrorrhagias. Int J Fertil 14:289, 1969

19

The Pathologic Process of Phenol-Mucilage–Induced Tubal Occlusion for Sterilization and the Causes of its Success and Failure

MO-YE CHEN

LIAN-CHENG XING

XUE-HUANG CHEN

HUI-GUO ZHENG

Since 1970, intraluminal injection of phenol-mucilage to produce tubal occlusion with consequent sterilization has been used in our hospital in a total of 4784 women. The success rate as reported previously was 85.3%, and in a more recent group of 448 women it went up to 97.77%. In this chapter we will describe the histopathologic changes occurring during the process of tubal occlusion, as observed in the specimens from 107 patients. On the basis of these pathologic changes, we have obtained knowledge regarding the causes of success and failure of this procedure.

MATERIALS AND METHODS

From August 1970 to April 1980, pathologists at the Second Teaching Hospital of Zhongshan Medical College examined 157 fallopian tubes taken from 107 patients who had received phenol-mucilage injections for sterilization. The main mucilage preparation consisted of liquid phenol (35 ml) tragacanth (5 g), glycerin (20 ml), and distilled water added to a total volume of 100 ml. The dosage was 0.10 ml to 0.15 ml for each tube.

The indications for laparotomy during which the tubes were removed were as follows:

Phenol-mucilage could be injected into only one of the tubes during the procedure, so that tubal ligation had to be performed subsequently. During the operation the tube already injected with phenol-mucilage was removed for pathologic examinations.

After the tubal injection the women became pregnant again, so tubal ligation was then performed. During the operation, one or both tubes were removed for the same purpose as given above.

Patients who developed pelvic inflammation after the mucilage injection had incomplete relief of symptoms after conventional treatment. To rule out the possibility of concomitant associated disease, exploratory laparotomies were performed in six women. During the operation the tubes were removed for examination. Other women who had a tubal pregnancy or an ovarian cyst were also operated on, and the tubes were also removed.

Some of the patients who were operated on for some other abdominal diseases voluntarily received an injection of phenol-mucilage 1 or 2 hours before the operation. The tubes were then removed for observation of early pathologic changes.

After the tubes were removed, one to three slices from the isthmus, as well as one slice from the ampulla, were taken for pathologic sections. All of the sections were stained with hematoxylin and eosin. Some were specially stained for reticulin and collagen fibers.

RESULTS

The pathologic changes after phenol-mucilage injection were mainly at the isthmus and may be divided into three stages:

In stage I there is tissue damage and inflammatory reaction. These changes could be clearly seen in the specimens about 1 hour after injection. The epithelial cells adjacent to the mucilage showed degenerative changes, disappearance of the cilia, and swelling of the nuclei, even to the extent of fading away of the nuclear structures.

In the specimens obtained 6 to 24 hours after injection, coagulation necrosis of the epithelial cells and detachment of the necrotic tissue could be seen. At the same time, congestion and edema were very conspicuous. Some neutrophils infiltrated into the lamina propria and also entered into the lumen.

In the specimens obtained after 3 or 4 days, the entire portion, or a large portion of the epithelial layer around the lumen, showed coagulation necrosis. The lamina propria was also involved. Many neutrophils, some macrophages, eosinophils, and lymphocytes were constantly seen in the inflammatory exudate. The tubal lumens were partially or completely obliterated by detached necrotic tissue and inflammatory exudate.

In stage II there is phagocytosis and foreign body granuloma formation. Congestion and edema had diminished in this stage. In the specimens 14 days after injection, proliferating histiocytes were present in the lamina propria and the muscular layer. Macrophages and foreign body giant cells were also seen. The histiocytes were present all around in the mucosal wall or only in part of it. At the same time, there was proliferation of fibrous tissue with scattered lymphocytes and eosinophils. The granulomatous tissue newly formed at this stage was foreign body granuloma. All of the pathologic changes described above were more common in the specimens seen 1 month to as long as 1 year postinjection.

As a result, the granulomatous tissue completely or partially occluded the lumen. In cases of partial occlusion, the granulomatous tissue protruded into the lumen but a cleft remained. Occasionally, there were some fibroblasts and lymphocytes in the mucosal layer, but no foreign body giant cells could be seen.

In stage III there is fibrous tissue formation. This usually occurred more than 1 year after injection. Foreign body giant cells and other inflammatory cells had greatly diminished, whereas fibrocytes were abundant and a large number of capillaries were seen in the newly formed fibrous tissue. As the fibrotic changes proceeded, the fibrous tissue became less vascular and eventually contained more collagen fibers. The fibrous tissue had completely or partially obliterated the tubal lumen, as in the granulomatous stage (stage II).

The granulomatous and fibrotic changes might be present separately at different sites of the same specimen, but in this study, it is the presence of the fibrous tissue that determines the stage to which it belongs (*i.e.,* stage III). Furthermore, it must be realized that there was no sharp demarcation between stage I and stage II as there is between stage II and stage III. We observed no definite time limit for each stage.

In the studies on the pathologic changes in the completely obliterated tubes, we found that among the 157 tubes removed for examinations, 50 were completely occluded, 23 were partially occluded, 10 were dilated, and 66 were practically normal. One of the completely occluded tubes was in stage I, whereas 49 tubes were in stage II or III.

Moreover, the muscle and serosa were not in direct contact with the mucilage but the intensity of the inflammatory reaction was about the same as that seen in the mucosa of the corresponding stage. It it noteworthy that the nature of the pathologic changes in the ampulla was the same as that in the muscle and serosa of isthmus, but the changes were less conspicuous.

The tubes removed from the 36 women in whom pregnancy occurred after mucilage injection were observed with special attention. In 4 patients only one tube was removed, while in the other 32 patients both tubes were removed. In the latter, 10 women showed normal tubes bilaterally, 15 showed a normal tube on one side and complete or partial occlusion or dilatation on the other side, and 7 women had the same pathologic changes on both sides, such as complete or partial occlusion or dilatation, but none of the women had complete bilateral occlusion.

Regarding the pathologic changes of the tubes removed from the patients with pelvic inflammation, most of them had some chronic inflammatory changes in the tubal walls, but only one patient developed adhesions between the tube and the ovary with the presence of granulomatous nodules. The lumens of the tubes were completely or partially occluded.

DISCUSSION

From the pathologic changes observed, we realize that tissue damage and inflammatory reaction, phagocytosis and foreign body granuloma formation, or fibrous tissue formation might be responsible for the tubal occlusion. Plugging of the tubes by inflammatory exudate and detached necrotic tissue, foreign body granuloma, and newly formed fibrous tissue could result in only temporary occlusion. It was only when the fibrous tissue had been transformed into old scar tissue without continuous clefts could permanent tubal occlusion be obtained.

The effectiveness of producing cellular proliferation around the encircling mucosa and muscular layer and the inward growth of proliferated cells into the lumen of the tube are probably determined by the chances of phenol-mucilage being in contact with all portions of the mucosa around the lumen. This is closely related to the concentrations of the drug, the site at which the drug is introduced, as well as the time of its contact with the mucosa. In the isthmus, the caliber of the tube is small and the mucosal folds are very shallow. Therefore, the lumen of the isthmus could easily be occluded, provided that the mucilage has definitely been introduced into this segment and has remained there long enough to cause necrosis.

From the pathologic point of view, the possible causes of failure are as follows:

The concentration of the drug was insufficient to produce necrosis; the inflammatory reaction was not intensive enough to produce a sufficient amount of substance to plug the lumen.

Although the mucilage may have filled the lumen, part of it had subsequently been absorbed or displaced.

The mucilage introduced could only affect a part of the surrounding mucosa, so that granulomas only developed from a portion of the mucosal wall and the tube became patent again after contraction of the granuloma.

The granulomatous tissue caused complete obliteration only after transformation into fibrous tissue. The granulomatous and fibrous tissues could contract and leave clefts that communicated with each other.

Study of the tubes removed when pregnancy occurred after mucilage injection suggests that failure might have resulted because:

The procedure had failed to introduce the mucilage into the tube, as indicated by lack of inflammatory reaction or other pathologic changes.

The mucilage had definitely been injected into the tubes, but it had been absorbed in one or both of the tubes or the tubes had recovered from the injury, as shown by the very little inflammatory reaction and the presence of only a small amount of fibrous tissue.

The hydrotubation test might have forced the tube to become patent, although tubal occlusion had already been accomplished after mucilage injection.

Some other general or local factors that might contribute to the failure require further study.

20

Discussion: Chinese Techniques for Chemical Sterilization

GERALD I. ZATUCHNI, MODERATOR

During the past 5 or 6 years, individuals interested in nonsurgical methods of female sterilization have been tantalized by published reports of work by Chinese scientists in this field. Two simple and promising techniques, using different approaches and materials, have been described in the preceding chapters, and Drs. Tien and Zheng supplied further details in the discussion summarized here.

HOW MANY INDIVIDUALS ARE DOING THESE PROCEDURES, AND HOW MANY PROCEDURES HAVE BEEN DONE UP TO THE PRESENT TIME?

At the Xin-Hua Hospital in Shanghai, two or three people perform the PAP instillation technique. By now, they have been doing it for several years and are able to achieve almost 100% successful tubal entry.

To date, there are 200 medical units located in 28 provinces of China where personnel have received training in instilling the PAP material, and in an effort to find out how many procedures had actually been done, Dr. Yu-Hau Wu visited 33 medical units, including the 10 in and around Shanghai. If one considers only the 10 Shanghai units, about 10,000 procedures have been done. Adding the 20,000 more done in other parts of the country, some 30,000 patients have had PAP instillations. The patients that have been followed for the most recent 2-year period have had 99% success, in terms of tubes occluded and no pregnancies.

At the Second Affiliated Hospital in Canton, every month about four or five nurses, physicians, and midwives receive training in the phenol-mucilage procedure. The midwives are allowed to do the procedure without supervision, and two nurses are also doing it on a regular basis at the hospital.

The Chinese government has just approved a visiting training program, through which Dr. Wu will travel throughout China, training people in the field with this technique. The Chinese government apparently has accepted it as a useful technique that is applicable to the needs of the Chinese people.

Panelists: Shueh-Ping Tien, H.G. Zheng. *Discussants:* Rohit V. Bhatt, Lee Bolduc, Jay M. Cooper, Philip A. Corfman, Amy D. Engineer, Enrique Guiloff, Douglas Huber, Miriam H. Labbok, Nargesh D. Motashaw, Robert S. Neuwirth, Ralph M. Richart, Lillian Yin, Itic Zighelboim

HOW LONG DOES IT TAKE TO BECOME EXPERT IN THE PAP INSTILLATION TECHNIQUE?

If a person can perform the procedure on 20 patients, that is, 40 tubes, he or she is considered to have mastered the technique. The length of training depends on whether the individual is a doctor or nurse, who can complete the training in about 2 weeks, or a paramedical person, who may require longer training.

HOW LONG DOES IT TAKE TO PERFORM THE PAP INSTILLATION, FROM THE TIME THE PATIENT GETS ON THE TABLE UNTIL THE PROCEDURE IS COMPLETED?

Generally, the entire procedure is completed in 15 minutes or less. Much depends on the position of the tubes. If the tube is easily located, it may take only 1 to 2 minutes for instillation, but if the orifice is somewhat difficult to locate, the procedure may take longer.

IN THE ROENTGENOGRAMS, SOME OF THE PAP WAS SEEN FLOWING BACK INTO THE CORNUAL AREAS; IS THIS A USUAL OCCURRENCE?

The material seen on the films flowing back into the uterine cornu was the excess PAP, which is expected when the cannula is withdrawn after the injection. However, only 0.1 ml to 0.15 ml per tube is required for successful blockage.

AFTER THE PAP INJECTION, DOES THE MATERIAL COMING BACK INTO THE UTERINE CAVITY PRODUCE IRRITATION OF THE ENDOMETRIUM, ADHESIONS, ASHERMAN'S SYNDROME, OR SIMILAR PROBLEMS?

A small percentage of the women complain of a yellowish, possibly serosanguineous discharge for about 3 weeks after the procedure, so apparently there is some endometrial irritation caused by the chemical, but it does not seem to last. The cannula may also produce some trauma. No cases of endometrial adhesions have developed post procedure.

DO PATIENTS HAVE A SIGNIFICANT AMOUNT OF PELVIC PAIN OR OTHER SIDE-EFFECTS FOLLOWING INSTILLATION OF THE PHENOL-MUCILAGE?

American investigators testing silver nitrate (an ion that is similar to phenol) stopped using the chemical because of the high proportion of patients who had significant pelvic pain.

In the phenol-mucilage studies, pain has not been a major complaint. Some patients complained of backache, but they did not require medication. They also had some feelings of abdominal bloating for about 3 weeks after the procedure. In one of the studies described, 40 patients had inflammation of the pelvis, probably secondary to chemical peritoneal irritation; 7 of the patients developed fever 1 or 2 hours after the injection and experienced the pain later. These 7 were observed in the hospital for 2 or 3 days. In the other 33 patients, the pain and fever, and an elevated leukocyte count, did not develop for 2 or 3 days, but none of these patients required hospitalization.

ARE THE COMPLAINTS ABOUT PAIN MORE SEVERE WITH THE CHEMICAL PROCEDURE THAN WITH STANDARD SURGICAL STERILIZATION PROCEDURES?

Making a comparison of a symptom that is subjective is difficult. The PAP patients do not complain much of pain and do not return to the hospital specifically because of pain, although when they come in for follow-up and are asked about pain, they say that they did have some.

WHAT PERCENTAGE OF PATIENTS ELECT SURGICAL STERILIZATION RATHER THAN CHEMICAL STERILIZATION?

Very few surgical sterilization procedures are being done now; most are non-surgical, and at the Xin-Hua Hospital the chemical sterilization procedure is recommended. It is highly acceptable because it is simple and does not require surgery.

WHAT IS CONSIDERED "SUCCESS" IN THE PAP PROCEDURE?

As long as there is no back-flow of the saline and there is no a positive result of the sodium saccharide test, then the procedure is considered successful. Failure means failure to identify the ostia in order to get the saline in or to have a positive result of the sodium saccharide test. In about 8% of cases, the operator fails to find the ostium on the first try, but in this case the woman is asked to return for a second treatment or more until the procedure has been completed.

HOW SUCCESSFUL ARE EFFORTS AT FOLLOW-UP IN CHINA?

There is almost 100% follow-up of these patients, so the 99% success rate with regards to pregnancy (or the 1% failure rate) is probably a very accurate figure. Once the patients leave Shanghai, however, they are not easily followed, even through vital statistics records.

21

Pharmacology and Toxicology of Methyl Cyanoacrylate

ROBERT E. KRALL

ROBERT S. NEUWIRTH

RALPH M. RICHART

The alkyl-2-cyanoacrylates, of which methyl cyanoacrylate (MCA) is a congener, are a homologous series of organic monomers that polymerize on and adhere to moist living tissue. MCA, the first congener of this series, was popularized as a tissue adhesive and as a hemostatic agent during the late 1950s and early to mid 1960s. It was not until the late 1960s, however, that MCA was considered as a possible candidate for the occlusion of the human oviduct. Its considerations as such seem to have stemmed from papers presented by Woodward[26] and one of us (RMR)[24] in 1969 at a conference on human sterilization.[9]

In this chapter the pharmacologic and toxicologic effects reported for MCA in the decade or so following the discovery of its tissue adhesive and hemostatic properties will be summarized. Some recent basic studies we have performed with our highly purified proprietary brand of MCA and radiopaque MCA will also be described.

TISSUE ADHESIVE ACTION

The adhesive action of MCA is accomplished through its polymerization, which is catalyzed by weak bases, such as hydroxyl groups, that are abundantly present within moist living tissues. Rapid polymerization, which is associated with considerable local evolution of heat,[5] can be retarded by incorporating acidic moities into the monomer. Bonding to biologic substrates such as dermal collagen provides bonds requiring 1000 to 2000 g/sq cm for disruption, which usually takes place by fragmentation of the collagen substrate.[26] Enthusiasm for the tissue adhesive properties of MCA had waned by the end of the 1960s, largely because of the intense local necrosis that develops at the site of application. It is this intense necrotizing or sclerosing effect of MCA that led to its recommendation as a possible tubal occluding agent.

TABLE 21-1. Bacteriologic Properties of Methyl Cyanoacrylate*

	ZONE OF INHIBITION (MM)	
BACTERIA	*MCA-MONOMER (0.02 ML)*	*MCA-POLYMER (10 MG)*
Staphylococcus aureus	14.7 (6.0)	
Proteus	41.9 (6.0)	Trace
Pyocyaneus	29.0 (6.50)	Slight trace
Escherichia coli	32.7 (6.0)	Trace
Klebsiella	(5.80)	
Enterococci	16.1 (6.20)	Slight trace

*Number of trials = 5 each.

IN VITRO PHARMACOLOGIC EFFECTS

Since very small amounts of MCA are required when it is used as a tissue adhesive, there has been a paucity of interest in assessing its pharmacologic effects in nonliving systems. From a strictly *in vitro* point of view, perhaps the bacteriologic properties of MCA are the only ones worth noting.

Heiss studied the bacteriologic properties of MCA and a number of higher cyanoacrylate homologs.[7] The results of his work are summarized in Table 21-1.

In further work performed in conjunction with Linzemeier, Heiss showed wide inhibitory zones after application of the adhesives on agar plates that had been previously infected with pure cultures of *Staphylococcus aureus, Proteus, Pyocyaneus, Escherichia coli, Klebsiella,* enterococci, and pneumococci.[7] The inhibitory zones were especially marked for MCA, which corresponded to the size obtained with 20μg chloramphenicol.

The bacteriologic properties of liquid cyanoacrylates, including MCA, have also been reported by others.[2,6,14] According to Lehman and associates, the bacteriotoxicity of MCA may be due, in part, to products such as formaldehyde and cyanoacetate, which are formed as a result of aqueous degradation of the polymers.[14] The hypothesis advanced by Fassett and co-workers[6]—namely, that the MCA monomer is self-sterilizing—was subsequently discredited by Page and his associates,[19] who showed that various fungi and bacterial spores were able to survive under a layer of MCA monomer.

IN VIVO PHARMACOLOGIC EFFECTS

A number of reports have appeared dealing with the pharmacologic effects of ingredients normally employed in the synthesis of polymeric substances. For the most part, however, these reports deal with industrial health problems, especially those resulting from the inhalation of such substances. Polymerized cyanoacrylates, such as poly-methyl-2-cyanoacrylate, are soluble in only a few organic solvents and therefore have few measurable pharmacologic actions. The principal action appears to be hemostasis.

To compare the hemostatic effects of MCA and other (n-butyl and neo-pentyl) α-cyanoacrylates, Herrmann and associates sprayed the monomers of these substances on the cut surfaces of the liver in ten adult beagle dogs to control hemorrhage, following resection of tips of various liver lobes (Table 21-2).[8] Temporary occlusion of vessels supplying the hepatic pedicle was applied; following this, methyl, n-butyl, and neo-pentyl α-cyanoacrylates were applied in succession to sections of liver lobes. Polymerization was rapid, especially with n-butyl, and blood loss was only moderate. Hemostasis and blood loss were scored 0 to 4 plus. Employing n-butyl and neo-pentyl monomers, a single spraying produced good hemostasis. Methyl, its *p*H intentionally lowered to increase its spreading properties, polymerized slowly and was the least effective hemostatic agent. Adhesions were graded 0 to 4 plus, and were not conspicuous at sacrifice, 7 or 14 days later. At both 7 and 14 days, surfaces sprayed with methyl were inflamed and vascular. Little of the polymer was identified even at 7 days, but its pyogenic effects, including continuing accumulation of neutrophils and development of a wide zone of granulation tissue were obvious. In contrast to the other two polymers, the MCA polymer did not elicit a foreign-body response. These polymers were in close proximity to hepatic cells. Unlike methyl, n-butyl and neo-pentyl deposits did not appear to undergo appreciable resorption within 2 weeks.

IN VITRO TOXICITY

Tissue culture systems consisting of mouse fibroblast strain L-929[21] and HeLa cells and initial growths of embryonal bovine skin cells[7] have been used to study the cytotoxicity and histotoxicity of MCA. A summary of these *in vitro* findings is presented below.

TABLE 21-2. Results of Spraying Cyanoacrylate on Cut Surface of Livers in Dogs

	METHYL	N-BUTYL	NEO-PENTYL
Surface areas (sq cm)*	3.60	3.53	3.30
Polymerization times (sec.)*	28.2	3.64	6.11
Blood loss (a)†	33.5	20.00	16.00
Hemostasis (a)†	16.0	29.5	34.5
Adhesions at sacrifice (b)†	23.0	29.5	22.0

*Mean values, ten determinations.

†Sums of scores, ten resection sites; higher values indicate greater blood loss or more effective hemostasis: (a) $p \leq 0.001$ by xr^2, (b) $p \leq 0.10$ by xr^2

TABLE 21-3. Average Cytotoxicity Zone Size in Millimeters

COMPOUND	1 HR	2 HR	4 HR	6 HR	12 HR	24 HR	36 HR
Methyl	1.5	2.5	3	4	6.5	12	15
Isobutyl	0	0	0	0.5	1	2	3
n-Octyl	0	0	0	0	0.5	1.5	2

CYTOTOXICITY

The cytotoxicity of methyl, isobutyl, and n-octyl cyanoacrylate monomers was measured by the agar diffusion method of Guess. Cytotoxicity was exhibited by the rupture of cell membranes, resulting in the leaching-out of a stain (neutral red) that had been introduced evenly into the cells. In order to have some basis of comparison, we measured the zone of cell damage for each of the cyanoacrylates and recorded following exposure periods of 1, 2, 4, 12, 24, and 36 hours. The average zone size in millimeters is shown in Table 21-3.

After 1 hour of exposure, it was possible to observe zones of toxicity in response to MCA, whereas isobutyl and n-octyl cyanoacrylate caused no observable reaction until after 6 to 12 hours' exposure. After exposure periods of 12, 24, and 36 hours, the toxic zones surrounding the MCA spread rapidly.

The zones surrounding the disks were not always concentric, which may be explained by the fact that the polymer on the disks was degraded at different rates and also by the fact that areas of the disks may have contained different concentrations of the polymer. It was interesting to note, however, that no appreciable differences were observed between the disks exposed before polymerization and those exposed after polymerization.

The results of this study indicate that all the cyanoacrylates tested demonstrated definite cytotoxicity. The occurrence of cell injury was a great deal more severe in the case of MCA than with either of the other two compounds.

The chief undesirable property of MCA is its tendency to cause local inflammation and tissue necrosis. The intensity of the response is dependent on the bulk of material used and on the length of the monomer chain. It has been shown, for example, that the longer the chain, the less is the necrosis and the milder is the inflammatory response. Leonard and associates have suggested that the histotoxicity of these compounds results from the release of toxic degradation products and that the histoxicity would, therefore, vary with the rate of polymer degradation.[15] Previous investigation has also shown that MCA polymer degrades more rapidly *in vivo* than any of the other cyanoacrylates thus far tested, and therefore exhibits a greater degree of histotoxicity. The degradation products believed to be responsible for this toxicity are formaldehyde and cyanoacetate. It should be noted, however, that the presence of either of these two chemicals has not been demonstrated *in vivo*.

The possible effect of the heat of polymerization on the coagulation necrosis observed has also been questioned. Woodward and colleagues found a mean temperature rise of 4°C for MCA,[27] whereas the higher homologues exhibited lower temperature rises, probably because of slower polymerization rates. It was thought that, although the temperature rise was small, the possibility of tissue injury by the heat of polymerization could not be dismissed.

It is possible that the heat of polymerization, together with the products of degradation, may contribute to the initial toxic response. Of the cyanoacrylates tested, the occurrence of cell injury was a great deal more severe in the case of MCA, which tends to limit its use as a tissue adhesive but, fortunately, which increases its usefulness as an effective sclerosing agent for occluding the oviduct.

HISTOTOXICITY

Cultures of HeLa cells and initial growth of embryonal bovine skin cells were chosen by Heiss to test the *in vitro* toxicity and histocompatibility of MCA and higher homologs of the cyanoacrylates.[7] In these tests, the histocompatibility of MCA was found to be less than that of butyl cyanoacrylate. Animal experiments in rats fed pulverized MCA for 100 days at the rate of 150 mg/kg showed no significant difference in the histocompatibility of these substances. An estimation of the LD_{50} was not successful when given orally. Pulverized adhesives suspended in water were tolerated up to amounts of 1.4 g MCA; larger amounts caused vomiting.

As in the case of the studies performed to assess cytotoxicity, studies performed to determine the mechanism of action of the histotoxicity of MCA have failed to elucidate a specific mode of action.

IN VIVO TOXICITY

The toxicologic effects of MCA have been determined using the methods traditionally used with drugs and ones more aptly described as *in situ* histotoxicity methods. Of the two types of methods, only the latter ones have produced meaningful information in terms of the principal intended use of MCA with the FEMCEPT system, namely, as a sclerosing agent to block the human oviduct.

GENERAL TOXICITY

The acute toxicologic effects of MCA reported in the literature were determined by way of the oral, intraperitoneal, and subcutaneous routes of administration (see Table 21-4).[7,18] Interestingly enough, it was not possible to actually deliver an LD_{50} by any of these routes of administration.

TABLE 21-4. Acute Toxicity of Methyl Cyanoacrylate in Rats

ROUTE OF ADMINISTRATION	FORM OF MCA USED	COMMENTS
Oral	Polymer	Rats tolerated doses up to 1.4 g/kg. Larger doses caused vomiting.
Intraperitoneal	Monomer	An LD_{50} of 6.7 ml/kg was arrived at by calculation rather than by direct dosing.
Subcutaneous	Monomer	Administration of doses up to 1.0 ml failed to produce any acute systemic effects.

The vomiting induced by the extremely large doses of a suspension of pulverized MCA polymer is probably best explained as resulting from an irritant effect on the gastric mucosa, rather than as being an indication of a demonstrable systemic effect. Indeed, the lack of untoward systemic effects strongly suggests that MCA apparently does not release degradation products to the immediate biologic environment or into the bloodstream in concentrations sufficient enough to elicit demonstrable pharmacologic or toxic effects.

We have performed a series of studies with our highly purified proprietary brands of MCA and radiopaque MCA. Studies have included both the monomeric (liquid) and polymeric forms of both types of MCA. To obtain the latter form, the monomer was allowed to polymerize, following which it was pulverized in a special mortar and pestle and suspended in cottonseed oil. Appropriate control groups were included in all studies. Table 21-5 contains data obtained in mice and rats for two routes of administration (subcutaneous and intraperitoneal) for both the monomeric and polymeric forms of MCA and radiopaque MCA.

SHORT-TERM STUDIES

Oral administration of MCA was undertaken over a 90-day period to male and female Sprague-Dawley weanling albino rats. Groups of 16 animals each received 0, 50, 100, and 200 mg/kg MCA daily in their diets.

No toxic pharmacologic effects were noted. Weight gains and survival rates were normal. No untoward clinical findings were observed in hematologic, transaminase, blood urea nitrogen, or blood glucose values or in the results of urinalysis. Histopathology was generally unremarkable. Increases in terminal ovary weights and respective organ/body weights in females, and thyroid weight increases in male and female animals, were interpreted as coincidental statistical phenomena.[20]

Oral feeding of MCA was carried out over a 90-day period in 6- to 8-month-old beagle dogs. Groups of four animals each (two male and two female) received 0, 50, 100, and 200 mg/kg daily in the diet.

TABLE 21-5. Results of Studies in Mice and Rats with Subcutaneously and Intraperitoneally Administered Monomeric and Polymeric Forms of MCA and Radiopaque MCA

SPECIES	MCA MONOMER LD_{50} (G/KG)	RADIOPAQUE MCA MONOMER LD_{50} (G/KG)
Subcutaneous route		
Mice	15.85	15.85
Rats	6.46	7.94
	MCA POLYMER LD_{50} G/KG)	RADIOPAQUE MCA POLYMER LD_{50} (G/KG)
Intraperitoneal route		
Mice	500.0	583.0
Rats	354.0	229.0

No hematologic changes were noted, nor were there any changes in the transaminase, blood urea nitrogen, blood glucose, and urinalysis values.

LONG-TERM STUDIES

A single subcutaneous injection into Sprague-Dawley rats of 0.1 ml and 0.4 ml MCA was carried out. No untoward effect on growth was noted over 19 ½ months. Of the animals receiving 0.4-ml injection, 13% showed tumor development at the sites of the polymer mass remaining.[20]

A single subcutaneous injection of 0.1 ml and 0.4 ml MCA thickened with polymer was given to eight mongrel dogs. No adverse effect on body weight was noted over a 2-year period. At necropsy, no polymer remained and no lesions were found at the injection site. Findings by gross and histologic examination of organs were unremarkable.[20]

BIODEGRADATION

It has been demonstrated by Kulkarni and associates that perhaps 5% of the cyano groups in MCA may be liberated *in vivo* as cyanide anions that are immediately converted to thiocyanate.[12] In this study, 100 mg of the monomer was introduced subcutaneously into 12 rats and 1000 mg of the monomer was similarly implanted into a dog. One week before implantation, and daily thereafter for 4 weeks, urinary thiocyanate levels were monitored. The results of this study are summarized in Table 21-6.

However, these results are challenged by a later study in which the thiocyanate content of the urine was measured in rats receiving 1500 and 3200 mg/kg of the monomer orally and intraperitoneally. There was no increase found in the urinary thiocyanate levels of treated animals versus untreated controls. This was interpreted as indicating there was no release of free CN radicals associated with the degradation process of MCA.

The ultimate fate of implanted MCA, or of MCA polymerized *in situ,* has been well established as a result of several studies using MCA monomer tagged with carbon 14. When this substance was applied to intact oral mucosa of rats (0.05 ml) or introduced into the stomach via tubes (100 mg MCA), about 34% of the original radioactivity appeared in the urine and feces by the fourth day, as a result of absorption from the digestive tract.[17] Similarly, when implanted subcutaneously in rats (0.5 ml) as the monomer[4] and in guinea pigs (3 mg MCA per centimeter of incision),[23] radioactivity was completely absent from the initial sites after 154 and 107 days, respectively. All of the radioactivity could be accounted for when the respiration elimination

TABLE 21-6. Metabolic Degradation of MCA by way of Urinary Thiocyanate

SPECIES	DOSE OF MCA (MG)	PATTERN OF THIOCYANATE (DAY OF PEAK EXCRETION)	URINARY EXCRETION (DAY EXCRETION BECAME NORMAL)
Rat	100	30	50
Dog	1000	7	20

TABLE 21-7. Elimination of Radioactivity by Guinea Pigs Treated with MCA Tagged with Carbon 14

ANIMAL	DAYS TO SACRIFICE	% DOSE RECOVERED				
		URINE	*FECES*	*RESPIRATORY CO_2*	*SCAB*	*TOTAL*
1	4	65.3	4.6	1.7	5.0	76.5
2	18	90.9	12.1	2.5	1.7	107.2
3	24	78.7	7.7	2.1	7.4	95.8

route is monitored, in addition to examination of the urine and feces (Table 21-7). These studies indicate that MCA is entirely biodegradable, since no radioactive entities were found remaining in the tissues and vital organs.

HISTOTOXICITY

The reaction of various types of tissue to the application of MCA monomer and subsequent polymer formation has been studied primarily in dogs, although studies in virtually all types of experimental animals, including primates, have been reported. Although slight variations in the tissue reaction have been noted, the reaction over time is essentially similar for most types of tissues. One of the most comprehensive studies demonstrating this fact is summarized below.[10] In this study in 31 dogs, MCA was used in conjunction with sutures to achieve anastomoses of the carotid and femoral arteries (four anastomoses/dog). Vessels from each of three different dogs were examined microscopically after intervals of 12, 24, 48, and 72 hours; after 4, 5, 6, and 7 days; and after 1, 3, 4, and 6 months. The histologic findings over time were summarized as follows:

> The application of MCA resulted in a marked initial acute inflammatory response in the immediate area of application with coagulation necrosis occurring distally.
>
> The acute inflammatory response, which persisted until fragments were removed by phagocytosis, changed gradually to a chronic one, showing fibroblastic organization.
>
> After 6 months, the chronic inflammatory reaction to MCA and around the sutures were similar in duration and inflammatory cell response.
>
> Necrosis with MCA was much greater than with sutures alone but did not result in any problems of infection or aneurysm formation.

CARCINOGENICITY

The carcinogenic potential of man-made plastics was first reported in 1941 by Turner[25] and was further elaborated on over a decade later by Oppenheimer and associates.[16] As a result of the latter experimental information, it was concluded that imbedding plastic film in rodents resulted in the production of fibrosarcomas in a high percentage of animals studied. Similar results have been reported since Oppenheimer's observation, but in all such

TABLE 21-8. Carcinogenic Studies of MCA

SPECIES AND STRAIN	AMOUNT & HOW MUCH GIVEN	DURATION OF STUDY (MONTHS)	SUMMARY AND CONCLUSIONS
Mice[11] C-311 Swiss Albino C-57 Black	0.3 ml; subcutaneously	6	Subcutaneous injections of MCA into mice with varying susceptibility to carcinogenesis did not produce tumors after 6 months, even in highly susceptible animals.
Rats[19] Sprague-Dawley	0.1 and 0.4 ml into a shallow pocket on the dorsal subcutis	19 5	Study indicates that a carcinogenic effect is evident in the rats that had a large aggregate of MCA polymer in the subcutis for more than 11 months.
Not specified[7]	0.01 to 0.5 ml injections (SC, IM, and IP) in liquid, solid, and pulverized form	17 to 24	Hard lumps of adhesive were present after 6 months in animals given large doses but gradually disappeared. Traces of local tumor formation could not only be found in any of the animals treated with MCA and observed for periods up to 24 months.
Dogs[19] Not specified	0.1 and 0.4 ml into a shallow subcutaneous pocket on thigh	24	MCA was degraded more rapidly in dogs than in rats and there were no visible lesions at the implant site after 24 months.

cases the imbedded plastic material was in the forms of discs or films.[3,13] Of considerable import is the observation that if the solid body implant is made smaller,[1] or is used as a powder, the incidence of tumor formation decreases greatly or becomes nonexistent in rodents.

An equally important observation in assessing carcinogenic potential of plastics is that the likelihood of cancer decreases when species other than rodents are employed. For example, Page and co-workers found no visible lesions in dogs 2 years after the injection of 0.1 ml or 0.4 ml of MCA monomer "containing 20% polymer" into shallow subcutaneous pockets.[20] The observation by these investigators that MCA "appeared to be more rapidly degraded in dogs than in rats" also is not without significance (Table 21-8). It should be noted that the BioNexus brand of MCA contains no polymer whatsoever.

From the above, it can be concluded that, in addition to the species used in studying the induction of tumors and the rate at which the plastic material is degraded *in situ,* the physical state of the imbedded plastic is perhaps the single most important fact in determining causal relationships between MCA and tumor formation. In this regard, the following findings have been shown through the use of radioactive Carbon-14 tagging:[23]

The polymerized material, 4 days after being imbedded, appeared not to be solid sheet or film, but seemed to be perforated.

After 8 days, the holes had enlarged and the continuity of the polymer had been disrupted.

By 16 days, only small clusters of powderlike material remained in the lower dermis.

No radioactivity was detectable after 107 days.

On the basis of the above experimental findings, it appears that MCA has a negligible carcinogenic potential in higher animals, including humans (where tumors from this material have yet to be reported), because of its rapidly changing physical characteristics in tissue and its relatively rapid absorption and complete biodegradation. Additionally, the BioNexus brand of MCA also possesses the favorable attribute of purity.

REFERENCES

1. ALEXANDER P, HORNING ES: Ciba Foundation Symposium on Carcinogenesis. Boston, Little, Brown & Co, 1959
2. AWE WC, ROBERTS W, BRAUNWOLD NS: Rapidly polymerizing adhesive as a hemostatic agent: study of tissue response and bacteriological properties. Surgery 54:322, 1963
3. BERING EA JR, MCLAURIN RL, LLOYD JB et al: The production of tumors in rats by the implantation of pure polyethylene. Cancer Res 15:300, 1955
4. CAMERON JL, WOODWARD SC, PULASKI EJ et al: The degradation of cyanoacrylate tissue adhesive. Surgery 58:424, 1965
5. COOVER HW et al: Chemistry and performance of cyanoacrylate tissue adhesives. Soc Plastics Engineers J 15:413, 1959
6. FASSETT DW et al: Microbiological growth from Eastman-910-Monomer and adhesive. Cohesive News 1:3, 1961
7. HEISS WH: The use of synthetic polymeric materials as suture substitutes and their place in pediatric surgery. Prog Ped Surgery 1:99, 1968
8. HERMAN JB et al: In Woodward SC (ed): Tissue Response to Polymeric Implants.
9. HUMAN STERILIZATION: A conference sponsored by the International Institute for the Study of Human Reproduction, College of Physicians and Surgeons of Columbia University, and Center for Population Research, National Institute of Child Health and Human Development. October 28–31, 1969, Cherry Hill, New Jersey
10. JACOBSON JH, MOODY RA, KUSSEROW BK et al: The tissue response to a plastic adhesive used in combination with microsurgical technique in reconstruction of small arteries. Surgery 60:379, 1966
11. JUST VIERA J et al: Bal Assoc Med Puerto Rico 62:181, 1970
12. KULKARNI RK, HANKS GA, PANI KC et al: The *in vivo* metabolic degradation of poly(methyl cyanoacrylate) via thiocyanate. J Biomed Mater Res 1:11, 1967
13. LASKIN DM, ROBINSON IB, WEINMANN JP: Experimental production of sarcomas by methyl methacrylate implants. Proc Soc Exp Biol Med 87:329, 1954
14. LEHMAN R, WEST RL, LEONARD F: Toxicity of alkyl-2-cyanoacrylates: II. Bacterial growth. Arch Surg 93:447, 1966
15. LEONARD F et al: Synthesis and degradation of poly(aklyl alpha cyanoacrylates). J Appl Polym Sci 10:259, 1966
16. OPPENHEIMER BS et al: Surg Forum 672, 1954
17. OSTERHOUT DK et al: Digestive tract absorption of alkyl alpha-cyanoacrylate-beta-14-C. Oral Surg 27:410, 1969
18. OTA K et al: Current status of tissue adhesives in Japan. In Matsumato T (ed): Tissue Adhesives in Surgery, p 341. New York, Medical Examination Publishing Co, 1972
19. PAGE RC: Contamination and recovery of bacterial spores from methyl-2-cyanoacrylate monomer. Arch Surg 94:162, 1967
20. PAGE RC et al: Chronic toxicity of MCA in dogs and rats. Prog of Symp on Physiological Adhesives. Austin, Texas, Univ Texas Press, 1966, p 11

21. PANI KC: Histotoxicity of cyanoacrylate plastics. Proc of Symp on Physiological Adhesives, Austin, Texas, Univ of Texas Press, 1966
22. REYNOLDS RC, FASSETT DW, ASTILL BD et al: Absorption of Methyl-2-cyanoacrylate-2[14]C from full-thickness skin incisions in the guinea pig and its fate *in vivo.* J Surg Res 6(3):132, 1966
23. RICHART RM et al: Experimental studies of fallopian tube occlusion. In Richart RM, Prager DJ (eds): Human Sterilization, p 360. Springfield, Illinois, Charles C Thomas, 1972
24. TURNER FC: Sarcomas at sites of subcutaneously implanted bakelite disks in rats. J Natl Cancer Inst 2:81, 1941
25. WOODWARD SC: Tissue responses to polymeric implants: The cyanoacrylates. In Richart RM, Prager DJ (eds): Human Sterilization, p 264. Springfield, Illinois, Charles C Thomas, 1972
27. WOODWARD SC, HERRMANN JB, CAMERON JL et al: Histotoxicity of cyanoacrylate tissue adhesive in the rat. Ann Surg 162:113, 1965

22

Histologic Findings Following MCA Application to the Fallopian Tubes

RALPH M. RICHART

ROBERT S. NEUWIRTH

Methyl cyanocrylate (MCA) is one of a family of cyanoacrylates that differ from one another principally in the length of the side chain. The family includes methyl, ethyl, isobutyl, and isopropyl cyanoacrylate, and each differs slightly in its properties, with regard both to its adhesiveness and to its ability to produce epithelial damage. The cyanoacrylates were used initially in medicine as a suture substitute, particularly for closing small linear wounds such as incision lines in the skin, gingiva, cornea, or other sites at which speed of closure and cosmetic results are important considerations. In general, the degree of inflammatory response is greatest in cyanoacrylates with short side chains and least in those with longer side chains, with methyl cyanoacrylate having by far the greatest degree of local reaction.

Because MCA generally produced extensive local tissue necrosis and a local inflammatory response so intense as to break down the suture line to which it was applied, it was abandoned as an incision-closing agent at an early stage in its development, and cyanoacrylates with longer side chains were developed, studied, and improved so as to have far better properties for suture application. In fact, methyl cyanoacrylate was not used again in a medical application until 1964, when Corfman, Richart, and Taylor applied the material to the fallopian tube as part of a comprehensive screening program studying potential chemical tube-closing agents.[1] Although the local inflammation-producing properties of MCA are inimical to its utility as a suture substitute, they are precisely the properties required for a tube-closing agent. This paradox has produced certain problems when investigators discuss these materials with members of regulatory agencies and review committees, who are unaccustomed to the concept that production of the local necrosis and inflammation is a useful property of a therapeutic agent.

MCA has been studied in monkeys, rabbits, rats, and humans,[2] and the histologic events that accompany its tube-closing properties are reasonably well defined.[3] The material analyzed for this chapter was derived from our own experiments using animal material and from hysterectomy specimens obtained by Stevenson in his studies of MCA and kindly supplied to us for analysis.[4]

RESULTS

When MCA first enters the tube, it does so as a monomer; but as the flow proceeds toward the distal fimbriated end, the monomer is rapidly changed to a polymer and the material adheres to the tubal epithelium. Polymerization initially takes place at the flowing border of the MCA that is adjacent to the tubal epithelium. The central portion of the MCA initially remains liquid or semiliquid, but gradually increases its viscosity and polymerizes toward the center, until the entire bolus has become converted into a brittle, plasticlike material. Polymerization also routinely occurs at the advancing front of the bolus as it moves through the fallopian tube, and by the time the fimbriated end is reached (if it is reached), the advancing border of the MCA has a thin film of polymerized MCA between the liquid MCA and the peritoneal cavity. It is this property of an outward-to-inward polymerization pattern that protects the peritoneal cavity from injury by MCA, even if (as apparently rarely occurs) some of the material spills into the peritoneal cavity from the fimbriated end.

After polymerization has taken place, the fallopian tubes become rigid because of the plasticlike stent that now occupies the lumen. Following a FEMCEPT/MCA application in which the tubes are filled with MCA, the rigid rodlike material can easily be palpated through the thin tubal walls; and if the tubes are manipulated, the MCA can be semipulverized and a gritty sensation easily appreciated. At the time the MCA is polymerizing, the heat of polymerization is considerable;[5] and can blister the skin if touched.

Histologically, the MCA is a highly refractile material. It lies within the tubal lumen and generally is intimately juxtaposed to the tubal epithelium and insinuated between the tubal folds and plicae. There is little, if any, discernible histologic change in the first 12 hours following MCA application. Subsequently, increasingly severe cytologic and histologic alterations occur in the tubal epithelium, including obvious cell death with epithelial detachment and a gradually increasing inflammatory response. This response accelerates over the next 2 days, until most of the epithelium has desquamated and lies within the tubal lumen in an admixture with the polymerized MCA. Over the course of the next 4 weeks, the MCA is gradually degraded by macrophages, and the tubal lumen, the immediately subjacent lamina propria, and, occasionally, the tubal musculature as well become infiltrated with a mixture of polymorphonuclear leukocytes, lymphocytes, and macrophages. Areas of epithelial regeneration appear during the first week, but they become necrotic again in the region of MCA degradation. In regions not intimately juxtaposed to the MCA, regeneration and repair continue. These changes are sometimes accompanied by squamous metaplasia, which may be focal or widespread. Gradually, the tubal epithelium becomes totally absent, principally in the interstitial and isthmic tubal segments, as does the lamina propria, and the lumen becomes filled with a mixture of inflammatory debris, fibrin, and degrading MCA (Fig. 22-1). This material is eventually replaced by fibrous tissue, between 3 and 4 weeks following MCA application, extending in from the musculoluminal junction until the entire lumen has been converted to fibrous scar tissue (Fig. 22-2). The scar tissue initially is composed of young fibroblasts with large numbers of new blood vessels and a sprinkling of in-

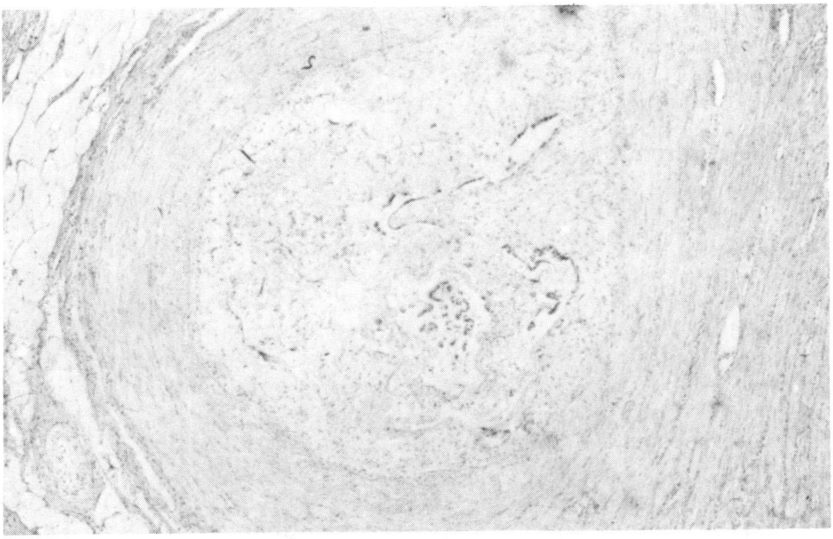

FIG. 22-1. Section of isthmic fallopian tube 3 weeks after application of MCA. Most epithelium is necrotic, and portions of the lining epithelium have been shed into the tubal lumen. There is mild chronic inflammation, and fibroblasts have begun to insinuate on the lumen.

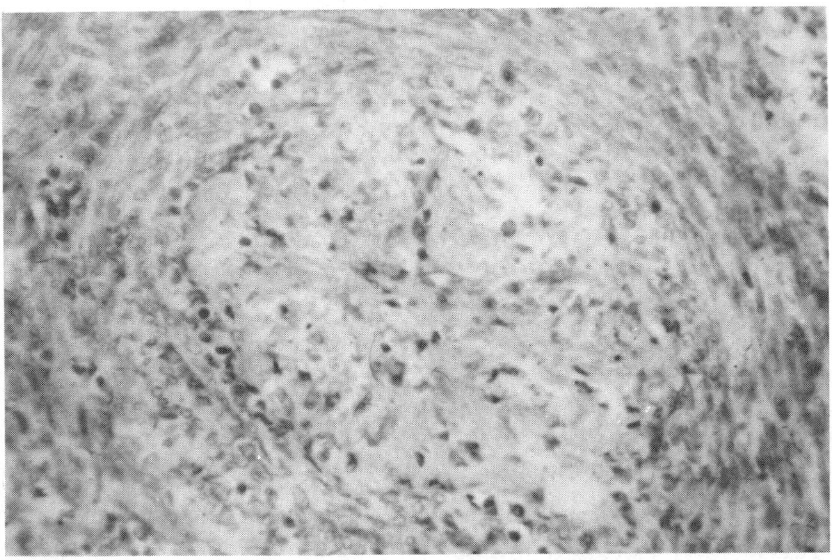

FIG. 22-2. Section of interstitial fallopian tube 4 weeks after application of MCA. Epithelium is no longer present, and lumen has been replaced by young fibroblasts.

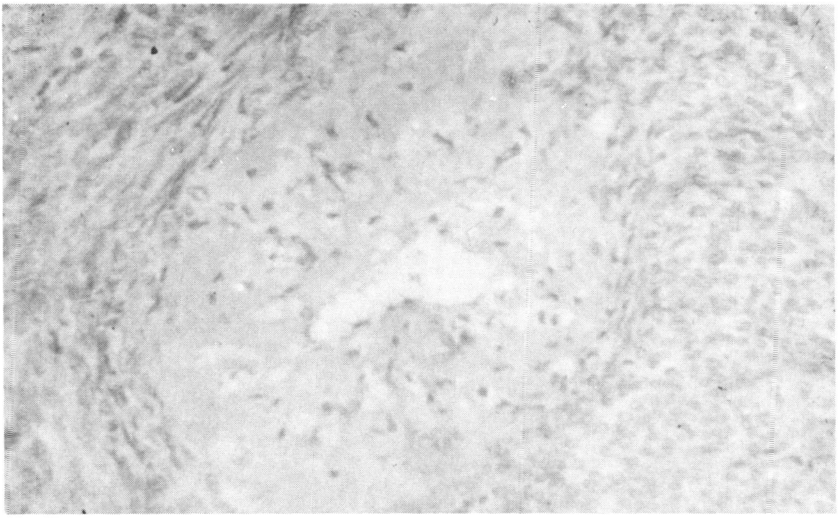

FIG. 22-3. Section of interstitial fallopian tube 16 weeks after application of MCA. The young fibroblasts are being replaced by dense collagen. There is a pinpoint lumen in this section, but the tube is totally closed more distally.

flammatory cells, but with time this material converts to dense scar tissue, inflammatory cells gradually recede, and the tubal lumen is totally obliterated (Fig. 22-3). By 12 weeks, polymerized MCA is no longer detectable in the fallopian tube, as it has been degraded and eliminated through mechanisms that have been described previously. By 6 to 12 months, the isthmic portion of the fallopian tube has diminished considerably in diameter (Fig. 22-4), and in many cases the interstitial portion of the fallopian tube can no longer be detected at all. The scar from the tubal replacement is indistinguishable from other small scars that may be present in the myometrium.

In the endometrium, the small amount of MCA that remains following the FEMCEPT application polymerizes on the surface of the endometrium, and endometrial epithelial necrosis occurs; but because the endometrium is considerably thicker than the fallopian tube, the superficial necrosis produces only a superficial wound, rather than complete ablation of the epithelium as it does in the tube. Local inflammation and epithelial damage in the endometrium also occur only superficially. Even if adhesions should form between the anterior and posterior uterine walls, they are endometrial rather than myometrial and inconsequential, since they are sloughed at the next menstrual period. There are no known long-term effects of MCA on the endometrium.

In some women in Stevenson's early experiments using large volumes of MCA, polymerized MCA leaked from the uterine cavity into the vagina.[4] Although it produced a gritty sensation and was found to be less satisfactory than lubrication for sexual intercourse, it produced no long-term vaginal sequelae because it was expelled with other vaginal secretions.

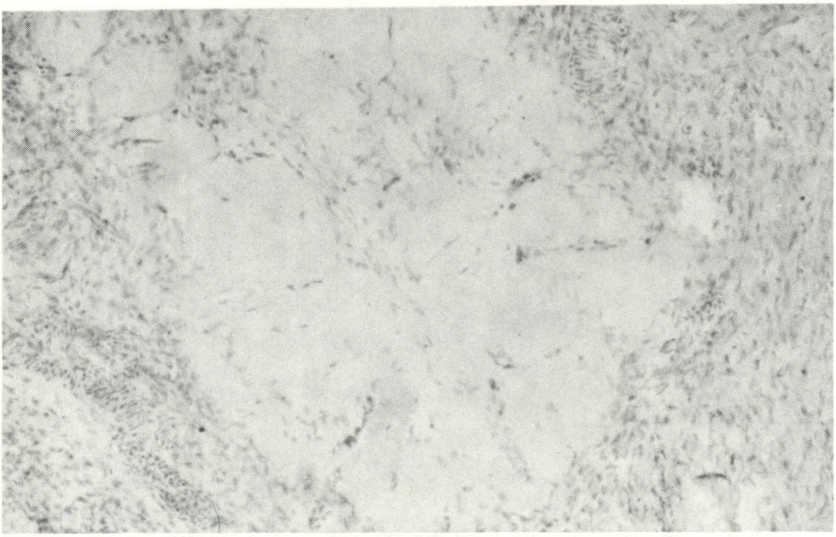

FIG. 22-4. Section of interstitial fallopian tube 6 months after application of MCA. The lumen has been completely replaced by dense collagen. No epithelial cells remain.

The effects of MCA on the peritoneal cavity are similar to those found in the fallopian tube and the endometrium. There is local inflammatory response with superficial tissue necrosis, and the extent and distribution of the change is proportional to the amount and distribution of the MCA. Although peritoneal spill has not been studied in women, its action would probably be similar to that seen in animals, and no long-term effects would be likely unless the volume of MCA application were considerable. Should the MCA enter the peritoneal cavity through the fimbriated end and produce adhesions on adjacent peritoneal surfaces, we would expect only a few adhesions to form in the lower pelvis, probably no more than are found following conventional tubal ligation procedures.

DISCUSSION

MCA has many properties that make it ideally suited to be used as a tube-closing agent: it is a low viscosity liquid in its monomeric form, its viscosity and polymerization time can be controlled within reasonable limits, and it produces a chronic inflammatory response that is limited in depth and severity. It is apparent from other studies that chronicity is of critical importance in closing the fallopian tubes, and this property of the MCA, occurring over its long degradation time, is apparently of greatest importance in producing tubal closure. Histologic changes that accompany MCA application and degradation are those that would be expected—tissue necrosis and a chronic inflammatory response resulting in fibroplasia and dense scar formation. These features occur in virtually any site to which MCA is applied. When they are localized to a small lumen, they are highly effective in producing closure. Because MCA is totally degraded and eliminated from the body, there are no residual long-term effects and the acute inflammatory response, once its course has been run, disappears. Thus, long-term sequelae due to the MCA are unlikely.

An acute inflammatory response that extends through the epithelium and lamina propria to the inner portion of the muscularis would be expected to produce clinical side-effects. The patient has, in essence, an iatrogenically produced acute mucosal salpingitis, which is gradually converted to a low-grade chronic salpingitis and results in tubal closure. Any agent that produces tubal necrosis and inflammation is likely to be accompanied by side-effects, and MCA is no exception. As would be expected, these changes are accompanied by low-grade pelvic pain, fever, and uterine tenderness in patients in whom applications have been made; but as would also be expected these signs and symptoms gradually resolve and the patients appear to have no residual side-effects. The FEMCEPT/MCA system appears to be safe, and promises widespread applicability in the field of contraception.

REFERENCES

1. CORFMAN PA, RICHART RM, TAYLOR HC: Response of the rabbit oviduct to a tissue adhesive. Science 148:1348, 1965
2. RICHART RM: Female sterilization using pharmacologically active agents. In Zatuchni GI (ed): Research Frontiers in Fertility Regulation, vol 1, No. 5, December 1981 Chicago, Program for Applied Research on Fertility Regulation
3. RICHART RM, TAYLOR HC, NEUWIRTH RS: Experimental studies of fallopian tube occlusion. In Richart RM, Prager D (eds): Human Sterilization, pp 360–367. Springfield, IL, Charles C Thomas, 1972
4. STEVENSON TC, TAYLOR DS: The effect of methylcyanoacrylate on the human fallopian tube and endometrium. J Obstet Gynecol 79:1028, 1972
5. WOODWARD SC, HERRMANN JB, CAMERON JL et al: Histotoxicity of cyanoacrylate tissue adhesive in the rat. Ann Surg 162:113–122, 1965

23

Design Objectives for the FEMCEPT Device

LEE R. BOLDUC

ROBERT S. NEUWIRTH

RALPH M. RICHART

The primary objective in developing the FEMCEPT* system was to provide a sophisticated transcervical chemical technique for female sterilization that is applied on an outpatient basis without anesthesia or operative entry into the peritoneal cavity. The instrument was designed to be safe, effective, relatively inexpensive, and simple to operate. The aim was a self-contained instrument that would not require complicated mechanical assembly prior to use, outside power sources such as electricity or compressed gases, or complex manual procedures.

Construction design called for the use of inexpensive materials that would lend themselves to large-volume production methods, such as injection molding.

The instrument was designed to be disposable, thereby eliminating the problems of disassembly, cleaning, and maintenance in the field. It was essential that it not be dependent on a unique technique that could be mastered only by skilled physicians and that it be potentially usable by trained paramedical personnel.

The FEMCEPT device is shown in Figure 23-1. It has three phases of operation: (1) sealing, (2) fluid delivery, and (3) pumping; all three occur in less than 2 seconds.

The device is constructed of inexpensive plastic materials, a latex rubber balloon with a bonded Dacron mesh, and three metal component parts: a spring, a hypodermic needle, and an aluminum sleeve to attach the balloon. Limiting the number of metal parts reduces cost, an important consideration in a disposable instrument. A cannula cover is provided to protect the cannula and fragile balloon. The balloon is made of soft rubber to conform to the uterine cavity and is reinforced by Dacron mesh attached to its backside to prevent herniation through the cervix. The balloon is coated with a lubricating oil to help ensure its shelf life of 2 years from date of manufacture and to ease entry through the cervical canal. The cannula is 4 mm in diameter, is semirigid, and is designed to deform, or collapse, if excess stress is applied, so as to minimize the possibility of uterine perforation. Two opposing fluid

*FEMCEPT is a registered trademark for BioNexus, Inc, Raleigh, North Carolina.

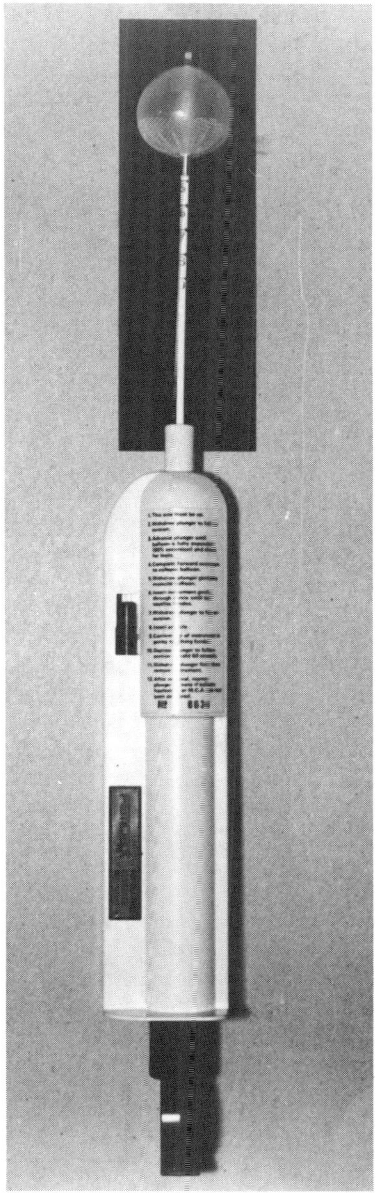

FIG. 23-1. The FEMCEPT device with the balloon in the shape it takes within the uterus at the time the MCA is injected. (Courtesy of Population Research, Inc)

exit ports are located back a small distance to prevent them from being obstructed by the endometrium. In the handle assembly, there is an ampule with a volume of 0.6 ml, designed so that the ampule can only be inserted cap end first.

The actuating plunger telescopes into the air piston, where it is held to its farthest extension by a preloaded compression spring designed to be as linear as possible; the force needed to compress it is approximately the same throughout its 2 inches of travel.

When the actuating plunger is compressed, that force is transmitted by the spring to the air piston without a rigid mechanical connection. As the actuating plunger is pushed forward to its full excursion and held in place, the dispensed fluid is pumped into the fallopian tubes by the balloon and the balloon becomes larger to occupy the space formerly occupied by the fluid. In some applications, the uterine muscles may relax, allowing the balloon to expand farther, but the air piston moves forward to maintain a constant pumping pressure. If uterine contractions occur, the increased air pressure in the balloon is transmitted back down the cannula to the air cylinder, forcing the piston back against the pressure-regulating spring and again maintaining a constant, safe pumping pressure.

The ampule plunger is attached by a ramp to the actuating plunger. In use, it travels part of the way forward and then disengages after it has pushed the ampule forward onto a hollow needle that punctures a rubber diaphragm at the cap end of the ampule. The ampule plunger continues to move forward against the ampule piston, forcing the fluid out of the ampule through a Teflon transfer tube to the two exit ports located at the end of the cannula. The fluid hole in the hollow needle is small and restricts the flow of fluid through it. This functions hydraulically to limit the speed at which the actuator plunger can be depressed. When the actuating plunger is disengaged from the ampule plunger, however, it is free to travel forward at a faster rate and pushes the spring-loaded air piston past a vent hole located in the cylinder. This accounts for the very rapid expansion of the balloon in the uterine cavity after the fluid is delivered and is necessary for division and positioning of the fluid in the cornual area.

In addition to its operating sequence, the instrument is designed to have a venting mode to test the integrity of the balloon and inflating mechanism in the field before use. When the actuating plunger is pushed 90% of the way forward, the balloon expands to its maximum capacity and can be tested. Pushing the plunger the additional 10% of the way forward to its full excursion will allow the air to escape from the balloon, and slow withdrawal of the plunger (approximately 1.5 inches) creates a vacuum in the balloon, causing it to cling to the cannula, reducing its diameter and making it easier to introduce through the cervical canal. The vented mode will function only when the fluid-filled ampule is not in the instrument. When the ampule is in place, the venting mode is mechanically blocked, allowing the plunger to be pushed all the way forward and held. The balloon can then go to high pressure and not collapse.

DISCUSSION

The FEMCEPT device has evolved through 14 models to its present configuration. It has performed to expectations in the latest series of clinical trials, and the design objectives appear largely to have been met. The "plunger" incorporates sophisticated engineering designs that automatically monitor pressures and control flow rates, thus removing the need for complicated decision making from the clinician. This has resulted in tubal closure rates that are remarkably similar from center to center, provided the operator follows the protocol.

Although the instrument, as currently manufactured, is designed to pump low-viscosity fluids, and the ampule to accept no more than 0.65 ml, it is possible to redesign the system to pump more viscous materials and higher volumes using the same engineering principles used in this design. Whether the need will arise for such new designs is speculative.

SPECIFICATIONS OF THE FEMCEPT DEVICE

1. Diameter of cannula at aluminum balloon-retaining ring is 4 mm.
2. Cannula length is 6 inches.
3. Length of device in shipping or venting mode is 17 inches.
4. Device weight is approximately 7 ounces.
5. Handle material is ABS plastic.
6. The device is sterilized with ethylene oxide gas prior to shipping in the inner container only. The outer foil envelope is added after sterilization to protect the balloon from light and ozone gas.
7. Shelf life of instrument, if contained in protective package, is 2 years from date of manufacturer.
8. Storage temperature should not exceed 100°F (37.8°C).
9. Volume of ampule is 0.6 ml.
10. Volume of fluid delivered to uterine cavity is approximately 0.5 ml, with approximately 0.2 ml delivered to each tube.
11. Viscosity limitation of fluid to be delivered is 30 centipoise.

24

Nonsurgical Sterilization Using Methyl Cyanoacrylate With a Fertility Regulation (FEMCEPT) Device

MANOEL BOMFIM DE SOUZA FILHO

ELSIMAR M. COUTINHO

Voluntary sterilization of the female, unlike that of the male, is widely accepted as a legitimate method of fertility control in Latin America. In this area of the developing world, modern techniques of sterilization, such as laparoscopic sterilization and minilaparotomy, are being introduced, but tubal ligation carried out during cesarean section remains the most widely used procedure. In Brazil, intrauterine injection of phenol has been used for many years by midwives as an alternative to the surgical procedure that they were not qualified to do.[6] The technique was widely used in the big cities, but intrauterine synechiae and intraperitoneal adhesions resulting from the sclerosing action of phenol on the endometrium were common and many patients developed amenorrhea following treatment. In order to restrict injection of the occluding agent to a small segment of the fallopian tubes, a new device (FEMCEPT) was developed, which operates with a balloon that is inflated inside the uterine cavity, protecting the endometrium from spillage.[4,5,7] Methyl cyanoacrylate (MCA) tissue adhesive is used as the occluding agent. We report here the use of this device in 112 subjects who desired nonsurgical tubal sterilization.

MATERIALS AND METHODS

Multiparous women aged 21 to 40 years were selected from a large group of candidates for tubal sterilization who opted for nonsurgical tubal closure. Patients were randomly assigned to three groups. In group I, 38 women were submitted to a single injection of MCA. In group II, 33 women had a single injection, preceded by intrauterine flushing with 10 ml saline. In group III, 41 women were subjected to two applications at a 4-week interval.

Before injection, presterilized disposable FEMCEPT devices were tested to ensure proper balloon expansion. The balloon was then collapsed and the device loaded with 0.65 ml MCA. The uterus was sounded, and the cannula of the device was inserted into the uterus until its tip touched the uterine fundus. The device was maintained in position by pulling the uterus with the help of a tenaculum. The plunger of the device was depressed, activating the expansion of the balloon and the injection of MCA. After 1 minute, the plunger was withdrawn, in order to deflate the balloon, and the device was removed. Following removal, the device was tested again by inflating the balloon and inspecting it for leaks and for distribution patterns of MCA on its surface.

The patients agreed to use contraception until bilateral tubal occlusion could be documented by hysterosalpingography and to be available for follow-up for 2 years thereafter. Except for six women who were injected after day 16, injection was done between days 7 and 10 of the menstrual cycle, in order to rule out early pregnancy.

RESULTS

Hysterosalpingography carried out at 4 months following the injection of MCA revealed bilateral occlusion in 28 subjects (74%) of group I, in 23 (70%) of group II, and in 36 (88%) of group III.

Occlusion of only one tube occurred in two subjects of group I (5%), in four of group II (12%), and in only one of group III (less than 2%). These results are summarized in Table 24-1. The distribution of occlusion, according to the phase of the menstrual cycle when the injection was made is shown in Table 24-2. Following a single application between days 7 and 10, bilateral closure was 72% in group I and 65% in group II. In group III, bilateral closure occurred in 83% of the subjects. All six subjects injected with either one or two applications after day 16 had bilateral occlusion (100%).

Bilateral occlusion in subjects whose uterine length was between 7 cm and 9 cm was 73% for group I, 71% for group II and 90% for group III. The occurrence of occlusion according to uterine length is shown in Table 24-3.

TABLE 24-1. Summary of Clinical Results in MCA Studies

RESULT	GROUP I—SINGLE APPLICATION (N = 38) NO. PATIENTS	%	GROUP II—UTERINE LAVAGE + SINGLE APPLICATION (N = 33) NO. PATIENTS	%	GROUP III—TWO APPLICATIONS (N = 33) NO. PATIENTS	%
Bilateral closure	28	74	23	70	36	88
Bilateral patency	8	21	6	18	4	10
Unilateral patency (right)	2	5	1	3	0	
Unilateral patency (left)	0		3	9	1	2

TABLE 24-2. Bilateral Closure and Date of Injection Since Onset of Menses

DATE	GROUP I—SINGLE APPLICATION		GROUP II—UTERINE LAVAGE + SINGLE APPLICATION		GROUP III—TWO APPLICATIONS	
	NO. PATIENTS	%	*NO. PATIENTS*	%	*NO. PATIENTS*	%
Day 0–6	6/7	86	2/4	50	5/5	100
Day 7–10	18/25	72	15/23	65	20/23	83
Day 11–15	2/4	50	5/5	100	8/9	89
Day 16+	2/2	100	1/1	100	3/3	100

The influence of uterine position on closure is shown in Table 24-4. When a single application is performed, the highest rates of tubal closure seem to occur in uteri positioned on the midline.

Side-effects and complications included pelvic pain (4%), abdominal tenderness (5%), and hyperthermy (2%) following the procedure. One subject developed cervical stenosis 1 month after the injection of MCA. Three women required hospitalization. Two patients had uterine perforation, and one patient had excessive pelvic pain. The incidence of side-effects in the various groups is shown in Table 24-5.

TABLE 24-3. Bilateral Closure and Instrument Depth

DEPTH	GROUP I—SINGLE APPLICATION		GROUP II—UTERINE LAVAGE + SINGLE APPLICATION		GROUP III—TWO APPLICATIONS	
	NO. PATIENTS	%	*NO. PATIENTS*	%	*NO. PATIENTS*	%
4–6 cm	3/4	75	1/1	100	1/1	100
7–9 cm	24/33	73	22/31	71	35/39	90
10–12 cm	1/1	100	0/1		0/1	

TABLE 24-4. Bilateral Closure and Uterine Position

POSITION	GROUP I—SINGLE APPLICATION		GROUP II—UTERINE LAVAGE + SINGLE APPLICATION		GROUP III—TWO APPLICATIONS	
	NO. PATIENTS	%	*NO. PATIENTS*	%	*NO. PATIENTS*	%
Anterior	3/5	60	1/2	50	3/3	100
Midline	20/24	83	18/23	78	29/34	85
Posterior	5/9	56	4/8	50	4/4	100

TABLE 24-5. Side-effects of MCA Sterilization, All Protocols

SIDE-EFFECT	MONTHS FOLLOWING TREATMENT	NO. PATIENTS %
Pelvic pain	1	5/130 (4)
	3	0/31
Fever	1	3/130 (2)
Hospitalization*	1	3/30 (2)
Uterine stenosis	1	1/130 (1)
Uterine tenderness	1	6/130 (5)

*Two patients had uterine perforation; one had excessive pain.

Four subjects conceived before the radiologic evaluation of tubal patency. Four other women conceived after hysterosalpingography suggested bilateral tubal occlusion. Reevaluation of their hysterosalpingography plates indicated that interpretation of bilateral tubal occlusion may have been wrong.

DISCUSSION

The present report confirms previous experience with the FEMCEPT device and indicates that nonsurgical sterilization may be developed into a practical and safe method of fertility control. MCA produces effective closure of the fallopian tube in 88% of the subjects when it is applied twice. Although this percentage of successful closures is substantial, further improvement appears to be necessary before the technique receives worldwide acceptance. One possible area of investigation is suggested by our finding, in that in a small number of patients, closure is readily accomplished when application is made after day 16, probably after ovulation has taken place. It seems that relaxation of the tubal isthmus that occurs under progesterone domination facilitates the penetration of MCA, resulting in effective closure. If failures result from spasm of the uterotubal junction or of the tubal isthmus, we should indeed achieve a greater success rate by pretesting the patient with a progestin, an oral contraceptive, or a tubal relaxant. We have shown that tubal spasm may be promptly neutralized by several treatments preceding injection of a contrast medium for hysterosalpingography.[1–3] Prostaglandin synthesis inhibitors, α-adrenergic receptor blockers, β-adrenergic agonists, or prostaglandin antagonists may be considered as tubal relaxants to be used in conjunction with injection of MCA with the FEMCEPT device.

The greatest advantage of this method over laparoscopic sterilization is its noninvasiveness. Transcervical tubal closure simplifies the sterilization, making it practical as an office procedure. However, the two cases of uterine perforation recorded in our series indicate that this new method should not be used by inexperienced doctors or paramedical personnel. Its use without the back-up of the services available at a hospital should not be encouraged for the time being, certainly not before the risk of uterine perforation is further reduced.

REFERENCES

1. COUTINHO EM: Motility of the human fallopian tube. In Persianinov LS, Chervakova TV, Presl J (eds): Recent Progress in Obstetrics and Gynecology, pp 576–582. Amsterdam, Excerpta Medica, 1974
2. COUTINHO EM: Physiologic and pharmacologic studies of the human oviduct. Fertil Steril 22:207, 1971
3. COUTINHO EM, MAIA H: The contractile response of the human uterus, fallopian tubes and ovary to prostaglandins *in vivo.* Fertil Steril 22:539, 1971
4. RICHART RM, GUTIERREZ-NAJAR AJ, NEUWIRTH RS: Transvaginal human sterilization: A preliminary report. Am J Obstet Gynecol 111:108–110, 1971
5. RICHART RM, NEUWIRTH RS, BOLDUC L: Single application fertility regulating device: Description of a new instrument. Am J Obstet Gynecol 127:86–90, 1977
6. SALGADO C: Sterilization induced by caustic injections. Am Brasil Genet 503:121, June 1941
7. STEVENSON TC, TAYLOR DS: The effect of methylcyanoacrylate tissue adhesive on the human fallopian tube and endometrium. J Obstet Gynecol 79:1028, 1972

25

Transcervical Tubal Occlusion Using Methyl Cyanoacrylate: The Two-Application Technique

NARGESH D. MOTASHAW

R. TALATI

The technique of female sterilization has achieved major importance as a means of fertility regulation during the past 3 decades, first with the laparotomy procedure and later with a minilaparotomy or laparoscopy. Despite improvements in anesthesia, surgical training, and equipment, operative procedures carry a small but significant mortality. In developing countries, mortality is in the range of 10 to 20 deaths per 100,000 procedures.

When discussing sterilization, family planning personnel must contend with several barriers to acceptance, one of which is the word "operation." A nonoperative technique of tubal occlusion performed as an office procedure is likely to be more readily accepted by women all over the world than an operative method requiring hospitalization. With this in mind, investigators in many centers are carrying out research on transcervical chemical methods of female sterilization.

Workers have sought a suitable chemical that would destroy the tubal epithelium and yet be safe to the peritoneum and devoid of any systemic effects. One of the more promising agents is methyl cyanoacrylate (MCA). A suitable system has been studied in depth by bioengineers, and their efforts have resulted in the production of the FEMCEPT device.[3] A study evaluating a two-application technique is described in the following sections.

MATERIALS AND METHODS

Fifty healthy parous women desiring permanent control of their fertility were selected, according to protocol; patients with medical disorders such as heart disease, diabetes, hypertension, or tuberculosis were excluded. In a few cases, a chest roentgenogram was taken, because of the high incidence of tuberculosis in the city. Patients who had undergone recent abortions or who had delivered a child a few weeks prior to being seen were counseled to return after two normal menstrual periods. A woman who had used an IUD was enrolled 4 weeks after the removal of the device.

The details of the technique were explained to the patients, and a social worker emphasized the necessity of a second instillation and the need for continued contraception, regular follow-up visits, and later a hysterosalpingogram. A routine clinical examination was done, a Papanicolaou smear was taken, and the uterocervical length was measured. Those patients with uterine length under 7 cm or over 10 cm were excluded.

All the procedures were carried out at the office within 5 days of the termination of menses. A few patients who were using oral contraceptives did not menstruate and underwent the second instillation after the result of a pregnancy test was negative. The procedure was done with all aseptic precautions, exactly as recommended. The volume of MCA injected was 0.6 ml.

Dilatation of the cervical canal was necessary at the time of the first injection for 7 patients and at the time of the second injection for 5 patients; one patient required dilatation for both occasions. In all cases, a 4-mm cervical dilator was used.

COMPLICATIONS

Pain is a subjective variable phenomenon that is always difficult to assess. In this small series, the private patients from a higher socioeconomic level complained more frequently of minimal discomfort than did those women from the lower socioeconomic group.

Hospitalization was necessary in only 1 patient (No. 015), who experienced abdominal pain and vaginal bleeding 3 weeks after the procedure. A small 3 × 3-cm swelling was palpable in the right fornix. The woman responded well to antibiotic therapy, and her hysterosalpingogram 4 months later revealed bilateral patent tubes. The pelvic inflammatory disease may not have been due to the procedure.

No serious complication has occurred.

RESULTS

Forty-seven of the 50 patients have had the nonradiopaque MCA injected twice. Hysterosalpingograms 4 months after the second application have been obtained in 41 patients. The dye used was water-soluble meglumine iothalmate injection 60% W/V containing 280 mg iodine in combined form in each milliliter (Conray 280). Three patients, one of whom has had a hysterosalpingogram, did not return for the second treatment. Of the 41 patients undergoing hysterosalpingograms after completing two instillations, 39 were shown to have bilateral closure and one had bilateral patency. One patient had a unilaterally patent tube.

For various reasons, the roentgenographic interpretation is not always easy, and the radiologist and the clinician may disagree on findings. Two patients were reevaluated for doubtful patency of the right tube. One patient (No. 007) had a laparoscopy under general anesthesia; methylene blue test revealed tubal blockage. A second patient (No. 020) had a repeat hysterosalpingogram, which showed a bilateral closure. Patient No. 015, with bilateral tubal patency, had only one application of MCA and thus was truly out of the two-injection protocol.

DISCUSSION

The method of transcervical injection of MCA using the FEMCEPT device to produce tubal blockage must be compared with laparoscopy and minilaparotomy, the two methods of sterilization now in vogue. Being a nonsurgical procedure, the MCA technique is free from anesthesia, does not invade the peritoneal cavity, is simple to execute by medical and paramedical personnel, and does away with sophisticated expensive instruments. The patient spends only 30 to 60 minutes at the clinic. No mortality has occurred to date, and no life-threatening complications have been reported. In India, sterilization can be legally performed without the partner's permission, however custom dictates that the woman must have her husband's consent. If he refuses, she must accede to his decision and she must continue to bear children; having either a laparoscopy or a minilaparotomy procedure without his knowledge is impossible, since scars, albeit small, are visible. By the transcervical technique, however, a patient has the option of electing sterilization without divulging that fact to anyone other than the operator.

The disadvantages of this method are the frequent need for two applications, the long waiting period before effective blockage can be proved, the high failure rate, and the doubtful reversibility of the procedure.

A repeat procedure is difficult to implement in developing countries, and the continuous use of contraception for 4 months following the procedure is a serious drawback. Further, if the closure rate is shown to be related to the day of injection following the onset of menses, the procedure would have a limited application in camp situations, for when a patient is motivated for sterilization, postponement for any reason has a negative impact; once a patient has come to the clinic for sterilization, she wants to have it done right away so that she can return home. In many cases, waiting even for a day or so is unacceptable or impossible.

Surgical sterilization by laparoscopy or minilaparotomy is a one-time procedure. It is quickly executed, immediately effective, and possibly reversible, if the tube is not extensively damaged. These procedures necessitate physician training and skill, and in the case of laparoscopy, expensive equipment. In addition, these techniques are invasive procedures requiring anesthesia, local or general, with a small but significant mortality and morbidity. An analysis of the data from two major teaching institutions in Bombay for a 5-year period (1975–1979) revealed a mortality of 8.6 per 100,000 laparoscopic sterilizations.[2]

Ectopic pregnancy is a notorious late complication of sterilization. Cheng and associates, analyzing the data of a coordinaated study conducted by the International Fertility Research Program, found 15 ectopic pregnancies and 1,979 intrauterine pregnancies in 23,600 women who had undergone surgical sterilization by various techniques.[1] The occurrence of ectopic gestation after chemical sterilization is not known.

REFERENCES

1. CHENG CI, LAUFE LE, ATWOOD RJ: Ectopic pregnancy following female sterilization procedures. In Wynn RM (ed): Advances in Planned Parenthood. Amsterdam, Excerpta Medica, Association of Planned Parenthood Physicians, 1981
2. MOTASHAW ND: Some aspects of tubal sterilization. In Semm K, Mettler L (eds): Proceedings of III World Congress 421, Berlin 1981. Amsterdam, Excerpta Medica, International Congress Series No. 551, 1981
3. RICHART R, NEUWIRTH R, BOLDUC L: Single application fertility regulating device: Description of a new instrument. Am J Obstet Gynecol 127:86, 1977

26

Clinical Experience with Radiopaque Methyl Cyanoacrylate

ITIC ZIGHELBOIM

WIKTOR SZCZEDRIN

The study described in this chapter was performed at the Concepcion Palacios Maternity Hospital in Caracas, Venezuela. This is an unusual institution in that during 1981, 39,231 female patients were hospitalized there. Of this total, 29,944 delivered at or near term, and of these deliveries, 79% (23,757) occurred in multiparous women. The Family Planning Service of the Maternity Hospital provided 33,908 consultations during this same time period.

There is an increasing demand for irreversible contraception by patients in such an overcrowded institution with limited facilities. This has led us to consider methods that will permit us to fulfill the needs of the patients as well as the requirements of the hospital. An ideal method should be easily performed on an ambulatory or semiambulatory basis, with a low incidence of complications and side-effects, and should not require specially trained personnel or sophisticated equipment.

No presently available procedure meets all these criteria. Therefore, we have looked at some of the drugs and chemicals now being applied by transcervical injection as an alternative for tubal sterilization. We performed a clinical trial with radiopaque methyl cyanoacrylate in 87 volunteers, and the results of this ongoing trial, which was begun on October 10, 1981, are discussed here.

MATERIAL AND METHODS

All 87 patients were enrolled on a voluntary basis and were aware of the experimental nature of the procedure. The procedure was explained to them by the social worker of the Family Planning Service and one of the authors. All patients were of proven fertility and desirous of an irreversible sterilization procedure (Table 26-1).

Complete physical examination, routine laboratory tests, and gynecologic examination, which included Papanicolaou smear and uterine sounding, were performed on each woman before her enrollment in the study.

The procedure was performed as previously described after cessation of the menstrual period, no later than 8 days after the first day of bleeding. Since radiopaque MCA was used, a flat plate of the inlet of the pelvis was obtained prior to and after MCA application.

TABLE 26-1. Obstetrical History of 87 Patients Undergoing MCA Instillations for Sterilization

CHARACTERISTIC	MINIMUM	MAXIMUM	AVERAGE
Age	23	39	32
Gravity	2	11	5
Parity	2	9	4
Living children	2	9	4

RESULTS

Of the 87 patients, only 43 have had hysterographic confirmation of tubal patency. The results were analyzed according to radiologic and clinical observations.

RADIOLOGIC OBSERVATIONS

The radiopaque MCA findings on the postapplication flat plate are shown in Table 26-2. The radiopaque material could not be visualized on the flat plate in 11 cases, and in 18 cases, it was visualized in only one tube. The visualization of this material was more frequent in the left tube than in the right.

Both in bilateral and unilateral visualization, there was a wide variance in radiologic images. This variation was dependent on the extent to which the acrylate material penetrated into the tube (Fig. 26-1).

Of the 43 hysterograms performed, 32 showed bilateral tubal occlusion, demonstrating a success rate of 74%. In five instances there was closure of one tube only. A hysterogram of a bilateral patency is shown in Figure 26-2, and a unilateral patency is demonstrated in Figure 26-3.

CLINICAL OBSERVATIONS

The primary complaint during the application of MCA was pain (Table 26-3). This pain was described as moderate or severe in only 14% of the patients. Patients could get up from the table between 4 and 6 minutes after injection and were able to leave the hospital facilities within 14 minutes, on the average, with extremes of 5 to 25 minutes postprocedure.

TABLE 26-2. Visualization of MCA on Postinjection Roentgenogram

VISUALIZATION	NO. CASES	%
Bilateral	58	66.7
Left tube	11	12.6
Right tube	7	8.0
Not localized	11	12.6
Total	87	99.9

Side-effects were experienced by 16 patients after leaving the table: 11 women had a minor vasovagal reaction; 2 had pain of moderate intensity in the lower abdomen; 2 had pain radiating to the one leg; and 1 had pain and vomiting. All these symptoms disappeared with the administration of mild analgesics and antiemetics.

DELAYED SIDE-EFFECTS

During the month following the MCA application, some complications and side-effects were observed. Pain in the lower abdomen was observed in 16 instances (17%), but the women responded well to customary dosages of acetylsalicylic acid. Pain and fewer in seven cases (8%), fever in three cases (3%), endometritis in two cases, one case of urinary tract infection, one case of amenorrhea for 3 months, and two cases of pelvic inflammatory disease were also observed.

DIFFICULTIES RELATED TO THE FEMCEPT PROCEDURE

In seven patients (9%), the cannula was difficult to pass through the internal cervical os; dilatation with the uterine sound was required in two of these patients. In two patients, withdrawal of the inserted cannula was difficult.

In four patients (5%), the balloon was visible during MCA application. In these cases, hysterography has not yet been performed, therefore the effect on tubal occlusion is not known.

Finally, in one patient, the MCA vial became obstructed in the reservoir of the device, and a new FEMCEPT had to be used.

DISCUSSION

The cyanoacrylates are tissue adhesives, and owing to their necrotizing and pyrogenic action, they can be used as tube and deferens occlusives, as stated by Woodward,[4] who by adding some acid moieties succeeded in reducing local heat production during their transformation from monomer to polymer.

In experimental studies in rabbits, the cyanoacrylates have consistently produced tubal occlusion by destroying the epithelium.[1] The methyl derivative was tested by Stevenson and Taylor, with an ingenious but troublesome lavage technique, showing its effect as a tissue adhesive on the human fallopian tube and endometrium.[3]

Further, Stevenson has shown that by 24 hours, there is necrosis of the tubal epithelium touched by the polymer, and invasion of the stromal tissue by polymorphs and lymphocytes.[2] After 1 to 2 weeks, the necrosis reaches its maximum; and at the end of 24 weeks, the fallopian tubes are totally transformed into fibrous cords. Stevenson was able to demonstrate by means of hysterograms that a 70% bilateral occlusion had occurred in 41 procedures.

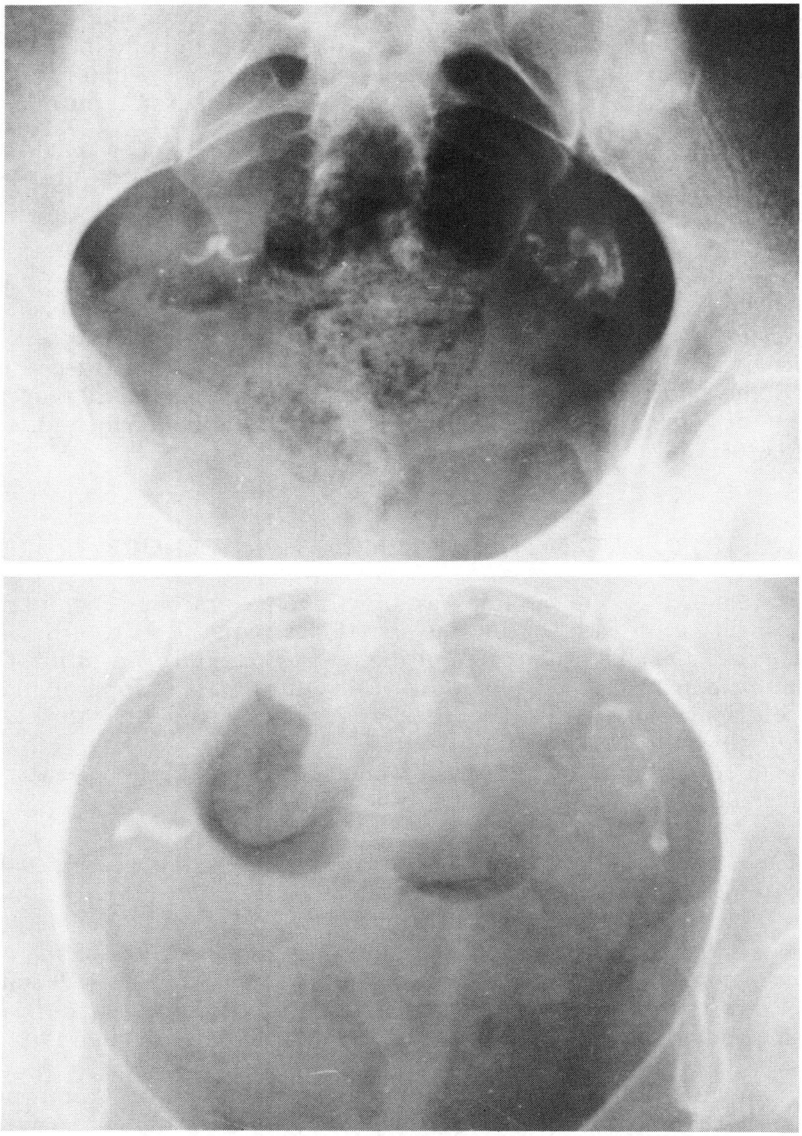

A

B

FIG. 26-1. Plain roentgenograms after MCA injection. (*A*) Left tube has been totally injected and the right tube has been injected only in the interstitial portion. (*B*) Right tube is totally visualized; MCA is spilling from the left tube into the peritoneum. (*C* and *D*) Entries in right and left tubes, respectively.

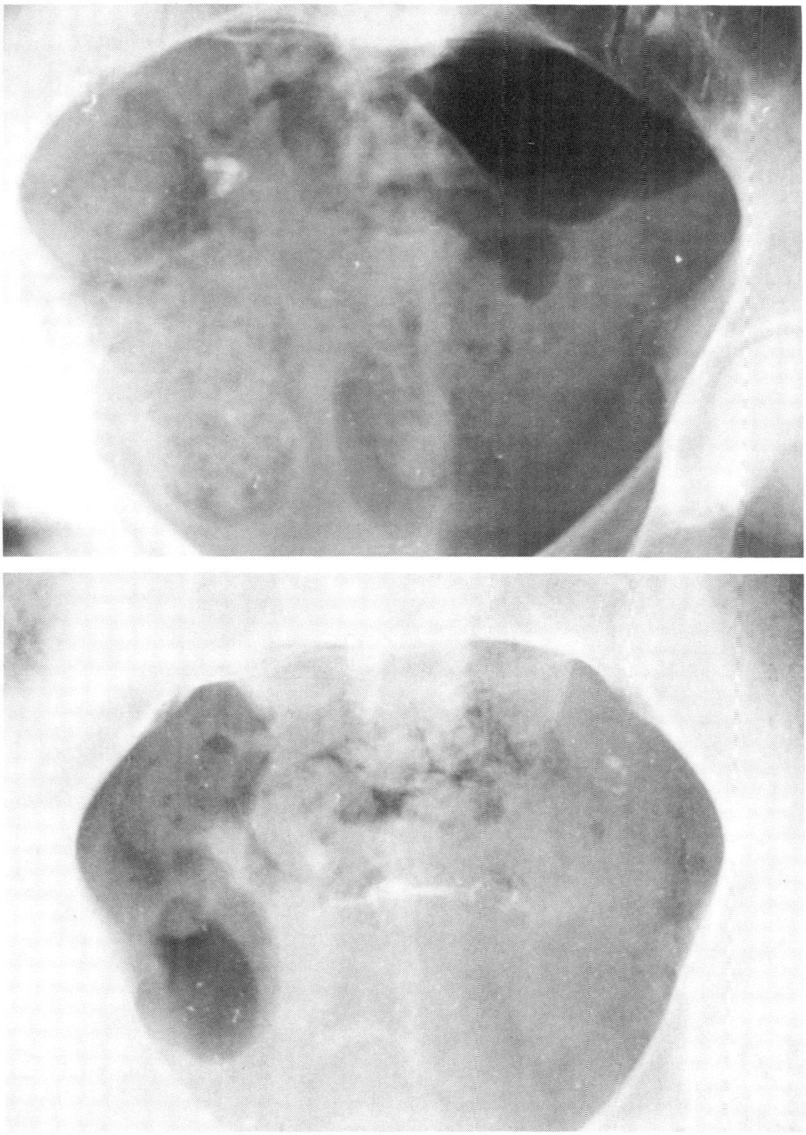

C

D

SUMMARY

In the present ongoing study, to date 87 patients have been treated with radiopaque MCA by transcervical injection by means of the FEMCEPT device. After application of the radiopaque material, a bilateral entrance could be visualized in 66.6% of these patients. Of 43 hysterosalpingograms, 32 showed bilateral tubal occlusion and 5 showed unilateral occlusion. The main

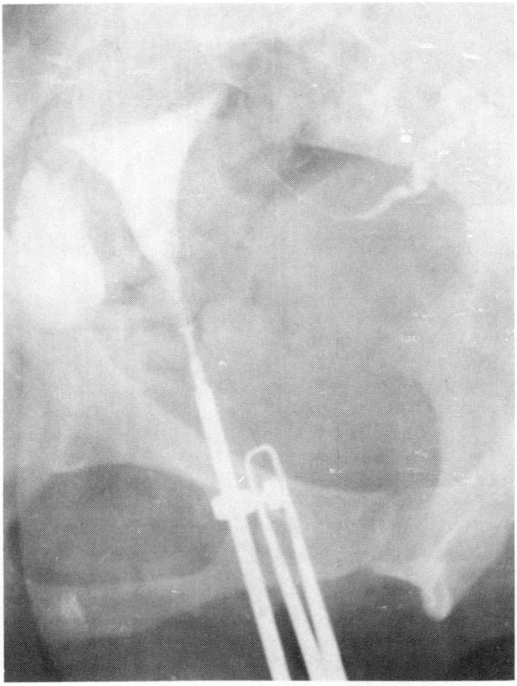

FIG. 26-2. Hysterogram showing bilateral patency.

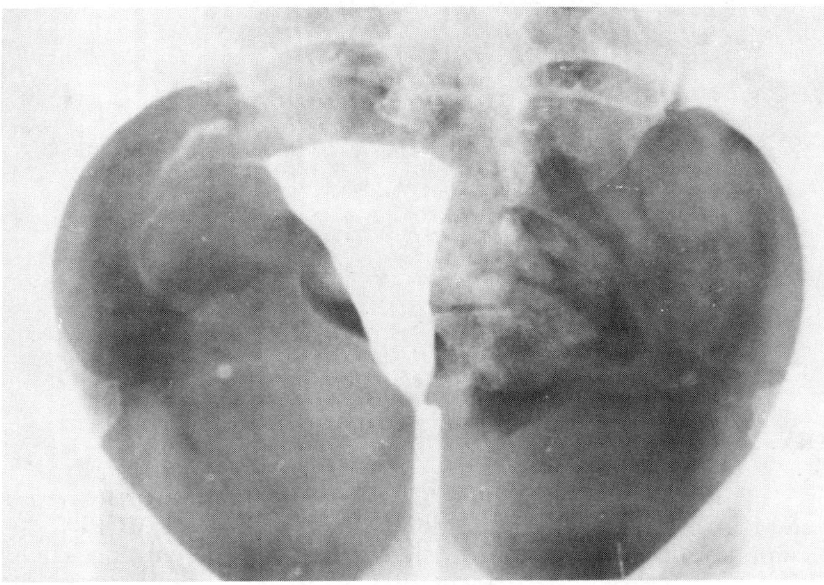

FIG. 26-3. Hysterogram showing patency of the right tube.

TABLE 26-3. Pain During MCA Injection

TYPE	NO. CASES	%
None	29	33
Mild	46	53
Moderate	6	7
Severe	6	7
Total	87	100

immediate side-effects were pain in the lower abdomen and vasovagal reactions. No patient required hospitalization.

We consider the use of MCA to be a promising new method for female sterilization.

REFERENCES

1. RICHART RM, NEUWIRTH RS, TAYLOR HC JR: Experimental studies of fallopian tube occlusion. In Richart RM, Prager DJ (eds): Human Sterilization, pp 360–367. Springfield, IL, Charles C Thomas, 1972
2. STEVENSON T: Methyl cyanoacrylate (MCA) for tubal occlusion. In Sciarra JJ, Droegemueller W, Speidel JJ (eds): Advances in Female Sterilization Techniques, pp 216–229. Hagerstown, MD, Harper & Row, 1976
3. STEVENSON TC, TAYLOR DS: The effect of methyl cyanoacrylate tissue adhesive on the human fallopian tube and endometrium. J Obstet Gynaecol Br Commonw 79:1028–1039, 1972
4. WOODWARD SC: Tissue response to polymer implants: The cyanoacrylates. In Richart RM, Prager DJ (eds): Human Sterilization, pp 264–275. Springfield, IL, Charles C Thomas, 1972

27

The Effectiveness of the FEMCEPT Method and Preliminary Experience With Radiopaque MCA to Enhance Clinical Acceptability

RALPH M. RICHART

ROBERT S. NEUWIRTH

PER AGNAR NILSEN

JACQUES RIOUX

ITIC ZIGHELBOIM

MANOEL BOMFIM DE SOUZA FILHO

RENE GUZMAN-SERANI

NARGESH D. MOTASHAW

The development of a widely applicable transcervical method of tubal sterilization remains an important yet elusive achievement for fertility control. In a previous communication an intrauterine balloon instrument system delivering methyl cyanoacrylate (MCA) for transcervical tubal sterilization was described.[2] Limited clinical experience has been reported, with small modifications of the instrument system, as well as with variations in the volume of MCA employed.[1] Tubal closure rates, as determined by hysterosalpingography 12 to 16 weeks following treatment, varied as modifications were made, but, in general, tubal closure improved from 64% to 78% after a single injection. As the system design was stabilized, the clinical techniques were changed in order to improve results further. In addition, a radiopaque MCA was developed. Preliminary experience with the iodinated radiopaque MCA will be described, as will the results of clinical trials.

MATERIALS AND METHODS

The FEMCEPT device in all these studies as the same model used in the previous report.[1] The instrument use was also unchanged, and 0.65 ml MCA was used in the ampule. Patients were randomly assigned, parous women with normal pelvic organs and regular menstrual function who desired sterilization and agreed to follow the protocol after counseling and consent.

In this study, three clinical protocols were designed for random assignment in six study centers. Although the system is simple to use, a clinical training session was held with each investigator at the outset of the study to ensure uniformity of technique and data collection.

In the first protocol, a single postmenstrual application of the FEMCEPT/MCA system was followed by a 4-month interval of barrier or oral contraception and then by a hysterosalpingogram. If the tubes were blocked, the patient was informed and then followed; she did not use other contraception. If one or both tubes were open, a repeat injection was offered and the sequence was repeated, or an alternative sterilization procedure was performed.

In the second protocol, a two-injection sequence was used, in which there was a one-cycle (30-day) interval between the injections. Contraception was then continued for 4 months until a control hysterogram was done. The protocol was otherwise identical to the first one.

In the third protocol, a single postmenstrual application was immediately preceded by a uterine lavage, using a Rubin cannula, with an olive 1 cm from the tip and 10 ml normal saline. The saline was irrigated gently over a 30- to 60-second period, after which the FEMCEPT/MCA system was applied. Following the MCA application, the protocol was identical to the other two.

In addition to the three-protocol randomized trials a fourth study was designed to evaluate the effectivity of a newly compounded MCA containing an inhibitor of MCA polymerization that is radiopaque. The physiochemical behavior of the MCA with radiopaque inhibitor was virtually indistinguishable from the nonradiopaque material. It was thought that this radiopaque property would allow the operator to determine whether the MCA had penetrated into the fallopian tubes, to measure the distance using a simple flat plate, and possibly to predict tubal closure prospectively. Following preliminary laboratory testing of the radiopaque material and its study in three patient volunteers using cinefluoroscopy immediately prior to hysterectomy, we used the material in ambulatory patients.

The radiopaque MCA clinical study was designed on the same basic pattern as the single postmenstrual application protocol, except that an inlet view pelvic flat plate was taken immediately prior to and following the MCA application (Fig. 27-1). The technique of application was identical to the nonradiopaque technique, except that the procedure in the first 20 cases was done under fluoroscopy. Following the application, the films were compared to study the distribution of the MCA. All patients used contraception, and a hysterosalpingogram was performed between 12 and 16 weeks postprocedure. The protocol was thereafter the same as in the nonradiopaque studies.

Computer-compatible data forms were developed for all four protocols, and the completed forms plus all flat plates were forwarded to the principal investigators for confirmatory reading and data analysis. The data included general information, gynecologic history and pelvic findings, device and adhesive identification, procedure characteristics, and follow-up history and physical findings at 1 month and 4 months postprocedure, and at 6-month intervals thereafter, in those patients whose fallopian tubes were bilaterally blocked on hysterosalpingography.

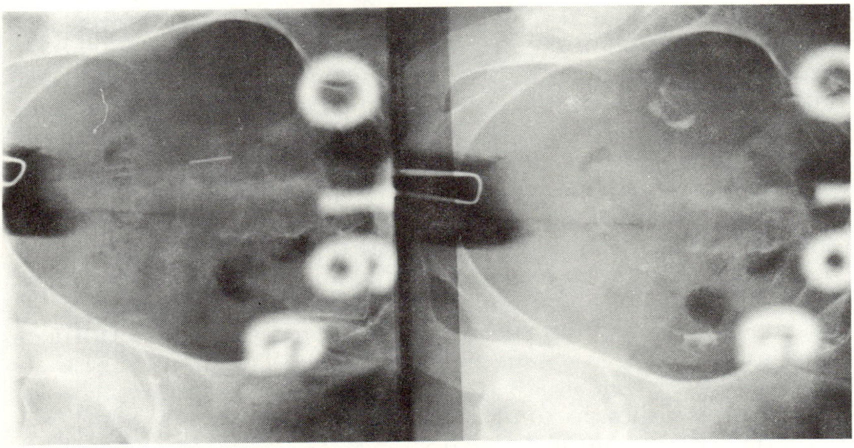

FIG. 27-1. Radiographic control of the injection of radiopaque MCA using the FEMCEPT device shows bilateral tubal entry.

RESULTS

RANDOMIZED TRIPLE PROTOCOL TRIAL

The data for the 295 patients studied in this protocol are summarized in Table 27-1. The bilateral closure rate by hysterosalpingogram after a single injection of MCA was 78% in the 102 cases so treated.

The bilateral closure rate was 68% in the 91 women studied under the uterine lavage protocol, and the combined unilateral patencies (18%) were about equally divided between the right and left sides. Because it was evident that the preliminary lavage of the uterine cavity was not improving the bilateral closure rate and may, in fact, have increased the overall patency rate, we have terminated this more complex protocol.

In the two-application protocol, the bilateral tubal closure rate was 87% in 102 cases. The bilateral patency rate was 5%, and unilateral patency rates were about equally divided at 4%. These data suggest that tubal entry is more

TABLE 27-1. Closure Rates With MCA in Randomized Protocol

	SINGLE APPLICATION		UTERINE LAVAGE		TWO APPLICATIONS	
RESULT	*NO. PATIENTS*	%	*NO. PATIENTS*	%	*NO. PATIENTS*	%
Bilateral closure	80/102	78	62/91	68	89/102	87
Bilateral patency	12/102	12	13/91	14	5/102	5
Right tube open	5/102	5	7/91	8	4/102	4
Left tube open	5/102	5	9/91	8	4/102	4

TABLE 27-2. Side-effects from FEMCEPT/MCA*

SYMPTOM	DURATION (MONTHS)	NO. PATIENTS (%)
Pelvic pain	1	138/622 (22)
Pelvic pain	3	11/262 (4)
Fever	1	34/622 (5)
Hospitalization	1	11/821 (1)
Uterine tenderness	1	42/622 (7)

*All protocols except radiopaque MCA

important to success than the effectivity of the adhesive in producing sclerosis.

The incidence of pelvic pain, fever, and hospitalization noted in the first or second follow-up report is summarized in Table 27-2. The data for this table was derived from 622 patients treated under all the MCA protocols since the inception of the project, except for the radiopaque studies. Hospitalization includes the 199 women treated to date with radiopaque MCA. Twenty-two percent of patients had reported pain between 1 and 3 months after the procedure. Unfortunately, there was no control baseline response to this question on the intake form nor was information gathered on the precise timing of the pain. Five percent reported fever within the first month; 1% were hospitalized.

Hospitalization for 6 of the 14 women (including 3 women treated with radiopaque MCA) was due to clinical signs or symptoms compatible with a low-grade pelvic inflammation. Three were treated with antibiotics, and the signs or symptoms were resolved. Two of these patients underwent laparoscopy; tubal inflammation was described, but no further surgery was performed. The other three patients were not treated and were discharged after a short hospitalization. The longest hospitalization lasted 7 days. Seven women were hospitalized for vagal reactions and released later the same day or the following day without treatment or with symptomatic therapy. One patient was hospitalized for heavy bleeding during the first menstrual period after the application, but she was released after 3 days with no therapy.

SINGLE INJECTION OF RADIOPAQUE MCA

We treated 199 patients with radiopaque MCA. In 62 patients, hysterographic control has been performed. In 87% of these patients, bilateral tubal blockage was evident on the hysterogram (Table 27-3). This is a significant improvement over the nonradiopaque MCA ($p < 0.05$). It is thought to be due to the faster spreading that is a characteristic of the radiopaque MCA monomer and may improve entry into the tubes. Of the 62 women in this group, 53 had preinjection and postinjection pelvic flat plates read. We found bilateral entry into the tubes in 75% of patients (40/53), and in 90% of these (36/40) the tubes were bilaterally closed on the hysterosalpingogram (HSG); 25% (13/53) did not have bilateral entry identified on the flat plate, but 77% of these

TABLE 27-3. Closure Rates With Radiopaque MCA

RESULT	NO. PATIENTS (%)
Bilateral closure	54/62 (87)
Bilateral patency	2/62 (3)
Right tube open	4/62 (6)
Left tube open	2/62 (3)

women had bilateral tubal closure evident on the HSG. The incidence of pelvic pain, fever, and hospitalization was not significantly different between those patients in whom radiopaque and nonradiopaque MCA were used, but the number of patients in the radiopaque group is still small.

REPEAT APPLICATIONS

The bilateral closure rates in 29 patients who were re-treated immediately after the first injection failed was 90%, as determined hysterosalpingographically. This re-treated group differs from the two-application series in that there is a longer interval between treatments (generally 4 or 5 months) and there is an intervening hysterogram. In those patients who elected to have a second MCA procedure directly after failure of the first, the bilateral closure rate was 98%.

Seventeen pregnancies are known to have occurred in the 821 women treated with MCA and subsequently exposed to a possible pregnancy. Twelve women became pregnant before the initial HSG was performed, or following an HSG in which one or both tubes were patent, but prior to a second sterilization procedure. In one instance the film was misread, but when it was reviewed after the pregnancy had occurred it showed a unilateral patency. Two women became pregnant after bilateral blockage was reported on HSG. Both pregnancies occurred within 6 months of the HSG. It is impossible to determine whether these failures followed a false-positive HSG, tubal spasm, or recanalization. In the 16th and 17th patients, bilateral closure was shown on the HSG, the patients were thought to be pregnant, but only decidua was found at the time of curettage for bleeding. No tubal pregnancies have occurred. The total number of women-months of patients followed to date, after closure on HSG, is 3629.

LONG-TERM FOLLOW-UP

To date, 291 women have been followed for 1 to 31 months following bilateral closure based on the hysterosalpingographic examination. These women have aggregated 3629 months of follow-up, and two pregnancies have been experienced, as reported above. Both pregnancies occurred in the early part of the follow-up, and whether these represent recanalization or false-positive HSGs is unclear. In any case, the population has remained pregnancy-free after 6 months and no ectopic pregnancies have been reported.

DISCUSSION

There has been a steady increase in bilateral tubal blockade following a single application of MCA since the clinical trials using the FEMCEPT/MCA system were first begun. Through a series of modifications in the delivery system in the MCA and in the clinical protocol, the closure rates have been improved from 64% in the early studies to 87% using the radiopaque MCA. It is clear that these rates are influenced as well by the care with which the clinician follows the protocol. The closure rates are highest when the system is used during the earliest phase of the menstrual cycle, and they are progressively lower in the luteal phase, when there is more mucus and a lush, delicate endometrium. It is also clear that the system is not effective in uteri that sound to greater than 9 cm or less than 6 cm, which is where the instrument is designed to operate. The instrument is also not effective in patients who have significant intrauterine anomalies (particularly bicornuate or deeply septate uteri) or in patients with significant distortions of the cavity owing to submucous leiomyomas or endometrial polyps. Deviations from the protocol, or the inclusion of patients with significant uterine pathology, will significantly diminish the closure rates.

One of the most promising aspects of the study has been that the procedure appears to be safe. The clinical side-effects are minimal and are related to the action of the MCA as a local inflammatory agent when associated with significant tissue destruction. As would be expected, some patients complain of low-grade pelvic pain and of fever; a small number of patients complain of significant pain, which may persist for weeks or months. These clinical sequelae do not seem to differ significantly from those associated with other methods of female sterilization. The hospitalizations have been related principally to conservative clinical care offered in association with the clinical testing of a new procedure. The majority of patients were hospitalized owing to vagal reactions, another group owing to a single heavy period, and the others because of varying degrees of pelvic pain. Two of the hospitalized patients had laparoscopically proven pelvic inflammatory disease, but in both cases the inflammation resolved after antibiotic therapy. Three of the six women admitted with possible pelvic infection were discharged without therapy after 1 or 2 days.

The addition of a radiopaque MCA to the FEMCEPT/MCA system promised to provide an opportunity to monitor the dynamics of the MCA application and its course in the upper female genital tract. It also appeared to have the potential for predicting those patients in whom tubal closure would occur, enabling the clinician to select out those patients who were prospective failures for re-treatment or sterilization by another technique. It has proved difficult to monitor the dynamics of the application *in utero,* because the present level of radiopacity is insufficiently radiodense to be seen easily in some patients.

A more disturbing finding, however, is that contrary to our previous belief based on our animal studies,[3] MCA does not always close the fallopian tubes if it enters them. There are a few patients in whom clear-cut bilateral tubal entry of radiopaque MCA extending well into the ampulla could be easily seen on the flat plate, yet one fallopian tube was shown to be patent on HSG. The converse situation, in which radiopaque MCA was not seen in the fallopian tubes but the tubes were nonetheless closed, can be explained in the following way. The MCA did not reach the ampullary segment where a sufficient concentration would provide enough radiopacity to be seen, whereas the thin column of MCA lying in the interstitial isthmic tubes might not be visible on the flat plate but still produced tubal closure.

The factors causing the MCA failure in occasional cases are unclear at this time. In spite of the finding that MCA does not always close the tube after entry, it does appear to produce permanent closure once the scar has been formed. The initial data indicate two or, at most, four pregnancies, in 3629 women-months following an HSG showing bilateral closure.

The most promising development is the observation that the bilateral closure rate on a single application is significantly greater in those patients treated with radiopaque MCA than with previous MCA formulations. This can probably be explained by the observation that the radiopaque inhibitor enhances the "spreadability" of the MCA, thus improving tubal penetration. It is likely that this property will likewise enhance the closure rates on a second application, and it is possible that rates of tubal closure approaching 100% can be generated by this blind transcervical technique in an appropriately designed two-application protocol.

REFERENCES

1. NEUWIRTH RS, RICHART RM, STEVENSON TC et al: An outpatient approach to female sterilization with methylcyanoacrylate. Am J Obstet Gynecol 136:951–956, 1980
2. RICHART RM, NEUWIRTH RS, BOLDUC LR: Single application fertility regulating device: Description of a new instrument. Am J Obstet Gynecol 127:86–90, 1977
3. RICHART RM, NEUWIRTH RS, TAYLOR HG JR: Experimental studies of fallopian tube blockade in human sterilization. Springfield, IL, Charles C Thomas, 1972

28

Future Developments in the FEMCEPT/MCA System

RALPH M. RICHART

ROBERT S. NEUWIRTH

The FEMCEPT device will consistently deliver nonpolymerizing, nonadhesive fluids of the viscosity of water to the fallopian tubes bilaterally after a single application, provided the plunger is fully depressed and kept in that position for a full minute at the time of the application.[5] Pressure by the preset piston, applied continuously for 1 minute, is sufficient to overcome the tubal spasm sometimes occasioned by cervical grasping and uterine manipulation, and the bilateral delivery rate is approximately 80% with free-flowing thin liquids in normal uteri. When methyl cyanoacrylate (MCA) is used with the FEMCEPT device, it begins to polymerize immediately after its application, and its viscosity increases rapidly with time. From cinehysterosalpingographic studies of radiopaque MCA, little, if any, progress in tubal entry appears to occur after 20 seconds, so prolonged application of additional pressure is futile.

The rate at which MCA enters the fallopian tubes has increased progressively during the life of the FEMCEPT project as we have developed more sophistication in manipulating the chemistry of this substance and enhancing its tube-entering abilities.[1,2,4] The most dramatic advance occurred when the successful radiopacifying of MCA was accompanied by an increase in its ability to flow (referred to as spreadability) and resulted in a significant increase in tubal entry and in bilateral tubal closure (see Chapter 27). Additional attempts to increase the spreadability and to control the adhesiveness and viscosity of MCA are likely to increase the rate of bilateral entry. It may be necessary to counterbalance improved spreadability by other changes in the FEMCEPT/MCA system, such as the volume of the application, however, since spreadability appears also to be accompanied by a deeper penetration into the fallopian tube and peritoneal spillage may be an undesirable side-effect. Our group is exploring changes in some of the inhibitor additives that will increase spreadability and potentially enhance entry rates.

Our operating hypothesis since the early animal experiments with MCA has been that if the chemical enters the fallopian tubes, it will produce closure.[6] This belief was derived from studies of MCA in the rabbit, rat, and monkey in our laboratory, and was confirmed in a limited number of monkey studies by the World Health Organization as well. Our belief, based principally on the experience in the People's Republic of China with phenol-based chemical occlusive preparations, was that the length of tubal entry would also be an important factor in determining tubal closure rates, a hypothesis that also was consistent with data derived from electrocoagulated fallopian tubes at the time of laparoscopic sterilization.[3] Our experience with radiopaque MCA now indicates that tubal closure does not always follow tubal entry, even when the MCA extends the full length of the fallopian tube (see Chapter 27). Thus, we are seeking a better understanding of the mechanisms through which MCA produces tubal closure, so as to be able to manipulate those factors that can be identified as important in enhancing the tube-closing ability of this substance. It is probable that certain additives will enhance the tube-closing effectiveness of MCA, as will certain changes in MCA handling and packaging.

It is evident that radiopaque MCA offers the possibility to study the dynamics of the system in clinical use. We plan to undertake additional studies using cinehysterosalpingography to determine the mechanism responsible for the failure of MCA to penetrate the tube and to correct the problem. We hope to obtain an MCA that is sufficiently radiopaque to permit consistent detection of tubal entry by means of a postapplication abdominal roentgenogram. Thus, if the tube-closing ability of the MCA can be improved sufficiently, it should be possible, at the time of the procedure, to distinguish those patients in whom bilateral closure is virtually ensured from those in whom tubal closure is unlikely. The latter group can then undergo a second treatment.

The ability to detect tubal entry and have it equivalent to tubal closure would vastly enhance the utility of the method, particularly in developed countries where access to radiologic facilities is widely available. Investigators are attempting to make the MCA more radiopaque, and preliminary studies suggest that at least a 50% enhancement over the prior product can be achieved (see Chapter 27).

Using the nonradiopaque MCA, we produced a 78% bilateral closure rate after a single application in 102 women. Using the radiopaque formulation, we increased the closure rate to 87%. The study of salpingitis spontaneously occurring in women, and animal data, indicate that the tubal closure rate is significantly enhanced by prolonged or repeated exposure to MCA. In an attempt to enhance the closure rates, we treated a series of patients with two applications of nonradiopaque MCA and produced a bilateral closure rate of approximately 87%. This rate was identical to the bilateral closure rate achieved with a single application of the radiopaque MCA.

In a further attempt to enhance the tubal closure rates, we changed the clinical protocol, rather than manipulating the FEMCEPT/MCA system. Patients who had experienced unilateral or bilateral failures after the first application elected to be re-treated, and a bilateral closure of 90% was achieved on the second application. This biased sample may not be representative of the patient population as a whole, however.

Theoretically, if the same closure rates achieved in this self-selected cohort would be achieved for all women treated with the FEMCEPT/MCA system, a bilateral closure rate of 98% to 99% would be expected after two applications. It was surprising, therefore, that a rate of only 87% was achieved in women who were treated with two applications 1 month apart. Possibly, the lower-than-expected bilateral closure rate was due to factors related principally to the interval that was chosen (1 month), as the theoretically calculated rate of 97% was achieved at a 4-month interval.

It can be argued that if the application is repeated after only 1 month, tubal edema, tubal inflammation, or, indeed, remaining polymerized MCA may prevent the new application of MCA from reaching the fallopian tubes and may thereby diminish effectiveness. It is also possible that the results of a second application would be enhanced by allowing the full measure of tubal fibrosis to occur prior to the second insult. These factors may account for the differences in the closure rates in the two series in which double applications were spaced by 1 month rather than 4 months.

In order to evaluate whether this is a real difference, we have planned a study in which women will be recruited *ab initio* to a two-application protocol that all participants would be expected to complete, thus eliminating the bias of self-selection. We also plan to vary the interval between applications on a consecutively assigned basis; one third of the study group will receive the applications at 2-month intervals, one third at 3-month intervals, and one third at 4-month intervals. With this protocol, we should answer the question of whether a prolongation of the intervals significantly enhances bilateral closure.

We also plan to continue the long-term study of patients treated with MCA who have bilateral tubal closure, by hysterosalpingography. The few pregnancies that have occurred thus far have all been intrauterine. Because of the time intervals involved, however, it is not clear whether these pregnancies resulted from open tubes that were not demonstrated by hysterosalpingography or from recanalization. We need additional data to be certain that the long-term effectiveness is as promising as the short-term results and that no deleterious sequelae will develop much later.

We are encouraged by the lack of significant morbidity or major side-effects in the large group of women treated by the FEMCEPT/MCA system. We are also encouraged that virtually all centers have attained statistically indistinguishable results, despite a very short-term training program (seldom exceeding 1 day). Also, the data seem not to change significantly with increasing experience. The procedure is simple to learn, simple to teach, and simple to apply. It can readily be accomplished on an outpatient basis after minimal training, and the result seems not to be operator dependent. Because it is a truly outpatient procedure, because it does not require sophisticated endoscopic or back-up techniques, and because it appears to be highly acceptable to women, we believe that even at the present levels of bilateral closure, it has a place in the "cafeteria" of contraceptive methods. The method has yet to reach optimal effectiveness, although the safety and convenience are now well established. A number of enhancements must be applied, and the bilateral closure rate must be increased significantly, to broaden the population to which the method is applicable. We believe that within the next several years, the method can be developed so that it will become one of the mainstays of family planning programs.

REFERENCES

1. NEUWIRTH RS, RICHART RM, BOLDUC LR: Clinical trials with the single application fertility regulating device. Am J Obstet Gynecol 129:348–349, 1977
2. NEUWIRTH RS, RICHART RM, STEVENSON TC et al: An outpatient approach to female sterilization with methylcyanoacrylate. Am J Obstet Gynecol 136:51–54, 1971
3. PHILLIPS JM, KEITH L (eds): Gynecological Laparoscopy: Principles and Techniques. New York, Stratton Intercontinental, 1974
4. RICHART RM: Female sterilization using chemical agents. In Zatuchni GI (ed): Research Frontiers in Fertility Regulation, vol 1, no 5, December 1981. Chicago, Program for Applied Research on Fertility Regulation
5. RICHART RM, NEUWIRTH RS, BOLDUC LR: Single application fertility regulating device: Description of a new instrument. Am J Obstet Gynecol 127:86–90, 1977
6. RICHART RM, TAYLOR HC, NEUWIRTH RS: Experimental studies of fallopian tube occlusion. In Richart RM, Prager D (eds): Human Sterilization, pp 360–367. Springfield, IL, Charles C Thomas, 1972

29

Discussion: Research and Clinical Experience With MCA

DEAN L. MOYER

ROBERT S. NEUWIRTH

JACQUES E. RIOUX, MODERATORS

IN THE TOXICOLOGY STUDIES OF MCA, IS FORMALDEHYDE AN INTERMEDIATE IN THE POLYMERIZATION PROCESS?

Formaldehyde is used to make the initial material, but only in the very early phase of organic synthesis, not in polymerization. There is no formaldehyde in the product used in the studies under discussion. For use as a medical product, MCA requires extensive purification, and at present the impurity level of MCA is only a half of a part per million.

WHAT ARE THE MUTAGENICITY AND TERATOGENICITY FINDINGS WITH MCA?

No one as yet knows how to run a meaningful mutagenicity test on MCA, even after 12 years of research to that end. As for teratogenicity, of the 5000 teratogenicity tests, none is known for MCA; however, no teratogenic effects have been observed clinically.

IN AN INTRAPERITONEAL SPILL, WOULD MCA CAUSE AN ACUTE REACTION SIMILAR TO THAT SEEN WITH QUINACRINE?

The intraperitoneal LD_{50} is in the same order of magnitude as quinacrine, and an intraperitoneal spill of MCA would have a similar acute effect. In the mouse, necrosis and fibrosis may occur, as with any intraperitoneal admin-

---

Panelists: Lee Bolduc, Manoel Bomfim de Souza Filho, Robert E. Krall, Nargesh D. Motashaw, Ralph M. Richart, Itic Zighelboim. *Discussants:* Ruben A. Apelo, David A. Blake, Jan Brundin, Jay M. Cooper, Elsimar M. Coutinho, Enrique Guiloff, Rene Guzman-Serani, Harrith M. Hasson, Douglas Huber, Miriam H. Labbok, Leonard E. Laufe, Suman Mehta, Per Agnar Nilsen, Tim H. Parmley, Earle W. Wilson, Gerald I. Zatuchni

istration, and because the bowel has so small a diameter, and the bowel wall is so thin, the viscus can be ruptured. But with any animal larger than a mouse, the wall is of significant size that the necrosis is only superficial and only a few adhesions occur, unless a bolus forms that is of sufficient size to erode through the abdominal wall. The reason is that MCA polymerizes, and once it becomes a spherule, it does not cause tissue adhesion.

Studies with intraperitoneal MCA administration performed under World Health Organization (WHO) auspices in 220 prehysterectomy patients resulted in only a few localized adhesions, usually fewer than occur with a surgical procedure, because cutting, tying, and burning are well-known producers of adhesions. Also, in these 220 patients, in only two or three instances did the MCA moisten the fimbria; in only one was there actually spillage—in a patient who was 65 years old, with tubes about 1 cm long.

In a study done in the Philippines, in which the abdomens of subjects were opened following treatment, there was one case of spillage of polymerized MCA into the pelvic cavity. The MCA looked like snowflakes on the surface of the uterus and bladder, and the flakes could actually be blown away; they did not adhere to the surface.

Certainly, the patients in whom peritoneal spill is known to have occurred should be carefully monitored for several years.

WHAT IS THE POSSIBILITY OF UTERINE PERFORATION WITH THE FEMCEPT DEVICE?

Actually, the instrument itself tends to protect against perforation. In the WHO studies, the tip of the instrument occasionally penetrated the superficial myometrium, and so there was deposition of the MCA into the muscle, but the device never completely penetrated the uterus.

However, even if the uterus were speared and the entire contents of the ampule were injected into the intraperitoneal cavity, only 0.3 ml of the material actually would be dumped, perhaps causing a few intestinal adhesions, especially of the sigmoid colon or cecum, and the possibility of intestinal adhesions among small bowel loops would exist. The problem comes not from penetration but from the local action of the material on the bowel wall. The dose is very small, however, and the action is limited by the instantaneous polymerization that occurs.

The risk of penetration with the device is probably in the same range as the risk of penetration of the uterus during an IUD insertion (approximately 1/1000). However, the perforation would presumably occur before the device had been actuated, and the device is also different from an IUD insertion in that the balloon provides resistance to the penetration.

The possibility of penetration was tested extensively with uterine specimens removed at hysterectomy, and when the investigator held the uterus and tried to perforate it with the device, considerable effort was required; a forceful stabbing motion was necessary for penetration, and usually the tip snapped off. The cannula is extremely flexible and was designed to snap off when too much pressure is put on it. In a postpartum patient, however, perforation probably would be fairly easily done.

UNDER WHAT CIRCUMSTANCES DID THE TWO PERFORATIONS REPORTED IN THE BRAZIL STUDY OCCUR, AND WHAT WERE THE CONSEQUENCES?

The two probable perforations occurred at the time the balloon was expanded, and the operator had the feeling that the device went further than the uterine fundus. The patients were kept in the hospital under observation and showed no untoward effects. No laparoscopic evaluation was undertaken at the time, so it was not proved that the perforations had in fact occurred. The two patients are being carefully followed, however.

The incidence of perforations with the FEMCEPT device will probably decrease with training, as is the case with the IUD. The two perforations occurred in the first group of 120 patients; in the second 140, there were no perforations.

HAS MCA BEEN ACCIDENTALLY APPLIED INTRAVASCULARLY?

In several patients, when radiopaque dyes were used, uterine intravasation occurred, but the material polymerized instantly and no sequelae were reported. The cyanoacrylates have been used intravascularly by vascular surgeons to stop bleeding, but use of methyl cyanoacrylate was discontinued, because once the bleeding stopped, the MCA produced tissue necrosis and eroded the vascular wall.

The difference between the intraperitoneal administration of this material and quinacrine is that the MCA stays in place; it does not circulate, the degradation is completely localized, and the elimination is rapid. There are no systemic effects, and no tissue levels are detectable.

WHAT ENDOMETRIAL LESIONS ARE SEEN FOLLOWING MCA INJECTION?

The effect of MCA on the endometrium has been studied by Stevenson and associates, who put 5 ml MCA (a very large amount) into the endometrial cavity and did subsequent serial studies of the uteri. These studies revealed only superficial necrosis, about five cells deep, and a local acute inflammatory response. No sequelae were histologically or clinically demonstrable.

In almost 1000 patients who have undergone hysterosalpingograms following instillation of MCA, no signs of injury, intrauterine synechiae, or peritoneal problems have been seen. In a limited number of patients having laparoscopy or laparotomy observation after an MCA application, no significant effects have been seen.

WHAT EFFECT WOULD MCA HAVE ON THE UTERINE CAVITY OF WOMEN USING INJECTABLE CONTRACEPTIVES—WOMEN WHO HAVE AN EXTREMELY THIN ENDOMETRIUM?

No significant effects on the endometrial cavity have been found in any patients. Whether high doses of progestin might potentiate the MCA effect by inhibiting epithelial regeneration is not known.

HAS THERE BEEN ANY PROBLEM IN REMOVING THE BALLOON FROM THE UTERINE CAVITY?

If the balloon collapses precipitously, it should be easily removed, because the balloon is coated with silicone oil and the MCA adhesive does not attach itself rapidly to the balloon. The MCA is a brittle material, and it can be pulled away quite easily. In four or five cases, apparently owing to a defect in the balloon, a little chunk of rubber may have remained inside the uterine cavity. However, in none of these cases were there any significant sequelae, and apparently the small piece of rubber subsequently was passed out of the uterus.

IS AN ALTERNATIVE CONTRACEPTIVE REQUIRED FOLLOWING INSTILLATION UNTIL FIBROSIS IS ASSURED?

It is not certain that an alternative contraceptive is necessary immediately following instillation. The MCA system has never been tested during the period of fibrosis. One would assume that if the material got into the tube at all, it would have formed a physical plug.

In programmatic terms, putting a patient on an interval means of contraception following treatment would be undesirable; the woman should be able to have the injection and then go home with the assurance that the procedure has been successful.

WHAT IS THE PROBABILITY OF DOING THE PROCEDURE ON A WOMAN WITH ASYMPTOMATIC SALPINGITIS?

In clinical studies, efforts to exclude such women have been made by means of history and pelvic examination, and thus far, no such case has been reported. Theoretically, it is possible; but based on present experience, it would be a rare occurrence.

IS THERE ANY DANGER OF DOUBLING THE DOSE OF MCA ON ONE SIDE IF THE BALLOON DOES NOT FORCE THE FLUID INTO THE SECOND TUBE?

There is no chance that the balloon will fail to force the fluid into the second tube and that all of the MCA will go into one tube, because the balloon moves forward so rapidly (it expands in 1/125th of a second), then tents up and isolates the fluid on either side. When one tube is blocked, the fluid simply stays in the cornu; it cannot cross over onto the other side. Then, once the balloon deflates, there is no more pressure, and by this time the material already has a skin of polymerization on it. In evaluation of the procedure, on over 200 salpingograms using cinofluoroscopy, no dose was doubled on one side.

HAVE ANY STUDIES LOOKED AT THE TISSUE RESPONSE TO MCA IN WOMEN WHO HAVE USED LONG-TERM CONTRACEPTIVE STEROIDS, EITHER THE ORAL COMBINED ESTROGEN-PROGESTOGEN PILLS OR THE INJECTABLES?

The tissue response has never been studied prospectively, but retrospectively the data have been evaluated on self-selected patients who have used oral contraceptives, IUDs, condoms and diaphragms, and long-term injectable contraceptives, particularly Depo-Provera. No significant differences in effectiveness or in side-effects have been seen in any of these groups.

WILL A CHEMICAL STERILIZATION TECHNIQUE THAT REQUIRES MORE THAN A SINGLE INJECTION BE ACCEPTABLE IN THE DEVELOPING WORLD?

In a hospital in Chile, where both the MCA/FEMCEPT technique and regular laparoscopic sterilization were offered, approximately 10 patients a day request laparoscopic sterilization, but a much larger number of patients request the nonoperative sterilization that does not require anesthesia, and at least twice the required number of patients volunteered to participate in an MCA/FEMCEPT study, even though it required two shots.

However the goal is to find a single-application technique that does not require follow-up and can be simply delivered in rural areas.

HOW USEFUL IS HYSTEROSALPINGOGRAPHY IN PREDICTING BILATERAL OCCLUSION?

Hysterosalpingography is expensive and discomforting to both the patient and the physician, and unfortunately, in some cases it may indicate occluded tubes but the patient still becomes pregnant. Of 53 women who had a radiopaque MCA application, and had flat plate roentgenograms immediately before and immediately after the instillation, 40 of the 53 (75%) showed bilateral entry of the MCA; of the 40 who showed bilateral entry, 36 (90%) subsequently were found to have closed tubes at hysterosalpingography; four patients who presumably had MCA blockage on both sides did not. Two investigators viewed the films, and neither was able to predict accurately in every case. When the investigators did not see the MCA in one or the other tube, 77% of the patients were subsequently found to have closure. Thus, although the hysterosalpingogram is reasonably reliable at showing occlusion, it is not adequately reliable.

Investigators hope to significantly improve the radiopacity of the MCA, so that it will show the key point of closure, the isthmus. In the patients in whom MCA was not seen in a tube and later the tube proved to be closed, the assumption is that the MCA could not be seen in the narrow portion, but was in fact effectively producing closure.

In a computer evaluation of covariables in over 1000 accumulated cases, investigators looked at the closure rates when hysterosalpingography was done at 1 month, 2 months, and up to 6 months after the procedure, and the closure rates went steadily up with time following the procedure; they never evened out. This suggests that hysterosalpingography itself may open up a number of tubes that were in fact closed, especially when it is done soon after the treatment, by "blasting" open some of the fragile granulation tissue. Importantly, it should be noted that "open" tubes do not necessarily mean functioning tubes.

The MCA/FEMCEPT method, when it becomes available in the field, will not use hysterosalpingograms as part of the clinical therapy. The hysterosalpingograms are only for the purposes of research protocol.

WHAT IS THE CLOSURE RATE WITH ONE APPLICATION VERSUS THE RATE WITH TWO APPLICATIONS?

Among the small number of patients (about 30) treated with two applications of radiopaque MCA, the bilateral closure rate was about 98%; with a single application, the closure rate was about 90%. The confidence level presently used for the two-application technique is 95%.

WHAT ARE THE PHARMACOLOGIC AND ENGINEERING CONSTRAINTS WITH THE PRESENT DEVICE FOR USING A GREATER VOLUME OF MCA OR ANOTHER INGREDIENT IN THE MIXTURE?

Originally, investigators were working with a total of 0.45 ml MCA, and they are now using up to 0.6 ml. As larger-scale clinical testing begins, if dose response becomes an issue, it will be possible to increase the volume of the material in the ampule until the most effective dose is established.

Several volumes have been evaluated, and not much difference in effect was seen; however, investigators are now using 0.6 ml, and this volume seems to be effective in filling the entire lumen. Even if a larger volume is used, and advances farther into the tube, because the MCA normally sets in 1 to 2 seconds, the polymerization is likely to occur at the same rate, thereby preventing the MCA from reaching the peritoneal cavity.

WHAT HAS BEEN LEARNED WITH DYNAMIC TESTS USING RADIOPAQUE MCA?

In one small ongoing project in Chile, investigators are using radiopaque MCA to improve the knowledge of the dynamics of this substance in the fallopian tubes. For that purpose, 10 patients meeting all protocol requirements were chosen. Following oral administration of 10 mg diazepam, the MCA/FEMCEPT radiopaque procedure was performed under fluoroscopy and taped on a videosystem.

With this dynamic system, the entrance of the material was shown to be instantaneous; and after 1 or 2 seconds, the rest of the fallopian tube became visible. Usually after about 20 seconds, the material is no longer moving. This is in contrast to some of the earlier studies using materials whose viscosity did not change, such as Sinografin and other radiopaque dyes, where the material flowed out of the tube.

Another point brought out by the dynamic study is that the material in the cornual areas may be affected by the withdrawal of the instrument, so it would appear that a 30-second interval prior to instrument withdrawal is desirable, even though entry is probably complete within seconds.

WHAT EFFECT WOULD ANTISPASMODIC AGENTS HAVE IN COUNTERING THE TUBAL SPASM RESPONSIBLE FOR SOME PROCEDURE FAILURES?

A multicentered study, performed under the auspices of WHO, looked at the FEMCEPT device used with Sinografin instead of MCA in 140 subjects, and bilateral tubal entry was found in 73% of cases. Conventional hysterosalpingography may give a discrepancy of perhaps 10%, but not 25% or 27% as in this case, so some of these failures might be considered procedure failures. In an attempt to overcome these procedure failures, the WHO investigators used tubal spasmolytic agents, especially glucagon, randomly allocated to control subjects (saline) for the relaxation of tubal spasm. The glucagon did not work; no difference was seen between the two groups. However, other compounds might be examined, either the nonsteroidal anti-inflammatory drugs, which block prostaglandin synthesis, or the β-sympathomimetic drugs, which act as uterine relaxants. Both of these have the programmatic advantage of being able to be taken orally and are effective within an hour of ingestion.

HOW CAN PAIN BE AVOIDED DURING MCA INSTILLATION?

Pain on uterine manipulation during the MCA/FEMCEPT method occurs at three points: (1) in negotiating the internal cervical os, (2) in touching the fundus, and (3) in the distention of the balloon. For the first two, topical uterine anesthesia might be useful. One investigator has used a simple method, which although not widely accepted, has been effective in preventing pain and postinsertion cramping following IUD insertion and in hysterosalpinography and dilation and curettage. With this method, 1 ml to 2 ml 2% lidocaine is held in the uterus for 4 minutes, the latency period of the drug, and is prevented from leaking out of the cervix with an acorn type of adaptor. This simple addition appears to lessen the pain associated with the MCA instillation.

CAN THE FEMCEPT DEVICE BE SAFELY APPLIED BY PEOPLE WHO ARE NOT PHYSICIANS?

The technique itself is easily mastered, but the careful selection of patients is crucial; the patient who has pelvic inflammatory disease or some other problem must not be treated with the MCA/FEMCEPT method, and whether the nonphysician could effectively make such diagnostic evaluations is not known. For now, the device should probably be applied only by physicians.

WHAT IS THE ANTICIPATED COST OF THE MCA/FEMCEPT DEVICE? WILL IT BE TOO EXPENSIVE FOR PROGRAMMATIC USE IN DEVELOPING COUNTRIES?

The manufacturers are attempting to keep the cost as low as possible; the device is made of a very inexpensive plastic, it is high-speed injection molded, and as volumes go up, the cost should come down rapidly. But at this time, the exact cost is not known.

Unless a disposable applicator can be developed, the present device will probably be too expensive for use in developing countries. The developers are pursuing a design in which the tip is detachable and can be disposed of. This should not only lower the cost but also facilitate cleaning. The cannula is plastic, and any solvents used to dissolve the MCA will also dissolve the cannula. A device with a disposable tip and a reusable handle will cost considerably less, but just how much will be highly volume dependent. Obviously, if millions of devices are made, with the plastic molding machine running night and day, the cost can be mere pennies, and if developing countries have the capability to assemble it, the component parts can be shipped to them, cutting the labor cost even more.

Another aspect of cost is malfunction of the device, so that more than one device is needed to complete a single treatment. With the present FEMCEPT device, of 125 procedures in one series, four FEMCEPT devices failed to work properly on the pretest and a second one was required.

HAS THE FEMCEPT DEVICE BEEN USED FOR OTHER APPLICATIONS BESIDES MCA INSTILLATION?

A modified version of the instrument has been useful in isolating and studying the tubes and measuring the pressures at the tubal openings, in the search for tubal relaxing agents. Tubal relaxing agents have been evaluated using cinefluoroscopy and measuring the number of frames between injection of the dye and the time of entry into both tubes.

The device could work also for delivering medications to the fallopian tubes. It has not proved useful for hysterosalpingograms, however.

WHAT IS THE EXPERIENCE WITH MCA IN CANADA?

In one series of 20 patients in whom two injections using regular MCA were planned, only one patient did not return for the second injection, because she said that the first one had been too painful. She accepted hysterosalpingography, however, and the tubes were closed.

In another 30 patients in whom the radiopaque MCA was used, the material was warmed beforehand, and because it was more fluid it seemed to go into the tubes more easily and effectively.

If the material were more radiopaque, patients could have the injection in the office, have a flat plate roentgenogram, and go home. Then if both tubes were shown to be satisfactorily injected on the flat plate, the chances of bilateral closure would be good and the woman would not need to return for a second injection.

The response of two patients with regard to pain was instructive; the women, nurses working in the same hospital, underwent exactly the same procedure, performed by the same operator, one after the other. One woman experienced no pain, and the other had pain sufficient to require meperidine. The difference in their responses to the procedure had not been anticipated.

WHAT HAS BEEN THE EXPERIENCE WITH MCA IN CHILE?

In comparative studies in Chile between MCA and quinacrine pellet insertions, 150 cases were done with quinacrine pellets and 197 cases were done with MCA (143 with nonradiopaque MCA and 54 with radiopaque MCA). In the Chilean experience, the MCA procedure was painful for the patients, and with the exception of the first three or four cases, analgesia was used (10 mg diazepam, 0.5 mg atropine, 50 mg meperidine intravenously, 10 minutes prior to application), which meant that women required at least 2 or 3 hours rest before they could go home. When the quinacrine pellets were used, the procedure was painless and the women could be discharged within a few minutes after completion of the procedure.

Regarding the management of the device used for each method, the insertion procedure of the quinacrine pellet, done with the simple plastic tubes similar to those used for insertion of an IUD, is simple and easily performed, even by paramedical persons. The FEMCEPT device used for MCA applications could be used only by physicians.

In the Chilean experience, the principal problem with the quinacrine pellet procedure has been that at least three insertions at 1-month intervals are needed for a good sterilization rate, which is a drawback in programmatic use. However, the Chilean investigators obtained over 98% of tubal occlusions with three insertions. With radiopaque MCA, using two applications, the rate was approximately 90%. Thus, the Chilean investigators concluded that the quinacrine pellet method was better, because it gave a better rate of tubal closure; it was less expensive, less painful, and more easily performed by a general practitioner or paramedical person.

WHAT IS THE EXPERIENCE WITH MCA IN INDIA?

The Indian experience with radiopaque MCA has been limited; as of the end of April 1982, only 66 subjects had been treated, all between the ages of 21 and 40, with 75% being between the ages of 26 and 35, the targeted group for making a demographic impact. Insertion was easily accomplished in 61 women (92.4%). Difficulty was encountered in six cases, when the woman had a retroverted uterus or when resistance was felt at the internal os.

In one woman, the balloon ruptured in the uterus and stuck to the uterine wall and considerable manipulation was necessary before the device could be removed. In six subjects, the balloon was visible in the cervical canal. These cases may be explained by the fact that the uterus is not a uniform organ and should be measured differentially—the endometrial cavity versus the cervical canal. For example, if the balloon is 2 cm or 2.5 cm and the endometrial cavity is less than that, then some of the balloon will be seen in the cervix. Also, the operator may not have inserted the device fully into the endometrial cavity—beyond the internal os.

In one center in southern India, where the temperature averages 100°F and the humidity is very high, the plastic of some of the FEMCEPT devices broke and gave way at the seams. Also, the color of the drug in some of the ampules has changed to yellow or pink. These effects may have resulted from the exceptionally high temperatures and humidity.

Postprocedure flat plate roentgenograms, which were taken in 66 cases, showed bilateral blockage in 66% of cases and unilateral blockage in 15%. Of the 17 patients who subsequently underwent hysterosalpingography, one patient was found to have a patent tube on one side and agreed to a second instillation; the other 16 patients had bilateral blockage.

In general, the investigators and the subjects have found the procedure simple and acceptable.

WHAT IS THE EXPERIENCE WITH MCA IN THE PHILIPPINES?

In a Philippine study performed over the past 2 years, MCA has been blindly injected by means of the FEMCEPT device in 66 women seeking permanent contraception, and many of the women have now completed 2 years of follow-up. Among the women, the results of the procedure have varied. The very first patient had only one tube occluded, and the second patient became pregnant even before the scheduled 4-month hysterogram. Then there were seven consecutive bilateral closures, and among the first 24 procedures the closure rate was 81%. Then, in a period of 2 weeks, seven consecutive patients had open tubes. After the 45th patient, the closure rate was 65%; and after 66 patients, it was 64.6%. One pregnancy followed what was at first interpreted on the hysterosalpingogram as bilateral closure but at a second reading showed one patent tube.

At the 12-month follow-up, another patient, who on hysterosalpingography was shown to have bilateral tubal closure, was found to have an unrelated adenocarcinoma. Histologic studies showed that one tube was open.

Among the 10 patients who agreed to have a second instillation, bilateral closure was 100%.

In the first 11 patients, no analgesia was required, but some patients complained of hypogastric discomfort and were easily relieved with mild medication.

The Philippine investigators feel the need for more information about the ideal time interval between instillations but indicate that if the closure rate can be maintained at 95% or above (using pregnancy as the criterion of success, not hysterosalpingography), this procedure should be applicable for programmatic use. Although the double application is not ideal, it will be acceptable until an equivalent rate of occlusion is achieved with a single instillation.

WHAT IS THE EXPERIENCE WITH MCA IN NORWAY?

Oslo investigators have had considerable experience with MCA, not only in terms of numbers of cases but also in length of time. During the past 3 years, 277 procedures with MCA have been performed in 250 patients, some having one instillation, some two, some preinjection uterine lavage, and some radiopaque MCA.

In one series of 103 procedures, 82 resulted in bilateral occlusion with one instillation, giving a success rate of 80% (82/103). Of the 14 patients who elected to have a second instillation, 12 achieved bilateral occlusion, raising the success rate to 91.2% (94/103). The remaining seven patients chose laparoscopic sterilization rather than a second MCA instillation; had they also accepted the second instillation, the closure rate would probably have risen to 98%, based on the other success rate.

Of the 42 patients treated with radiopaque MCA, 35 have been examined roentgenographically so far, and 28 (80%) have bilateral closure. Five of them had a second instillation, and three of the five obtained bilateral occlusion, increasing the success rate to 88.6%.

One interesting case involved a patient who on the first instillation clearly showed both tubes filled with radiopaque material, but nevertheless, the left tube was open on the hysterosalpingogram. With a second instillation, the left tube was properly filled, and this time bilateral closure was achieved. Why the woman did not respond the first time and did the second time is not known.

The acceptability of this method in Norway is good. It is rapid, requiring only a few minutes, and the woman can leave the hospital and go home. There are some side-effects and pain the first or second day, but there have been no serious adverse effects. An indication of the acceptability is that 50% of the patients with a failure elected to have the same method a second time. Some patients returned with friends who also requested the method, and some area physicians have also applied for MCA sterilizations.

30

Clinical Application of Hysteroscopic Sterilization Using Uterotubal Junction Blocking Devices

ABDOL H. HOSSEINIAN

WILSON A. MORALES

The clinical application of operative hysteroscopy to reach the uterotubal junction (UTJ) for sterilization purposes has been explored by a number of investigators.[1,4–7]

Electrocoagulation and chemical and mechanical occlusion of the tubal lumen have all been tested. Although the hysteroscopic techniques eliminate the need for general anesthesia, and they do not invade the peritoneal cavity or leave abdominal scars, the failure rates of such procedures have been unacceptably high. Minor and major complications have also been associated with some of the methods.[4]

During the past 8 years, we have been exploring the effectiveness of mechanically blocking the tubal ostia through hysteroscopy by means of UTJ blocking devices that can be implanted in or removed from the tubal ostia by a device carrier. The reversibility potential of the procedure has been one of the objectives of the project design. Since these experiments have been described elsewhere,[2,3] we will only briefly summarize them here.

MATERIALS

UTJ BLOCKING DEVICES

We have designed, manufactured, and used two types of devices (Fig. 30-1). The original device was made of polyethylene and measured approximately 10 mm in length, with a diameter of 1 mm at the tip and 2 mm at the base. Since the polyethylene plug was quite rigid and the possibility of tissue injury and tubal perforation was feared, we subsequently changed the composition of the plug to silicone rubber. The silicone plugs are cone-shaped, measuring 1 mm or less at the tip and increasing to about 2 mm at the base. The length of the device varies from 7 mm (small) to 9 mm (large).

Two metallic components are attached to the plugs: (1) Four anchoring spines, delicately made of elgiloy, serve to fix and keep the device in place by penetrating the adjacent myometrium; and (2) the assembly screw, made of stainless steel, attaches the anchoring spines to the plug and provides a grasping base for the device carrier.

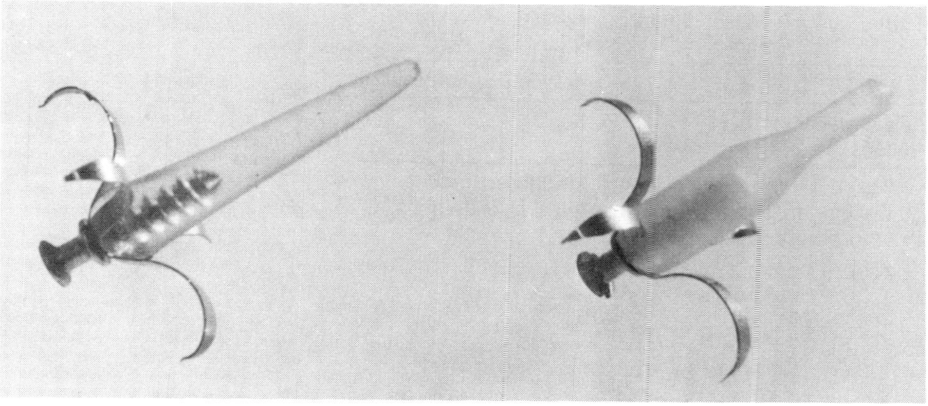

FIG. 30-1. Uterotubal junction blocking devices. (*Left*) Silicone device. (*Right*) Polyethylene device.

DEVICE CARRIER

The device carrier is also made of stainless steel and consists of three components: (1) tip with three grasping teeth, (2) shaft, and (3) handle. It is so designed as to carry a device through the hysteroscope and implant it in, as well as remove it from, the UTJs.

PRIMATE STUDIES

Hysteroscopic implantation and removal of the devices in primates has been described.[2,3] The efficacy of the device for contraception has been 100% in 21 baboons for a minimum of eight breedings (Table 30-1). The reversibility potential of our technique was tested by hysteroscopic removal of the device in 15 baboons. Eight animals became pregnant, achieving a total of 12 pregnancies (Table 30-2).

TABLE 30-1. Results of Hysteroscopic Implantation of Devices in 21 Baboons*

FACTOR	RESULT
Failures	1 (one-sided)
Duration of implantation	8–27 months
Pregnancies	None
Expulsions	
Polyethylene	None
Silicone	2 animals

*Polyethylene devices were implanted in 7 animals, and silicone devices were implanted in 14 animals.

TABLE 30-2. Reversal of Fertility After Hysteroscopic Removal of Devices From 15 Baboons*

TYPE OF DEVICE	NO. PREGNANCIES†
Polyethylene	3
Silicone	5

*Polyethylene devices were implanted in 6 animals and silicone devices were implanted in 9 animals. One to 18 breeding cycles were required.

†There were 12 pregnancies in 8 animals.

Since the fertility rate of baboons in our breeding colony has been estimated at 72%,* the reversal of fertility potential should be placed at 74%.

No early or late side-effects were noted in any of the animals, either after implantation of the devices or after their removal. The extent of tissue reaction around the plugs was minimal, with no difference between the polyethylene and silicone plugs. Conception after the removal of the devices progressed normally, and the offspring subsequently born were physically normal in all aspects.

CLINICAL TRIALS

PHASE I

Clinical trials have been conducted in two phases. During phase I, we investigated the capability of polyethylene and silicone plugs to occlude the UTJs and evaluated the extent of tissue reaction and the resumption of patency of the tubes after device removal. The technique and the detailed results of this phase of the study can be found in our previous report.[3] Since our 33 subjects were all scheduled for hysterectomy for various gynecologic conditions, we could observe the efficacy of the procedure for only a short time (2 to 6 months). Effective closure was achieved in 91% of the tubes; one pregnancy occurred.

All of the devices remained *in situ* for the entire period of the study. No side-effects were reported. In addition to expansion of the tubal lumen and flattening of the endosalpingeal cells, there was minimal to moderate tissue reaction around the anchoring spines. Ninety percent of the tubes regained their patency after device removal from 20 women. We encountered some difficulty in proper implantation of the devices in approximately 15% of the human subjects in whom the ostia were too laterally situated. This problem appeared to be related to our straight, rigid hysteroscope.

PHASE II

After completion of encouraging animal trials and acceptable preliminary short-term human trials, we investigated the long-term efficacy of the method

---

*Beluhan FZ, Director of Primate Colony, The University of Illinois: Personal communication, 1978.

in well-informed volunteers as a permanent sterilization procedure with reasonable reversibility potential. This phase of the project was carried out at Cook County Hospital, Chicago, Illinois. From January 1980 to January 1981, 11 volunteers underwent hysteroscopic device implantation.

During this phase, the procedure was performed under paracervical block by using 1% mepivacaine solution and preoperative intravenous administration of 5 mg diazepam and 50 mg meperidine. The procedure was performed in the follicular phase of the woman's cycle. For irrigation and expansion of the uterine cavity, 10% dextran in 5% dextrose solution was used in the first seven procedures. This solution provided better expansion of the uterine cavity and easier visualization of the tubal ostia. Because of a major complication (pulmonary edema) associated with its use in patient No. 7, this solution was replaced by 5% dextrose in water in the subsequent procedures. The difficulty in visualizing and entering the left tubal ostium in this patient made the procedure unusually long, necessitating excessive irrigation of the uterine cavity. This individual has so far been the only subject in whom the procedure was performed unilaterally. All of the others tolerated the procedure quite well and showed no early or late side-effects. The patients were ambulated shortly after the completion of the procedure and were allowed to go home after 2 hours.

Proper implantation of the device in some of the subjects was difficult, owing mainly to the rigidity of our hysteroscope. Proper implantation can be achieved only by bringing the device and the tip of the carrier in parallel with the tubal lumen at the uterine cornua (Fig. 30-2). Assumption of this position can be difficult or impossible if the tubal ostium is too laterally situated. To compare the efficacy of the two types of devices, we implanted the silicone plugs in the right and the polyethylene plugs in the left UTJs in the same subjects.

The patients used oral contraceptive steroids after the procedure for a period of 3 months, and the contraception was discontinued after hysterosalpingography confirmed bilateral tubal occlusion.

Five patients developed intrauterine pregnancy. Two of the patients did not follow the protocol and failed to take their contraceptive steroids (patients No. 3 and No. 10); they became pregnant before the condition of the tubes could be evaluated by hysterosalpingography. The failures in the other three patients (No. 5, No. 6, and No. 8) should be considered technical failures.

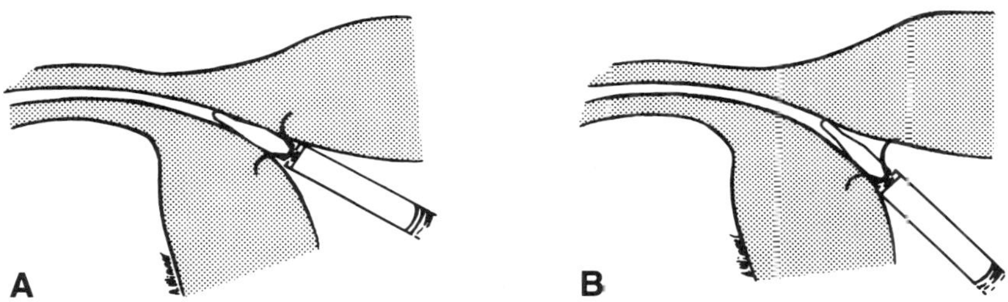

FIG. 30-2. Proper (*A*) and improper (*B*) alignment of the device and the tip of the carrier at the time of device implantation.

These three patients, despite bilateral tubal occlusion documented by hysterosalpingography, missed their menstrual periods somewhere from 9 to 16 months following the procedure. Subsequent tubal investigation in these patients revealed unilateral tubal patency (Table 30-3). Three of these pregnancies were terminated by suction curettage, and the other two patients chose to continue their pregnancies. These two pregnancies have since ended in vaginal deliveries. Although both of the infants were free of any congenital anomalies, they were both born approximately 6 weeks before term, one weighing 3 lb, 11 oz (patient No. 8) and the other weighing 4 lb, 3 oz (patient No. 10).

No significant differences were observed between the silicone and polyethylene plugs. Except in patient No. 3, who lost the left device after suction curettage, all devices were retained.

DISCUSSION

Despite the disappointing results of this phase of our study conducted in a small number of subjects, we feel that this method of sterilization should not be abandoned.

One of the impressive aspects of our method is its reversibility potential (74% in baboons), which has remained unmatched by any other sterilization procedure so far tested. The permanence of the other sterilization procedures commonly offered discourages some women from accepting them. The absence of untoward side-effects, a very short recovery period, and the noninvasive, nondestructive nature of the method are other advantages of our technique.

Efforts are being made to reduce significantly the present unacceptable rate of failures. Based on our animal experiments and limited clinical trials, we are convinced that proper alignment of the device and the tip of the

TABLE 30-3. Results of Clinical Trials: Phase II

PATIENT NO.	TUBAL OCCLUSION: *RIGHT*	TUBAL OCCLUSION: *LEFT*	PREGNANCY	SUBSEQUENT TUBAL INVESTIGATION IN PREGNANT PATIENTS: *RIGHT*	SUBSEQUENT TUBAL INVESTIGATION IN PREGNANT PATIENTS: *LEFT*
1	+	+	−		
2	+	+	−		
3	ND	ND	+ (SC)	+*	−
4	+	+	−		
5	+	+	+ (SC)	−	+
6	+	+	+ (SC)	−	+
8	+	+	+ (PVD)	+	−
9	+	+	−		
10	ND	ND	+ (PVD)		
11	−	+			

*Tubal occlusion. ND, Not determined; SC, suction curettage; PVD, premature vaginal delivery.

carrier with the tubal lumen at the cornua is the crucial key to proper implantation of the device, resulting in effective contraception. Improper device implantation not only results in a higher rate of tubal permeability but also can lead to an uneven device fixation and potential dislocation. This mechanism can explain the pregnancy in three patients in whom bilateral tubal occlusion was initially documented. Our technique proved 100% effective in 21 baboons, in terms of tubal occlusion as well as contraception, in some animals at 2 or more years of follow-up.

The uterine cavities in baboons were of much smaller dimensions, making the UTJs easily accessible for proper alignment and implantation through the rigid hysteroscope. In humans, however, when ostia are too laterally situated, alignment between the device and the tubal lumen through the rigid hysteroscope becomes technically difficult or impossible. Since the rate of failure is unacceptably high, with an overall tubal occlusion rate of 72.2% and a pregnancy rate of 50%, we feel that before any further clinical trials are performed, we must await the steerable hysteroscope, now under construction by Eder Instrument Company.

It would be easier to assume a proper position prior to device implantation in any shape uterine cavity through a suitable steerable hysteroscope. This should significantly reduce the chances for technical failures.

The exact mechanism causing premature labor in women with no past history of premature birth remains unknown. One can only speculate that the pressure of a plug, or its metallic components, may generate mechanical or electrical impulses, acting as a pacemaker, initiating uterine contractions before term, and leading to a premature delivery.

REFERENCES

1. DARABI KF, ROY K, RICHART RM: Collaborative study on hysteroscopic sterilization procedures: Final report. In Sciarra JJ, Zatuchni GI, Speidel JJ (eds): Risks, Benefits, and Controversies in Fertility Control, pp 181–101. Hagerstown, MD, Harper & Row, 1978
2. HOSSEINIAN AH, LUCERO S, KIM MH: Hysteroscopic implantation of UTJ blocking devices. In Sciarra JJ, Droegemueller W, Speidel JJ (eds): Advances in Female Sterilization Techniques, pp 169–175. Hagerstown, MD, Harper & Row, 1976
3. HOSSEINIAN AH, LUCERO S, ZANEVELD LJD: Hysteroscopically delivered tubal plugs. In Sciarra JJ, Zatuchni GI, Speidel JJ (eds): Reversal of Sterilization, pp 241–248. Hagerstown, MD, Harper & Row, 1978
4. ISRANGKUN C, PHAOSAVASDI S: Hysteroscopic sterilization in 296 cases. In Sciarra JJ, Droegemueller W, Speidel JJ (eds): Advances in Female Sterilization Techniques, pp 148–152. Hagerstown, MD, Harper & Row, 1976
5. QUINONES R, ALVARADO A, LEY E: Hysteroscopic sterilization: Follow-up of 800 cases. In Sciarra JJ, Droegemueller W, Speidel JJ (eds): Advances in Female Sterilization Techniques, pp 162–168. Hagerstown, MD, Harper & Row, 1976
6. REED TP, ERB RA: Hysteroscopic oviductal blocking with formed-in-place silicone rubber plugs: II. Clinical studies. J Reprod Med 23:69–72, 1979
7. RICHART RM, NEUWIRTH RS, BOLDUC LR: Single application fertility regulating device: Description of a new instrument. Am J Obstet Gynecol 127:86–90, 1977

31
Hydrogel Tubal Blocking Device: P-Block

JAN BRUNDIN

The isthmus of the oviduct constitutes the narrowest passage for obstructing sperm ascent and zygote transportation to the uterus. Thus, investigators have been attempting to occlude this region for many years.[1,2] The following report describes studies on an oviductal blocking device: the Mark 7 P-block.

MATERIALS

The Mark 7 P-block is a tubal blocking device with a 4-mm long and 1.2-mm wide hydrogel body fixed on a nylon 6 skeleton. It is shown in its dry and hydrated state in Figure 31-1. The 2-mm wide nylon "wings" prevent expulsion from the tube before hydratization, which requires about 30 minutes. The wings are flapped into a polyethylene catheter, the end of which is smoothly sealed by the nylon cup joining the two wings (Fig. 31-2). On cannulation of the intramural part, the P-block is held in position by a flexible plunger while the surrounding catheter (outer diameter, 2.05 mm) is removed.

Hydrogel is a polymeric compound of polyvinylpyrrolidone, a hydrophilic substance, and methylacrylate, a hydrophobic material. By adding liquid nylon 6 to the hydrogel, the compound becomes less fragile, and the swelling, on hydratization is reduced. The nylon 6 also improves the memory of shape of the end compound. The oviductal occlusive device, the Mark 7 P-block, is molded from a hydrogelic compound and copolymerized by γ-radiation. It is hydratized by the body fluids after insertion and retains a good memory of shape during swelling.

TOXICITY

Ophthalmologic experience with contact lenses made of hydrogel shows a low degree of toxicity to the eye tissue. In some patients attempting oviductal occlusion, the P-block device could be successfully placed only in one oviduct; after repeated attempts at occlusion of the second oviduct failed, the patients underwent surgical sterilization. Evaluation of the intramural portion of a tube removed 22 months after insertion of the P-block revealed ingrowth of tissue from the tubal wall into the porous surface of the P-block. A few giant

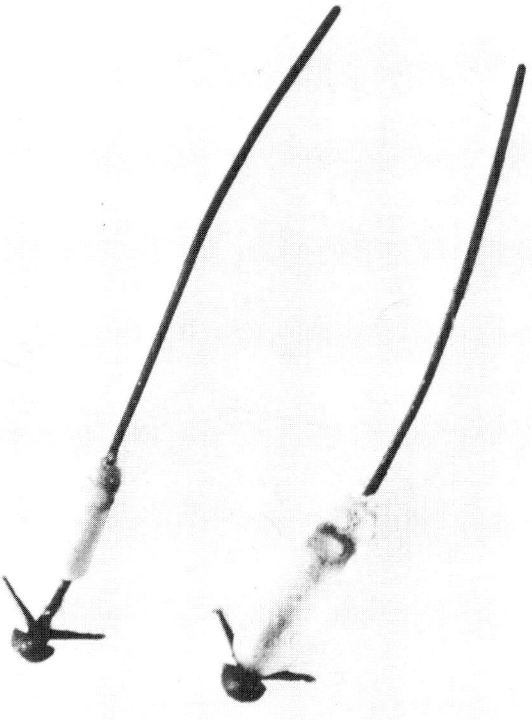

FIG. 31-1. Hydrogelic tubal blocking device. P-block in dry (*left*) and hydrated (*right*) state. Outer measures of hydrogelic body are width 1.2 mm and length 4.0 mm in dry state.

cells were seen in the surrounding tissues, and the capillaries, free from irritation, penetrated the tissue (Fig. 31-3).[3] This ingrowth augmented the retention of the P-block *in situ,* apparently without causing irritation to the surrounding tissues. The compressible nature of the P-block in its hydrated state produces an intimate contact between its surface and the tubal epithelial lining.

CLINICAL STUDY

Between September 1981 and April 1982, 35 women volunteered to undergo oviductal occlusion with the Mark 7 P-block as an alternative to surgical sterilization. To be included in the study, the women had to be parous with an apparent risk of becoming pregnant and they had to have regular periods and no history of salpingitis. After informed consent was obtained, the pa-

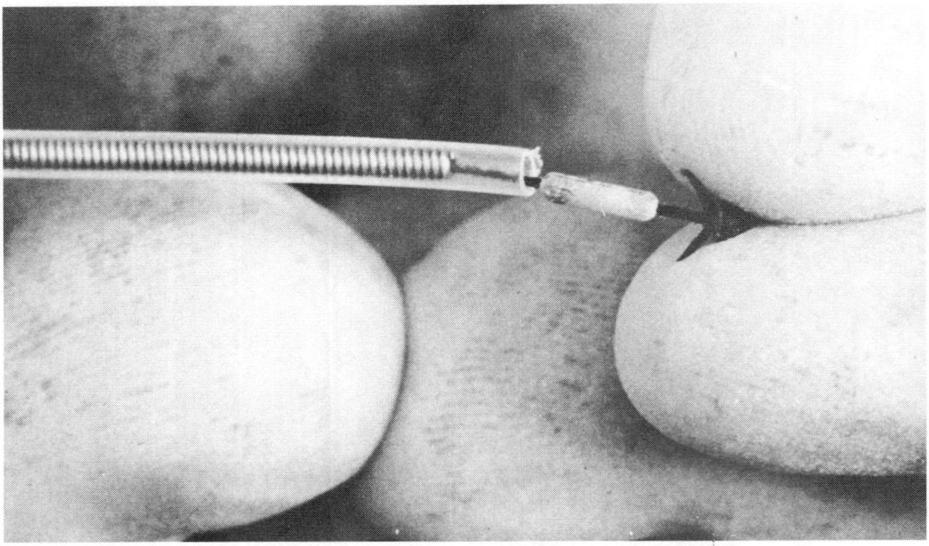

FIG. 31-2. Hydrogelic tubal blocking device. P-block with smooth end in polyethylene application catheter ready for insertion.

tients were admitted as outpatients to the Department of Obstetrics and Gynecology at Danderyd Hospital, Danderyd, Sweden, preferably in the postmenstrual phase.

The volunteers were given a paracervical block by mepivacaine hydrochloride without epinephrine, and the internal cervical os was dilated to Hegar 8. After intravenous injection of 0.25 mg terbutaline, an operative hysteroscope was inserted in the uterine cavity. The β_2-stimulant helped to relax the uterus during the distention by carbon dioxide. If anatomical conditions did not interfere, the tubal orifices on either side were inspected and cannulated with the P-block device. Application of P-blocks on both sides required 10 to 15 minutes. Following the procedure, the patient relaxed for 1 hour and then was permitted to leave the hospital. She was encouraged to use another barrier contraceptive until the hysteroscopic check-up 4 to 6 weeks later or until after her next menstruation.

RESULTS

Results of the attempts to occlude the oviducts with the Mark 7 P-block are shown in Table 31-1. In 15 of the 35 women, bilateral occlusion was achieved on the first attempt; and in 2 other women, a second procedure was necessary to produce successful occlusion of both tubes. One woman, who achieved satisfactory tubal occlusion, subsequently requested removal of the devices due to bleeding. In another 15 women, the Mark 7 P-block could not be inserted because of anatomical factors, such as too-narrow tubal orifices, sharply bent intramural portions of the oviducts, or a combination of these condi-

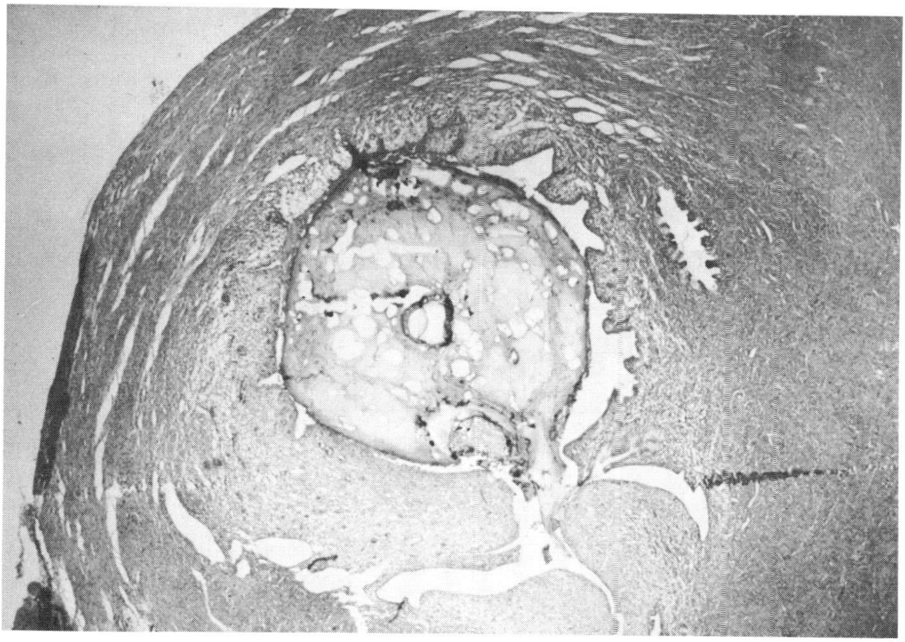

A

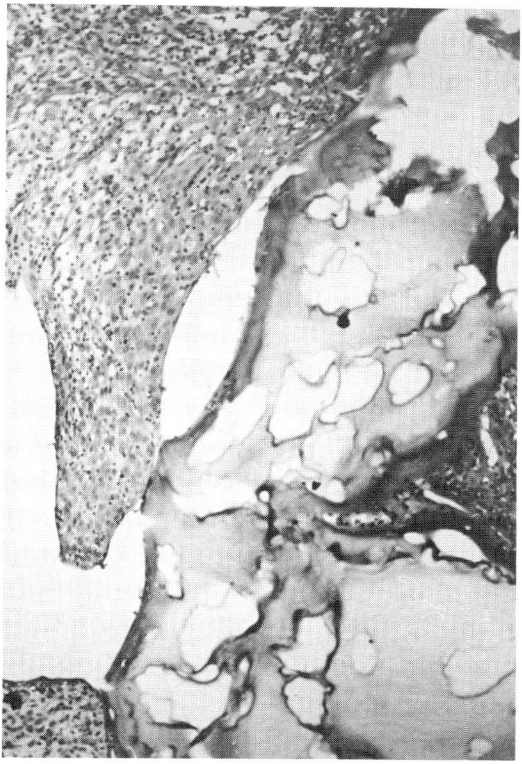

B

FIG. 31-3. (*A*) Transection of extirpated intramural part of human oviduct with hydrogelic P-block *in situ* for 22 months. (*B*) Detail shows tissue ingrowth in surface porosity.

TABLE 31-1. Results of Attempts at Oviductal Occlusion With the Mark 7 P-block, in 35 Volunteers (September 1981–April 1982) in Danderyd, Sweden

RESULTS	NO. WOMEN
Successful bilateral occlusion	15
First attempt	13
Second attempt	2
Subsequent pregnancy	4
Extraluminal placement of device	1
Unilateral expulsion	2
Rupture of P-block	1
Insertion impossible due to anatomical factors	15
Subsequent removal of device due to bleeding	1

tions. Four women subsequently had uterine pregnancies, which were interrupted by legal abortion combined with hysteroscopy. In one of these four women, sterilization was performed at the time of the abortion, revealing one P-block outside the lumen in the uterine muscle on one side. In another woman, the P-block device had fragmented. In all cases, the pregnancies occurred within 2 months after insertion.

Of the nonpregnant women, only one reported uterine bleeding and no woman experienced pain, genital infection, or extrauterine pregnancy.

At the follow-up hysteroscopy 4 to 6 weeks after insertion of the P-block device, bilateral occlusion was recorded in six patients. Four other women had not reported for follow-up examination at the time of this writing.

DISCUSSION

The Mark 7 P-block does not presently constitute an alternative to surgical sterilization, owing to the large number of cases in which the discrepancy between the size of the device and the uterine tubal orifice or other anatomical factors precluded insertion of the P-block. Also the failure (pregnancy) rate after bilateral occlusion is high. In those cases where pregnancy occurred, however, the P-block was not properly inserted.

Work is underway to reduce the size of the P-block so that it will better suit the tubal anatomy, will thereby be applicable to a larger number of women, and will be more easily put into place and retained in the oviducts. Certainly, the Mark 8 P-block (now being developed) holds promise as a safe, simple. nonsurgical means of female sterilization.

REFERENCES

1. BRUNDIN J: Intratubal devices in biodegradables and delivery systems for contraception. In Hafez ESE, van Os WAA (eds): Progress in Contraceptive Delivery Systems Series, vol 1, pp 123–137. Amsterdam, Elsevier, 1980
2. BRUNDIN J: Hysteroscopy for sterilization. In Hafez ESE, van Os WAA (eds): Contraceptive Delivery Systems, vol 3, pp 63–74. Amsterdam, Elsevier, 1982
3. BRUNDIN J, SANDSTEDT, B: Long-term toxicity of hydrogelic occlusive device in the human oviductal isthmus. Acta Obstet Gynecol Scand (in press)

32

Hysteroscopic Tubal Occlusion Procedure With Formed-in-Place Silicone Plugs: Instruments and Technique

ROBERT A. ERB

The use of Silastic tubal plugs for transcervical, nonincisional tubal occlusion involves a flow of catalyzed liquid silicone polymer into the oviduct through a silicone rubber obturator tip positioned at the tubal ostium. The formed-in-place plug becomes bonded to the tip. The resulting flexible structure is larger in the diameter at both ends than it is in the isthmus, and thus it remains in place to effect tubal occlusion.

This approach differs from other methods described in this volume in that it is not deliberately destructive of tissue (as are sclerosing agents and cryosurgery), it does not involve adhesion to the tissue of the tubal lumen, and its occluding member does not force the tissue to conform to its shape.

At the 1975 PARFR Workshop on Advances in Female Sterilization Techniques in Minneapolis, I presented an overview of the method for oviductal blocking with formed-in-place silicone rubber plugs as then developed.[9] Included in this early period of development are the following:

The concept of a formed-in-place silicone rubber plug by Braley and Helmer[1] and by Corfman and Taylor[2]

Experimental studies by Hefnawi, Fuchs, and Laurence (with rabbits)[15] and by Rakshit (with humans)[16–18]

The development of special instruments, material combinations, and techniques by Erb[8,9] to form effective plugs and to provide a practical procedure

Experimental studies with the improved technique reported by Erb and co-workers[11–13] and by Davis and associates[3–7] with rabbits and rhesus monkeys.

At the time of the Minneapolis conference the procedure was projected to be carried out under fluoroscopic guidance. (The fluoroscopic approach may indeed still find clinical application.) However, beginning in 1975, I was able to design miniaturized components so that the guide assembly with its ob-

This work was sponsored by RSP Laboratories, Inc., Stamford, Connecticut; earlier work was supported by Contraceptive Development Branch, NICHD, NIH

turator tip would pass through the operating channel of a standard hysteroscope,[10] and the hysteroscopic method became emphasized in the further development efforts.

Theodore P. Reed, III, MD, collaborated with me at Franklin Research Center beginning in 1977 in preclinical studies with the hysteroscopic procedure using extirpated organs.[14] Reed (Lankenau Hospital, Philadelphia) and Joris De Maeyer (Belgium) conducted the pioneering clinical studies, beginning in 1978.[19–22] The clinical program has since been expanded into a 1000-patient study (now moving into a 3000-patient study) with additional investigators and centers, under the sponsorship of RSP Laboratories, Inc.

This chapter will describe the instruments and technique for this method. The clinical aspects of the procedure and the results of the clinical test program will be described in Chapters 33 and 34.

THE GUIDE ASSEMBLY

The guide assembly is the system that conveys the liquid silicone composition through the operating channel of the hysteroscope, that provides communication to and obturation (sealing) at the tubal ostium, and that allows remote release of the preformed tip (and its bonded plug) from the other parts of the assembly.

The guide assembly (Fig. 32-1) consists of six main parts: (1) obturator tip, (2) inner polysulfone tube, (3) outer polysulfone tube, (4) pusher, (5) double-ended chuck, and (6) Luer fitting.

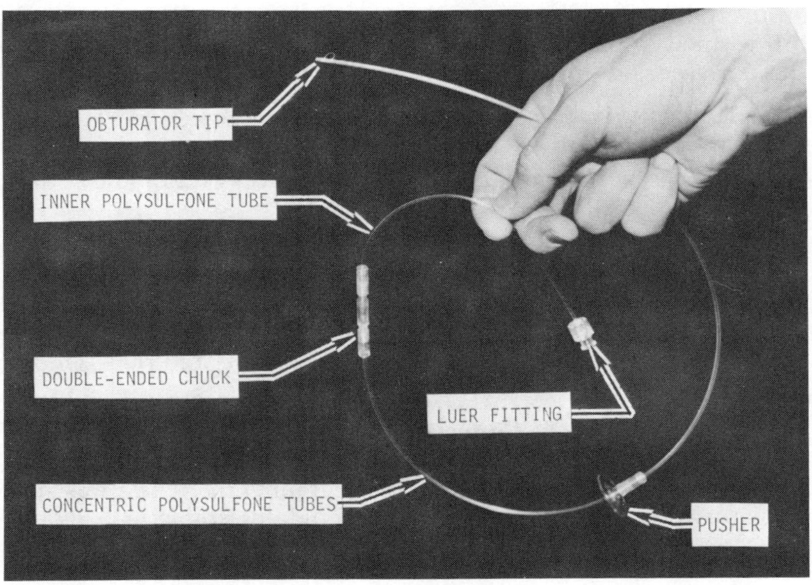

FIG. 32-1. The guide assembly.

The obturator tip is a very important component. By its sealing action at the tubal ostium and by its participation in the release step, it allows the formation of the plug to be carried out remotely. Because the bonded tip is larger in diameter than the oviductal lumen at the isthmus, it prevents intraperitoneal expulsion of the plug. The retrieval loop attached to the tip permits nonincisional removal of the plug if desired (*e.g.*, for replacement of improperly formed plugs or for restoration of tubal patency); if the plug breaks with pulling for removal, the distal end will fall out spontaneously with time into the peritoneal cavity. The distal portion may also be flushed out of the tubal lumen with saline solution through the use of a guide assembly.

The basic obturator tip is approximately 2 mm in diameter by 5 mm in length and is molded of silicone rubber (Dow Corning Silastic 382 Medical Grade Elastomer) (75%) and spherical silver powder (25%). The embedded retrieval loop is made of multifilament polyester thread. The silver powder is a radiopaquing agent.

Because of variations in anatomy in the cornual region, other configurations of tips have also been molded. The six types of obturator tips now in use are shown in Figure 32-2. The E-1 ("Erb-one") tip is the basic tip presently supplied with the guide assembly. The R-1 and C-1 tips were configurations requested by clinical investigators Reed and Cooper. The E-1, E-4, and C-1 tips will pass through a 2.3-mm operating channel. However, with E-2, E-3, and R-1 tips, the hysteroscope must be withdrawn, the replacement tip installed on the protruding guide, and the hysteroscope reinserted.

The inner polysulfone tube has a length of 750 mm and an inside diameter of 1 mm. It has a bonded polysulfone Luer fitting at one end and a ringed constriction at the other end to prevent tail formation and to promote cutoff of the cured silicone for release.

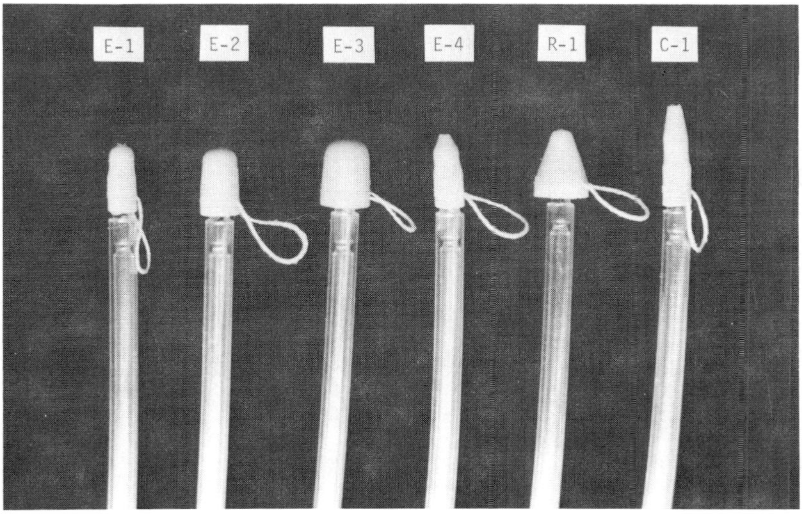

FIG. 32-2. Obturator tips shown with concentric polysulfone tubing.

The outer polysulfone tube (550 mm in length) provides the release function by the sliding arrangement with the inner tube. The inner and outer tubes are held, until the release step, in a fixed relation to each other by means of a double-ended collet device (double-ended chuck), injection-molded of polysulfone, through which the inner tube passes completely.

A pusher, attached to the outer tube with a collet fastener, allows the hysteroscopist to put an axial force on the guide and obturator tip, controlled with one finger. This is also injection-molded of polysulfone, which is used throughout the guide assembly because it is strong, transparent, and sterilizable by steam.

The guide assembly is supplied packaged and sterilized to the clinical investigators.

THE MIXER-DISPENSER

The non-air-entraining mixer-dispenser (Fig. 32-3) is an important element among the specialized instruments developed for the plug-forming procedure. It permits one to mix thoroughly a small quantity of catalyst with a very viscous material in a short time (35 seconds), without entraining any air, and then directly to dispense the catalyzed material, again without entraining any air.

The piston, mixing head, and shaft cap are injection-molded of polysulfone. In use the stannous octoate catalyst is added with a 100μl gas-tight syringe with hypodermic needle through the septum cap. The mixing head

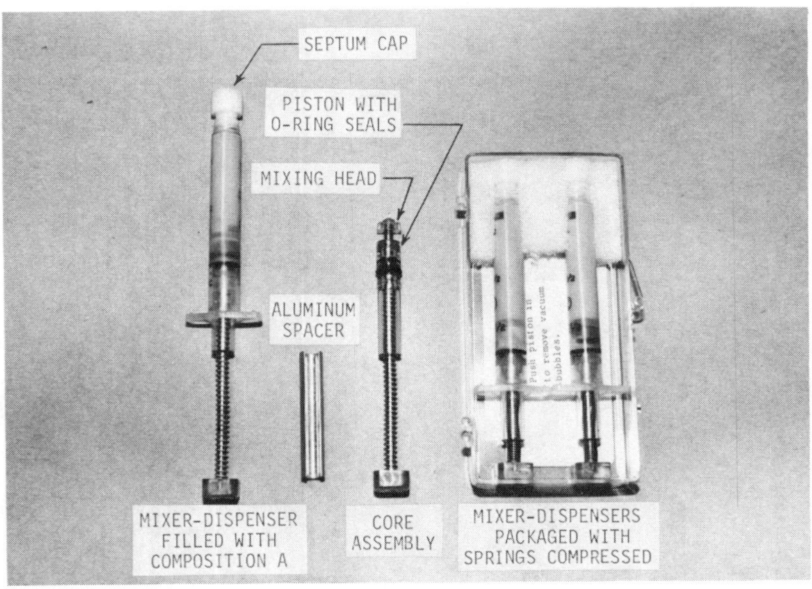

FIG. 32-3. The non-air-entraining mixer-dispenser.

is moved back and forth for 45 double strokes, with quarter turns. The aluminum spacer is inserted to convert the system for the dispensing function.

THE FLUID-FLOW ACTUATOR

The flow of the catalyzed silicone composition through the guide assembly cannot be accomplished by direct hand-holding of the mixer-dispenser syringe. This is because of the high viscosity of the fluid (about 10,000 times the viscosity of water), the narrow diameter and long length of the inner polysulfone tube, and the short time before flow-stopping gelling occurs (about 3 minutes after the addition of catalyst). The system as it is presently used is shown in Figure 32-4. It has a manually actuated screw drive with a driven force gauge pressing on the mixer-dispenser piston. The force gauge permits setting the pressure during flow. The plug is formed during a coasting phase. When the hysteroscopist sees the silicone reach the obturator tip, the turning of the screw drive is stopped; liquid-spring action in the silicone and other elastic behavior in the system cause the coasting. The force gauge allows the decay pressure to be followed to ensure that the plug cures under pressure. Curing under pressure has been shown to be important for properly holding open and filling the cross section of the oviductal lumen.

THE PUMP FOR HYSKON

The hysteroscopic visualizing fluid found most effective for this program has been 32% dextran 70,000 in 10% aqueous glucose solution (Hyskon, Pharmacia Laboratories, Inc.). A device for automatically pressurizing the Hyskon was designed; it allows the procedure to be carried out by two people, a

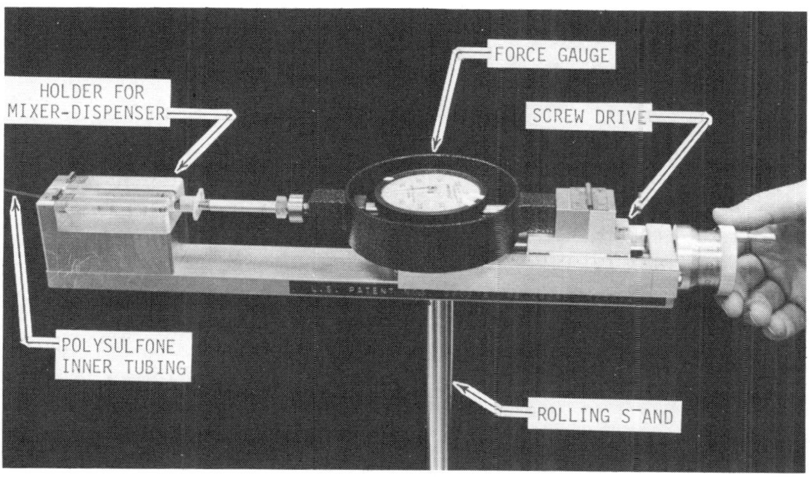

FIG. 32-4. The fluid-flow actuator.

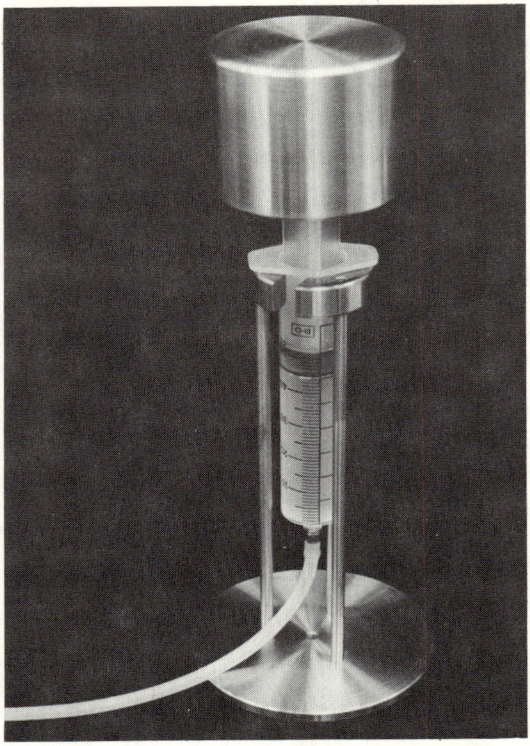

FIG. 32-5. The pump for dextran-solution hysteroscopic visualizing fluid.

hysteroscopist and one assistant. The pump (Fig. 32-5) consists of a support stand for a 50-ml disposable syringe and a weight for the piston such that it provides 150 mm Hg nominal pressure in the liquid. A light touch on the weight can provide a pressure increment when this is needed for visualization.

MISCELLANEOUS COMPONENTS

A special sealing cap (Fig. 32-6) has been made for the operating channel of the hysteroscope. It is molded of Dow Corning MDX 4-4210 silicone rubber and has three sealing rings, rather than the usual one. The aim of the design is to avoid damage to the delicate obturator tip that passes through the seal, while maintaining sealing action against the outer polysulfone tube.

An enlarging sheath for the hysteroscope (Fig. 32-6) has been fabricated to be used in cases where a patulous cervix causes excessive leakage of the Hyskon solution. This sheath, which has a sliding O-ring seal, will enlarge the diameter of Wolf or Storz operating hysteroscopes from 7 mm to 9 mm.

An aspirator tube has been designed and used for debris removal. It consists of a 750-mm piece of the larger-diameter polysulfone tubing, which is flared at one end and attached to a Tuohy-Borst fitting. It is used with a 30-ml disposable syringe.

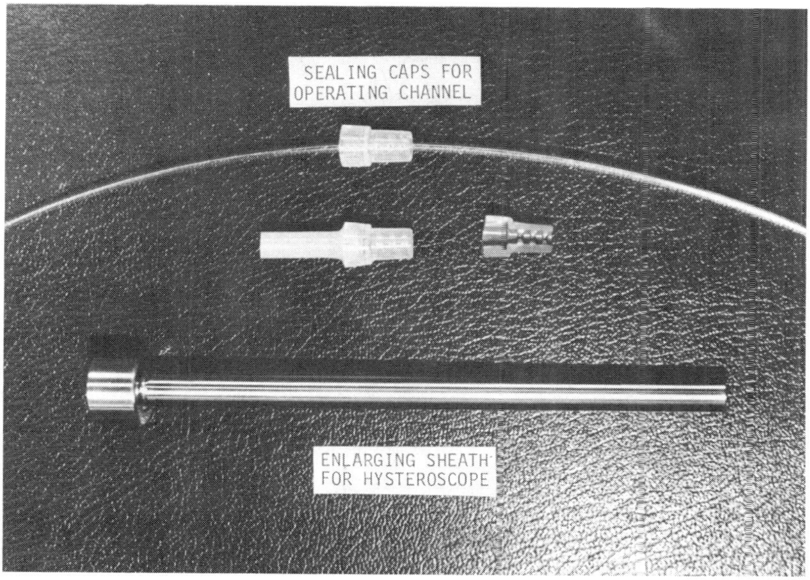

FIG. 32-6. Special items for the hysteroscope: sealing caps for operating channels and enlarging sheath.

MATERIALS

The materials system (designated as Composition A) used to form plugs consists of Dow Corning Silastic 382 Medical Grade Elastomer, 68%; Dow Corning 360 Medical Fluid (20 centistoke grade), 17%; and spherical silver powder (minus 400 mesh), 15%. This is the same materials system used in the animal studies with rabbits and rhesus monkeys. The Silastic 382 base material has had more than 20 years of use in applications in the human body. The 360 Medical Fluid is incorporated as a viscosity reducer, and the silver powder functions as a radiopacifier, permitting the clinical team to determine roentgenographically whether properly formed bilateral plugs exist.

The catalyst is stannous octoate, added in a quantity equal to about 1.5% of the Silastic 382 present. The curing reaction, producing a snappy rubbery solid in 5 minutes, involves cross linking of the silicone polymer. No sensible heat is generated in the reaction.

The Composition A is supplied to the clinical investigators in mixer-dispensers, which have been filled and degassed in a HEPA-filtered hood. The mixer-dispensers are packaged with the spring compressed (to reduce vacuum bubbles in cold storage by maintaining positive internal pressure) and stored and used at −15°C.

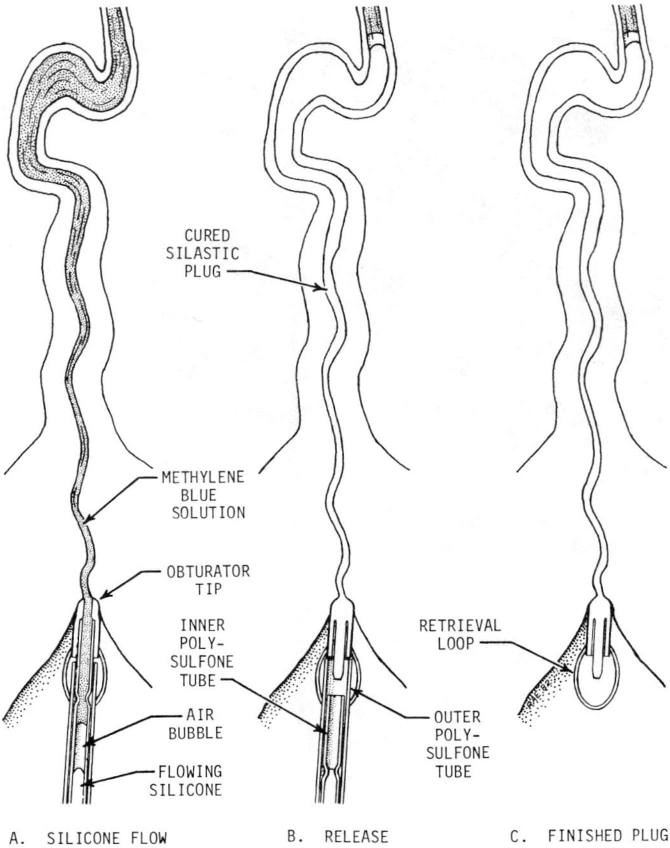

FIG. 32-7. Sequence in plug-forming procedure.

STEPS IN THE PROCEDURE

The guide assembly, while in its sterile bag, is attached to a 3-ml syringe containing 1:10,000 methylene blue solution (1% methylene blue diluted 1:100 in physiologic saline solution). The hysteroscopist feeds the guide through the Hyskon-lubricated sealing cap after the end of the hysteroscope is in the uterine cavity. The methylene blue solution may be used as a current tracer to help locate the tubal ostium. Its more important function is with the "push test," with the obturator tip seated in the tubal ostium. No resistance to flow indicates that communication with a patent tubal lumen has occurred. No reflux shows good obturation. At this point the sequence for plug formation begins:

1. The mixer-dispenser is removed from the freezer.
2. Catalyst is added through the septum cap, and a stopwatch is then started.
3. Mixing takes place: 45 double strokes, ending at 35–40 seconds.

4. The spacer is inserted, the Luer cap is removed, and a 0.4-ml sample is expelled onto a test plate for following the cure outside the body.
5. The Luer fitting on the guide assembly is removed from the methylene blue syringe and attached to the mixer-dispenser.
6. The mixer-dispenser is placed in the holder on the fluid-flow apparatus and the screw drive turned to reach and maintain a force of between 290 and 305 newtons.
7. The consistency of the material on the test plate is sampled with a probe to follow the transition from: "long" (strands forming); to "short"; to gelling (flow stops here, at about 3 minutes); to a soft slow-recovery rubber; to a "snappy" rubber (at about 4 minutes 45 seconds).
8. When the hysteroscopist sees the silicone come into view (usually an air bubble gets between it and the methylene blue solution), the command is given to the assistant to stop the screw drive. The stopwatch time should be about 2 minutes. This stage of the process is shown in Figure 32-7, *A*.
9. The time is recorded when pressure decay stops (when flow stops); the drive is turned, if necessary, to prevent the decay force from dropping below 50 newtons.
10. When a snappy cure is achieved, release is accomplished by loosening the rearward collet and withdrawing the inner polysulfone tube (Fig. 32-7, *B*). The outer polysulfone tube is then withdrawn to leave the finished plug in place (Fig. 32-7, *C*). The procedure is repeated for the other side.

CONCLUSION

Hysteroscopic tubal occlusion using silicone plugs has several attractive features: it is nonincisional; it is an office procedure, done under local anesthesia; it is less damaging to the oviduct than other tubal sterilization methods; and tubal patency can be restored without surgery. (The potential for reversibility exists, but this has not yet been demonstrated with humans.)

The procedure requires the learning of special skills by the physician's assistant, including learning to work efficiently with the materials and instruments under tight constraints of time. The hysteroscopist, too, must learn special skills in identifying the tubal ostia and being able to achieve sealing and alignment of the obturator tip with various uterotubal anatomies. Efforts have been continuing at The Franklin Institute, with the support of other investigators, to improve instruments and methods as needs become identified in the clinical program.

REFERENCES

1. BRALEY SA, HELMER JD: Method for sterilization of males. U.S. Patent 3,422,813, 1969
2. CORFMAN PA, TAYLOR HC: An instrument for transcervical treatment of the oviduct and uterine cornua. Obstet Gynecol 27:880, 1966
3. DAVIS RH, ERB RA, KYRIAZIS GA et al: Fallopian tube occlusion in rabbits with silicone rubber. J Reprod Med 14:56, 1975
4. DAVIS RH, ERB RA, SCHNEIDER HP et al: Chronic rabbit and rhesus monkey fallopian tube occlusion with polymer. Fed Proc 34:339, 1975

5. DAVIS RH, MOONKA DK, PLATT HA et al: Chronic occlusion of the rabbit fallopian tube with silicone polymer. Gynecol Obstet Invest 10:281, 1979
6. DAVIS RH, MOONKA DK, PLATT HA et al: Chronic occlusion of the rabbit fallopian tube with silicone rubber. IRCS Medical Science: Biomedical Technology; Physiology; Reproduction. Obstet Gynecol 6:142, 1978
7. DAVIS RH, PLATT HA, MOONKA DK et al: Chronic occlusion of the monkey fallopian tube with silicone polymer. Obstet Gynecol 53:527, 1979
8. ERB RA: Method and apparatus for non-surgical, reversible sterilization of females. U.S. Patent 3,805,767, 1974; reissue 29,345, 1977
9. ERB RA: Silastic: A retrievable custom-molded oviductal plug. In Sciarra JJ, Droegemueller W, Speidel JJ (eds): Advances in Female Sterilization Techniques, pp 259–271. Hagerstown, MD, Harper & Row, 1976
10. ERB RA: Apparatus and method for the hysteroscopic non-surgical sterilization of females. U.S. Patent 4,245,623, 1981
11. ERB RA, DAVIS RH, BALIN H et al: Device and technique for blocking the fallopian tubes: A method for reversible contraceptive sterilization. In Schima ME, Lubell I, Davis JE et al (eds): Advances in Voluntary Sterilization, Proceedings of the Second International Conference, Geneva, Switzerland, pp 336–337, 1973. Amsterdam, Excerpta Medica, 1974
12. ERB RA, DAVIS RH, KYRIAZIS GA et al: System and technique for blocking the fallopian tubes. Adv Plann Parent 9(2):42, 1974
13. ERB RA, DAVIS RH, KYRIAZIS GA et al: Device and technique for blocking the fallopian tubes. Contemporary OB/GYN 3(2):92, 1974
14. ERB RA, REED TP: Hysteroscopic oviductal blocking with formed-in-place silicone rubber plugs: I. Method and apparatus. J Reprod Med 23:65, 1979
15. HEFNAWI F, FUCHS A, LAURENCE KA: Control of fertility by temporary occlusion of the oviduct. Am J Obstet Gynecol 99:421, 1967
16. RAKSHIT B: Intratubal blocking device for sterilization without laparotomy. Med J (Calcutta) 65:90, 1968
17. RAKSHIT B: Attempts at chemical blocking of the fallopian tube for female sterilization. J Obstet Gynecol (India) 20:618, 1970
18. RAKSHIT B: The scope of liquid plastics and other chemicals for blocking the fallopian tube. In Richart RM, Prager DJ (eds): Human Sterilization, pp 213–221. Springfield, Il, Charles C Thomas, 1972
19. REED TP, ERB RA: Hysteroscopic oviductal blocking with formed-in-place silicone rubber plugs: II. Clinical studies. J Reprod Med 23:69, 1979
20. REED TP, ERB RA: Tubal occlusion with silicone rubber: An update. J Reprod Med 25:25, 1980
21. REED TP, ERB RA: Hysteroscopic female sterilization with formed-in-place silicone rubber plugs. In Phillips JM (ed): Endoscopic Female Sterilization—A Comparison of the Methods, pp 143–154. Downey, CA, American Association of Gynecologic Laparoscopists, 1982
22. REED TP, ERB RA, DEMAEYER, J: Tubal occlusion with silicone rubber: Update 1980. J Reprod Med 26:534, 1981

33

Study Protocol, Criteria, and Complications of the Silicone Plug Procedure

JAY M. COOPER

RICHARD M. HOUCK

A research and development program to design an improved system and application technique for a nonincisional method of blocking the fallopian tubes with medical-grade silicone rubber was initiated at the Franklin Institute Research Laboratories in 1971. In the course of this program, instruments were developed for the mixing and delivery of high-viscosity silicone to the fallopian tubes by hysteroscopic techniques. Effective instillations of oviductal plugs were made initially in New Zealand white rabbits by direct visualization. Prototype instruments were also developed for the human application of the procedure. Evidence from studies with extirpated human uteri and salpingography had indicated that the custom-fitted oviductal plugs could be instilled effectively.[1–5,7]

Once it was adapted to human use, this procedure was expected to have the following advantages over traditional sterilization methods:

- It is nonincisional.
- It is an office procedure, done with the use of local anesthesia.
- It is less damaging to the oviduct than other sterilization methods.
- Tubal patency can possibly be restored without the need for a traditional surgical procedure.

The initial human study consisted of a group of nine prehysterectomy patients who underwent plug instillation immediately prior to the surgical removal of the uterus and fallopian tubes. Subsequent histologic examination of the fallopian tubes revealed no abnormalities due to the instillation of the plugs. Therefore, in November 1978, investigators decided to proceed to plug instillation in patients without obvious uterine or tubal pathology who desired sterilization.[6,11] Approximately 200 patients had been studied by November 1980, when our group began its participation in this multicenter clinical investigation.

PROTOCOL

According to the protocol approved by the Food and Drug Administration, study objectives include investigation of the efficacy of tubal occlusion of both fallopian tubes by hysteroscopic instillation of Silastic plugs in women who are requesting sterilization and evaluation of tolerance to the plugs.

Criteria for admission to the study are as follows:

Patients should be women who are requesting sterilization, not temporary contraception.

Any patient must be of legal age. If the woman is married, consent of the husband should be obtained if required by state law.

The patient must have a history of "normal" menstrual cycles.

The results of a pelvic examination must be normal.

All patients who have a history of potential tubal disease (*e.g.*, pelvic infection, endometriosis, history of infertility) or a history of having used an IUD since their last pregnancy should have hysterosalpingography performed to confirm tubal normalcy.

Patients must agree to maintain their present means of contraception until permission to discontinue has been given by the investigator. Use of contraception should continue until the 3-month postprocedure roentgenographic examination. Also, the patient must agree to a 2-year postprocedure roentgenographic examination.

Results of a complete blood cell count, routine urinalysis, erythrocyte sedimentation rate, and Papanicolaou smear performed within the last 6 weeks must be normal.

PROCEDURE

The procedure requires close cooperation between the hysteroscopist and his assistant. The physician-hysteroscopist, wearing sterile gloves, carries out the following tasks:

1. Inserts speculum
2. Swabs vagina/exocervix with povidone-iodine solution
3. Attaches tenaculum
4. Injects local anesthetic
5. Inserts hysteroscope, dilating cervical canal if necessary
6. Identifies tubal ostia; calls for and inserts aspirator if needed
7. Feeds guide into and through the operating channel of the hysteroscope
8. Calls for the methylene blue "tap" and follows flow into the tubal ostium
9. Places the obturator tip in the tubal ostium, calls for the methylene blue "push," and readjusts the tip alignment as necessary to get free flow without reflux
10. Determines readiness to start catalyst mixing procedure

11. Reports when silicone flow reaches tip; holds tip in place until silicone is cured

12. Reports when tip snaps free from the guide as it should; removes guide

The assistant, not wearing sterile gloves, carries out these tasks:

1. Loads methylene blue in syringes, attaching these to guides in partly opened sterile packages

2. Loads Hyskon in syringe and attaches to the silicone rubber tubing.

3. Arranges rolling table with two three-well plates for following cure; catalyst syringe and its attached needle filled bubble-free; stopwatch; two spacers; mixer-dispenser in a freezer container; procedure-room record form; etc

4. Sets flow-actuation apparatus ready for use

5. Assists physician in getting sterile items when requested

6. Holds vial of lidocaine while physician fills sterile syringe

7. Fills in the procedure-room record form, with records of cure times, overall times, active and decay forces, and miscellaneous items of note

8. Starts Hyskon flow to hysteroscope by putting weight on Hyskon pump; gives "Hyskon push" for additional pressure when requested by physician

9. Operates aspirator syringe when requested by physician

10. Gives methylene blue "tap" and "push" as requested by physician

11. Gets mixer-dispenser from freezer container; adds and mixes catalyst

12. Controls stopwatch

13. Inserts spacer and puts sample on plate for cure following

14. Removes methylene blue syringe from Luer fitting of guide assembly and attaches mixer-dispenser

15. Places mixer-dispenser in Plexiglas holder, fits this on the fluid-flow actuator, and turns the mechanism to maintain the specified force range, stopping when directed by physician

16. Follows cure with retained sample and monitors elapsed time on stopwatch; makes decision when to release tip

17. Releases obturator tip from the guide

A brief chronological sequence of the procedure follows: The patient is placed in the dorsal lithotomy position, the cervix is visualized and washed with Betadine surgical prep solution and a paracervical block using 12 ml 1% lidocaine is administered. The standard operating hysteroscope with attached light source is inserted into the uterus. Hyskon (Pharmacia Laboratories, Inc.) is used to distend the endometrial cavity. Both tubal ostia are identified. A 3-ml syringe with methylene blue dye solution is attached to the guide assembly before the assembly is fed through the operating channel of the hysteroscope into the uterine cavity. The tubal ostium is cannulated. Good communication of the obturator tip with a patent tubal lumen is confirmed by pushing a small amount of methylene blue solution into the fallopian tube. Absence of resistance to or reflux of the methylene blue solution confirms good obturation. The mixer-dispenser is removed from the freezer, a prescribed amount of catalyst (stannous octoate) is added, and the stopwatch is started. Mixing takes place—45 strokes in 35 seconds. A small sample is expelled onto the test plate for following the curing reaction outside the body. The mixer-dispenser, having replaced the methylene blue syringe, is placed on the fluid-flow pump, and the screw-drive is turned to reach and maintain a force of 300 newtons. The hysteroscopist, seeing the silicone come into view, asks the assistant to stop the screw-drive. The consistency of the silicone material in the test plate is sampled with a probe to follow the transition from liquid to a snappy-rubbery state. When a cure is achieved, the assistant releases the catheter from the obturator tip, leaving a normal plug in place. The identical procedure is then repeated for the other side. At the conclusion of the procedure, the hysteroscope is removed from the uterine cavity, and the patient walks to the radiology department, where a single anteroposterior pelvic roentgenogram is obtained.

RESULTS

During a 17-month period (December 1, 1980 through May 1, 1982), 430 women had at least one attempted tubal occlusion procedure. Three hundred thirty-four procedures were bilaterally successful on the first attempt. Repeat procedures were undertaken in the majority of patients whose initial procedure was unsuccessful. A total of 528 procedures have been performed, and 372 women have had bilateral "normal" plugs placed. Five patients have had a unilateral "normal" plug and contralateral natural occlusion. Therefore, 88% of the study population has had a "successfully" performed procedure. Fifty-three women (12%) have had at least one unsuccessful procedure; 26 of these are planning to return for a repeat attempt.

Average procedure duration is 34.78 minutes, and average patient age is 30.54 years. Thus far, none of the women having roentgenographic confirmation of normal plugs at the 3-month postprocedure visit has conceived. This represents 1400 woman-months of sterilization without a pregnancy.

NORMAL VERSUS ABNORMAL PLUGS

No two patients will have identical plugs, owing to the unique method in which the plugs are formed. Therefore, it would seem difficult to differentiate a "normal" from an "abnormal" plug. Fortunately, there are valid hysteroscopic and radiologic characteristics that allow appropriate categorization of plugs (Figs. 33-1 through 33-3).

The major characteristic of the normal plug is a "dumbbell" configuration: continuity between a thick obturator tip at the ostium, a thinner isthmic portion, and a bulbous distal portion. A properly formed plug should preclude migration into either the uterine or the peritoneal cavity.

Abnormal plugs can be characterized as refluxed, extravasated, discontinuous, foreshortened, and slow-cure.

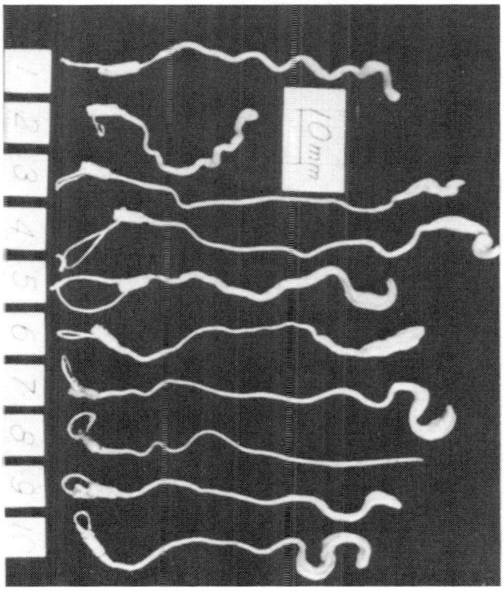

FIG. 33-1. Normal plug configurations, except for number 8.

REFLUXED PLUG

Of the abnormal plug types, the refluxed plug is the most common. Its detection and evaluation depend on both hysteroscopic and roentgenographic appearances. It can occur due to movement of the patient or operator or to failure of the operator to apply adequate pressure on the obturator tip during the instillation and flow of the liquid silicone. It may be a result of an unusually patulous tubal ostium, which prevents a proper seal between the ob-

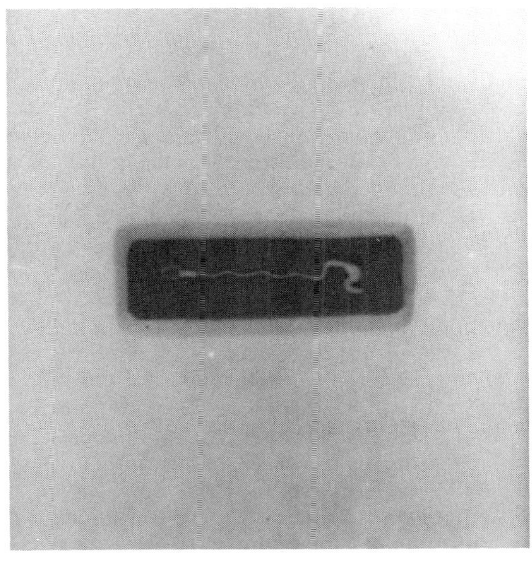

FIG. 33-2. Normal plug showing "dumbbell" configuration.

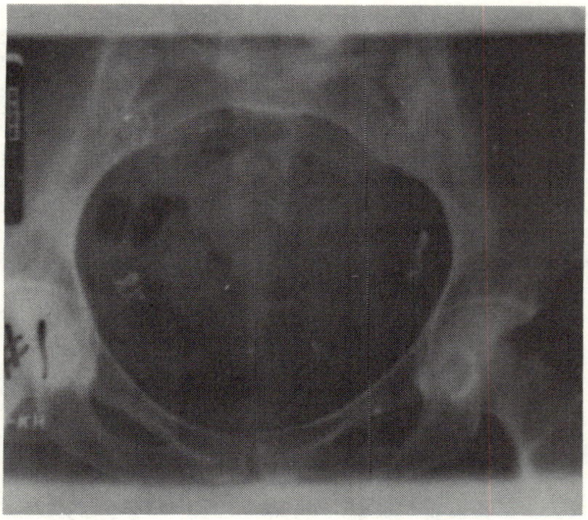

FIG. 33-3. Radiograph demonstrating bilateral normal plugs.

turator tip and the ostium. Tubal spasm, not allowing for proper "seating" of the obturator tip, may also be a cause. It is also a likely occurrence when the uterus cannot be adequately distended with Hyskon, as in the case of a patulous cervix or inadvertent uterine perforation. Most commonly, a refluxed plug results from inability of the physician to obtain parallel access between the obturator tip and the tubal ostium. The refluxed plug is not likely to be retained, because an inadequate volume of silicone, often at a reduced pressure, has flowed into the tube. Partial or complete migration into the uterine cavity is likely; therefore, it should be replaced with a normal plug (Figs. 33-4 and 33-5).

Case 1. P.C. is a 29-year-old single white female, gravida 3, para 0, AB-3, using condoms for contraception at the time of the initial hysteroscopic tubal occlusion procedure on day 10 of her cycle. The right tubal ostium was easily visualized, and the right fallopian tube was occluded without difficulty. The left tubal ostium was also identified; however, despite absence of reflux of methylene blue dye, there was significant silicone reflux at the time of plug formation. Although plug removal was attempted, only the proximal portion of the plug could be removed. A repeat procedure was scheduled 1 month later. A roentgenogram taken immediately prior to this second procedure demonstrated the previously placed normal-appearing right-sided plug, whereas on the left side the distal portion of the plug had now migrated into the peritoneal cavity.

Again, attempts to occlude the left fallopian tube were complicated by significant silicone reflux. As before, only the proximal portion of the plug could be removed, and a fourth roentgenogram showed additional distal silicone plug fragments in the peritoneal cavity. Two months later, a third attempt at tubal occlusion was made. On this occasion, the left fallopian tube was satisfactorily occluded (roentgenogram No. 5). A 3-month postprocedure film (roentgenogram No. 6) confirmed continued bilateral normal-appearing silicone plugs, as well as the multiple distal fragments of previously placed plugs in the peritoneal cavity.

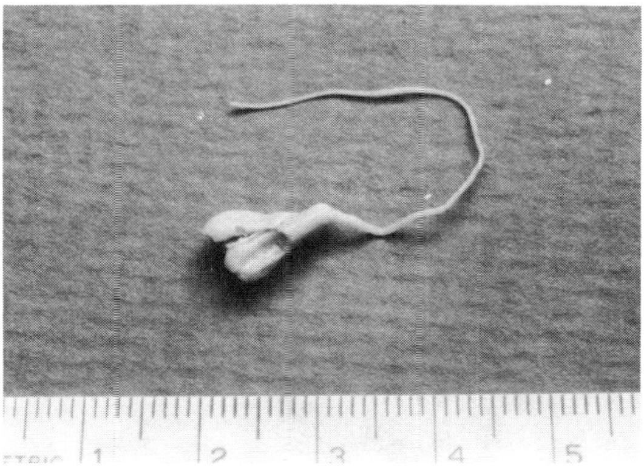

FIG. 33-4. Refluxed plug.

EXTRAVASATED PLUG

The second type of abnormal plug results from extravasation of silicone into the periosteal tissues and is more frequently encountered by the inexperienced operator. Occasionally, the hysteroscopist has no indication that the plug has formed. In some cases, unusual resistance to the flow of methylene blue solution prior to silicone infusion can alert the physician and the assistant that a problem exists. Inadequate uterine distention is often implicated; however, the common explanation is, again, improper alignment between the obturator tip and the tubal ostium. Often a "false pocket" or depression is created immediately adjacent to the true tubal ostium. The postprocedure roentgenogram shows filling of the myometrial outpouching adjacent to the tubal ostium. Obviously ineffectual and radiologically abnormal, an extravasated plug should be replaced with a normal plug (Fig. 33-6).

Case 2. J.C. is a 29-year-old married white female, gravida 3, para 2, using condoms for contraception, who underwent an intial hysteroscopic tubal occlusion procedure on day 10 of her cycle. The procedure was without complication. Postprocedure roentgenographic findings were a surprise, since there appeared to be an extravasated plug on the right side with a normal plug on the left. A 3-month postprocedure film revealed an identical picture. One month later the patient underwent

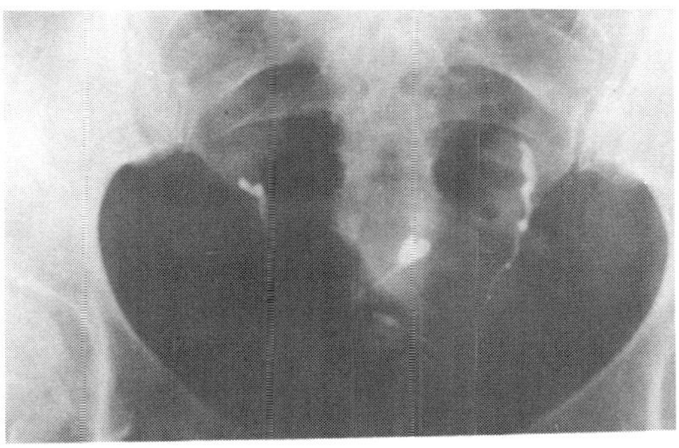

FIG. 33-5. Radiograph demonstrating refluxed plug (right).

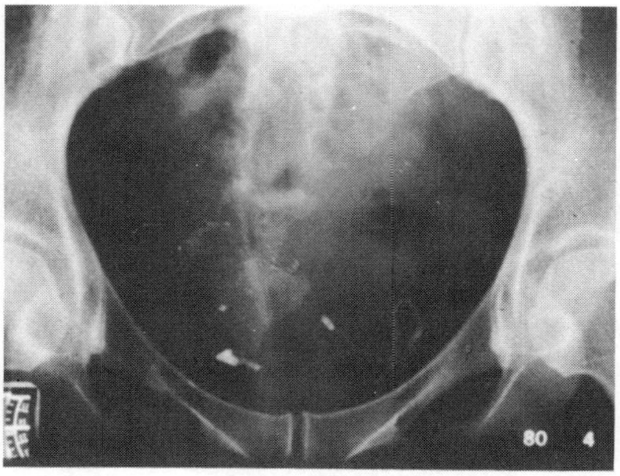

FIG. 33-6. Radiograph demonstrating extravasated plug.

an outpatient surgical procedure under general anesthesia. The plan was to attempt once more the tubal occlusion procedure, however if this was unsuccessful, to proceed with a laparoscopic sterilization. The tubal occlusion was successfully performed (roentgenogram No. 4). The immediate postprocedure view showed two normal-appearing plugs, as well as the extravasated silicone at the right cornua, as noted previously. The 3-month postprocedure roentgenogram has recently been obtained and is satisfactory.

Several steps can be taken to minimize the chances of getting a refluxed and extravasated plug:

Alteration of the curve of the catheter to allow for correct alignment and parallel axis at the tubal ostium

Alternative obturator tip designs, which will allow for different diameters of tubal ostia. After my design (J. M. Cooper), Dr. Robert Erb has developed a new obturator tip. The C-1 (Cooper-1) tip has increased length and flexibility, which allows for greater success in properly cannulating laterally placed tubal ostia and in tubal spasm.

A specially designed sheath to increase the diameter of the hysteroscope, which will minimize costly leakage of Hyskon from the patulous cervix. Adequate uterine distention will then allow better intrauterine visualization.

Intravenous administration of glucagon may counteract tubal spasm.

DISCONTINUOUS PLUG

The discontinuous plug usually occurs as a result of faulty technique. Improper silicone and catalyst mixing, or abnormal operation of the infusion pump or catheters used for silicone delivery, are sometimes implicated. Movement of the patient during silicone infusion may result in loss of plug continuity. The hysteroscopist may observe a peculiar "starting and stopping" activity of the infusing silicone.

Another common explanation for the discontinuous plug is difficulty with the guide assembly separation of the obturator portion of the plug at the conclusion of plug formation. The weakest portion of the plug exists at the newly formed junction between the obturator tip and the isthmic portions of the plug. Excessive tension on this newly created silicone bond will likely result in a broken plug. The roentgenogram will show loss of continuity between the obturator tip and the distal portion of the plug. Close scrutiny of the initial postprocedure roentgenogram, as well as of the 3-month post-procedure films, is necessary to suggest loss of continuity. Strict adherence to proper technique in mixing and dispensing silicone, as well as in minimizing patient anxiety and discomfort, will significantly diminish the incidence of this abnormal plug type (Fig. 33-7).

FORESHORTENED PLUG

The foreshortened plug may be the result of tubal disease, however it most often results from an inadequate volume of silicone entering a normal fallopian tube. A quick cure, usually precipitated by the addition of an excessive amount of catalyst to the liquid silicone, or slow delivery of the silicone-containing syringe to the infusion pump, is generally noted (Figs. 33-8 and 33-9).

Case 3. T. F. is a 26-year-old female, gravida 2, para 2, AB-1, using oral contraception at the time of the initial tubal occlusion procedure attempt on day 12 of her cycle. Difficulty in uterine distention secondary to a patulous cervix made visualization difficult. The left fallopian tube was successfully occluded using a C-1 obturator-tipped catheter. Attempt at right-sided tubal occlusion was complicated by premature curing of the silicone mixture. The postprocedure roentgenogram showed a shortened right-sided plug, confirming the suspicion that inadequate silicone had entered the right fallopian tube.

The patient returned for a repeat procedure 1 month later. The abnormally short right-sided plug was removed, using a flexible grasping forceps inserted through the operating channel of the hysteroscope. With tubal patency thus recreated, another plug was placed, this time with adequate flow-time of the silicone mixture. The postprocedure film demonstrated bilateral normal-appearing silicone plugs. A 3-month postprocedure roentgenogram has not yet been obtained.

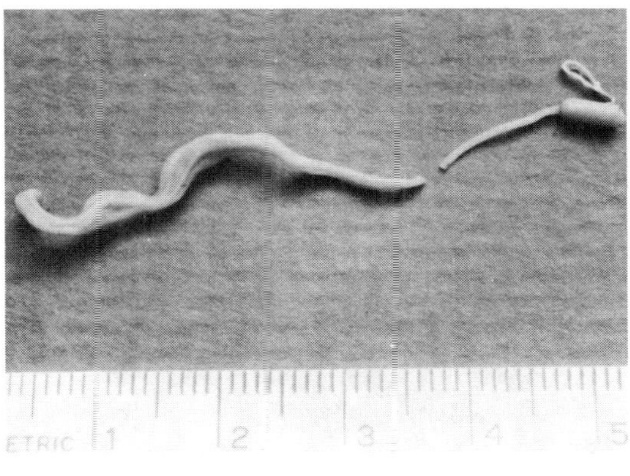

FIG. 33-7. Discontinuous plug.

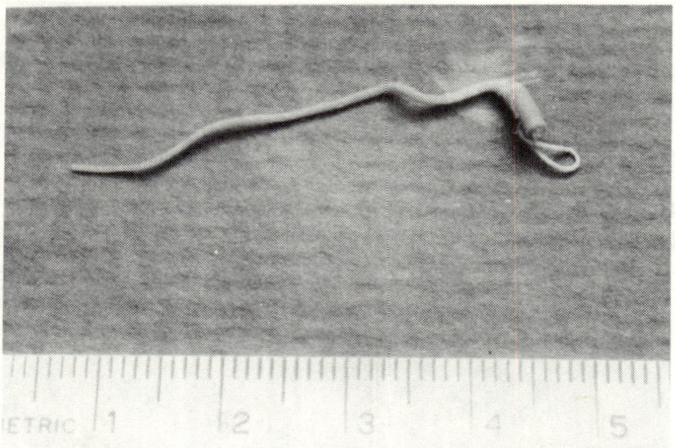

FIG. 33-8. Foreshortened plug.

SLOW-CURE PLUG

The slow-cure plug has no typical roentgenographic or hysteroscopic picture. However, placement of the intratubal silicone device is complicated by an abnormally slow cure of the silicone. The postprocedure film may show what are considered to be "normal" plugs. However, gross examination of these plugs under magnification has shown that isthmic and cornual portions are not symmetrically round. Rather, there is collapse of the plug to an ovoid shape, which is the result of loss of intratubal pressure during the liquid silicone infusion (Fig. 33-10).

Abnormal plug types result from problems with one or more of the key steps in the tubal occlusion procedure. These critical steps are:

1. Adequate uterine distention
2. Clear visualization of patent tubal ostia; avoidance or correction of problems caused by endometrial fragments, bleeding, or tubal spasm
3. Proper obturation of the tubal ostia
4. Free, uninterrupted flow of silicone into the tubal ostia
5. Properly timed curing of silicone plugs

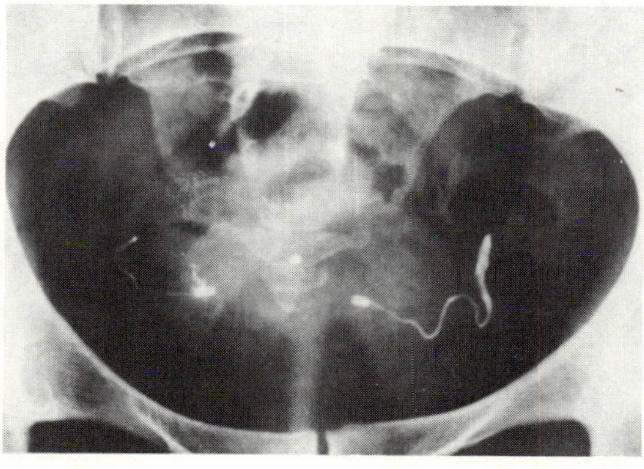

FIG. 33-9. Radiograph demonstrating foreshortened plug.

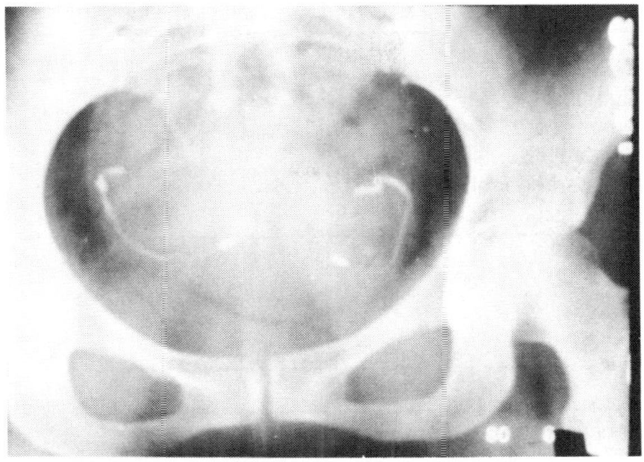

FIG. 33-10. Radiograph demonstrating "slow cure" plug.

6. Proper separation of the catheter guide assembly from the obturator tip portion of the formed-in-place plug

DISCUSSION

Experience to this point has allowed the following conclusions:

The major limiting factor in performing a successful tubal occlusion procedure, one that results in bilateral "normal" plugs, is the inability to properly cannulate the tubal ostia. Consistent tubal cannulization requires specialized training and considerable hysteroscopic experience to be performed properly.

In almost every case, there is hysteroscopic or radiologic evidence that clearly distinguishes the "normal" from the "abnormal" plug. Correct interpretation of the roentgenogram of the pelvis is a determining factor, minimizing the need for more expensive and time-consuming hystersalpingography

"Normal" plugs result from at least a 2-minute, uninterrupted flow of silicone into the fallopian tube under satisfactory pressure. Unusually viscous silicone is likely to flow slowly, cure quickly, and prevent adequate intratubal silicone for proper plug formation. In contrast, unusually liquid silicone is likely to flow rapidly and cure slowly, and may present controlled and adequate distention of the tubal lumen. Maintenance of pump pressure of at least 50 newtons is considered essential to proper plug formation.

Abnormal plugs, once recognized, can usually be removed and normal plugs placed. Normal plug migration or late separation is a rare event; however, a 3-month postprocedure roentgenogram is necessary to confirm plug continuity and proper placement.

Pregnancies have not occurred with "normal appearing," "properly formed" plugs.

An experienced hysteroscopist can expect to succeed with bilateral tubal occlusion in 85% to 90% of the selected patient population.

TABLE 33-1. Statistics for Tubal Occlusion Study, May 1, 1982

FACTOR	FINDINGS
Number of patients	430
Number of hysteroscopies performed	528
Bilateral normal plugs	372
Unilateral normal plug and unilateral natural occlusion	5
Successful procedure	88%

TABLE 33-2. Results With Silicone Plugs, May 1, 1982

RESULT	NO. PATIENTS
Successful procedure (normal plugs)	372
Bilateral abnormal plugs	1
Unilateral normal and unilateral abnormal plug	3
Incomplete (returning for repeat procedure)	22
Dropouts (not returning for repeat procedure)	27
Unilateral normal and unilateral natural occlusion	5
Total patients	430

TABLE 33-3. Average Patient Profile, Tubal Occlusion Study, May 1, 1982

FACTOR	FINDINGS
Age (years)	29.0
Gravida	2.1
Para	1.5
Day of cycle	10.0
Procedure duration (minutes)	32.0

TABLE 33-4. Comparison of the Tubal Occlusion Procedure With the Ideal Sterilization Procedure

	TUBAL OCCLUSION PROCEDURE		
CHARACTERISTIC	*THEORETICAL*	*ACTUAL*	IDEAL PROCEDURE
Safe	+	+	+
Effective	+	+	+
Applicable to ambulatory patients	+	+	+
Performed with local anesthesia	+	+	+
Simple to learn	+	−	+
Simple to perform	+	−	+
Socially acceptable	+	+	+
Inexpensive	−	?	+
Applicable to virtually all patients	−	−	+
Potentially reversible	+	?	+

Additional advances in technique may come with a better understanding of the interstitial or intramural portion of the fallopian tube. Its anatomical, physiological, and pharmacologic characteristics still remain only partially understood. The interstitial portion of the fallopian tube may describe one of several pathways as it traverses the uterine wall. It may follow a relatively simple, straight, or curved course to the superior surface of the fundus and then travel laterally for a short distance.[8] Alternatively it may take a tortuous or convoluted route.[13] The first convolution of the tube actually occurs in the uterine wall. These anatomical variations can make proper cannulization difficult.

Although anatomical valves or sphincters to prevent the movement of material from the uterus through the oviduct have been reported in other species, investigators have not yet found a structural arrangement that separates the extramural portion of the human tube from the uterine cavity.[10] Each of three muscular layers of the uterine wall is continuous with the tubal musculature. It may be that they act in some synergistic fashion to accomplish tubal closure or spasm. Our initial experience with glucagon to alleviate spasm at the uterotubal junction has led us to suggest its use to other clinical investigators.

Questions concerning the physiological influence of estrogen and progesterone on the myosalpinx have not yet been resolved. However, it is well known that there is a dense adrenergic innervation of the oviductal isthmus along with its prominent myosalpinx. This would suggest that this portion of the tube might act as an adrenergic sphincter. In addition, Koh reported that the contractile response of the isthmic musculature to epinephrine varied markedly with the ovarian cycle.[9] Tubal contractile activity is greatest at the time of the menses, which would implicate the prostaglandins. Antiprostaglandin administration would seem to minimize tubal or uterine muscular activity.

CONCLUSIONS

The ideal sterilization procedure should be safe as well as effective. It should be applicable to ambulatory patients with the use of local anesthesia or without anesthesia, since many of the complications that relate to sterilization procedures are complications that occur with the use of anesthesic agents. It should be simple to learn and simple to perform. It should be socially and personally acceptable; it should be inexpensive and applicable to large numbers of patients; and it should be potentially reversible, in the event of a change in desire for fertility potential on the part of the patient.[12] There is not yet a sterilization procedure that fulfills all of these requirements. The tubal occlusion procedure with formed-in-place silicone plugs satisfies a large number of these prerequisites. However, significant limitations exist that may prevent or delay widespread application of this promising sterilization procedure.

One major disadvantage is the need for sophisticated equipment and technology. Consequently, once marketable, the procedure is not likely to be inexpensive, although it is likely to cost considerably less than other traditional sterilization procedures, because hospitalization and general anesthesia will not be required.

Another limitation is the time demand on the physician and the assistant. The average procedure requires 70 to 90 minutes of assistant time and 30 to 50 minutes of physician time. Even when the operators have considerable experience, the procedure cannot be expected to be as routine as laparoscopic sterilization techniques.

Because the great majority of gynecologists have no personal experience with hysteroscopy, learning the procedure will require familiarization with a "new" endoscopic procedure. Improvements in instrumentation and teaching models will likely facilitate this learning process.

Of additional concern is the potential for inadvertent disruption of "normal" plugs at the time of a diagnostic dilation and curettage, should this be indicated at some later date. Perhaps preceding the dilation and curettage with a diagnostic hysteroscopy would obviate this possibility.

Clinical research to this point clearly supports the notion that the tubal occlusion procedure with formed-in-place silicone plugs is both safe and effective. However, even after "selecting out" women who would appear not to be good candidates (*i.e.*, those with fixed retroversion, history of endometriosis, pelvic infection) the procedure can be performed successfully in only 85% to 90% of the study population. No doubt, future instrumentation improvements, such as flexible catheters and endoscopes, will increase the incidence of successfully performed procedures.

One unforeseen advantage of the procedure has been its unique applicability to endoscopic teaching aids, such as teaching scopes and video documentation. This allows for the ultimate in physician-patient communication because the patient can visualize the actual performance of her sterilization procedure.

Potential for reversibility remains one of the most significant issues. Although the reversal procedure is not yet under clinical evaluation, the potential for reversibility would seem to be great. In fact, the design of the plug includes a nylon retrieval loop at the obturator tip portion of the plug, which would make the plug amenable to removal at hysteroscopy. Such a procedure could be accomplished in the physician's office with minimal risk and cost to the woman desiring restoration of fertility potential. Our limited experience has allowed the observation that plugs can be removed from the fallopian tubes with immediate restoration of tubal patency. Whether this would translate into restored fertility remains to be answered.

In conclusion, the tubal occlusion procedure with formed-in-place silicone plugs has both theoretical and practical significance. Further clinical investigation is warranted and should be encouraged.

REFERENCES

1. DAVIS RH, ERB R, KYRIAZIS GA et al: Fallopian tube occlusion in rabbits with silicone rubber. J Reprod Med 14:56, 1975
2. ERB RA: Silastic: A retrievable custom-molded oviductal plug. In Sciarra JJ, Droegemueller W, Speidel JJ (eds): Advances in Female Sterilization Techniques, p 259. Hagerstown, MD, Harper & Row, 1976

3. ERB RA, DAVIS RH, BALIN H et al: Device and technique for blocking the fallopian tubes: A method for reversible contraceptive sterilization. In Schima ME, Lubell I, Davis JE et al (eds): Advances in Voluntary Sterilization. Proceedings of the Second International Conference, p 336. Amsterdam, Excerpta Medica, 1974
4. ERB RA, DAVIS RH, KYRIAZIS GA et al: Device and technique for blocking the fallopian tubes. Contemporary OB/GYN 3:92, 1974
5. ERB RA, DAVIS RH, KYRIAZIS GA et al: System and technique for blocking the fallopian tubes. Adv Plann Parent 9:42, 1974
6. ERB RA, REED TP: Hysteroscopic oviductal blocking with formed-in-place silicone rubber plugs: I. Method and apparatus. J Reprod Med 23:65, 1979
7. HEFNAWI F, FUCHS A, LAURENCE KA: Control of fertility by temporary occlusion of the oviduct. Am J Obstet Gynecol 99:421, 1967
8. HERMSTEIN A, NEWSTADT B: Intramural portion of the fallopian tube. Z Geburtshilfe Gynaekol 88:431, 1974
9. KOK F: Peristalsis and anti-peristalsis of oviducts. Zentralbl Gynaekol 53:962, 1929
10. PAUERSTEIN CJ: The Fallopian Tube: A Reappraisal. Philadelphia, Lea & Febiger, 1974
11. REED TP, ERB RA: Hysteroscopic oviductal blocking with formed-in-place silicone-rubber plugs: II. Clinical Studies. J Reprod Med 23:69, 1979
12. SCIARRA JJ, DROEGEMUELLER W (MODERATORS) New developments in fertility regulation devices. In Zatuchni GI, Labbok MH, Sciarra JJ (eds): Research Frontiers in Fertility Regulation, p 322. Hagerstown, MD, Harper & Row, 1980
13. SWEENY WJ: The interstitial portion of the uterine tube. Its gross anatomy, course and length. Obstet Gynecol 19:3, 1962

34

Formed-in-Place Silicone Plugs: Improvements and Limitations

THEODORE P. REED, III

Over the past 5 years of laboratory and clinical investigation of the formed-in-place silicone rubber plugs,[1,3,4] improved and special techniques for the increased success of the procedure have been developed. Conversely, certain complications and limitations have been observed. Both of these aspects will be presented and discussed.

METHODS FOR IMPROVING LOCATION OF TUBAL OSTIA

Proper identification and location of tubal ostia, as well as perfusion of the fallopian tubes, are obviously essential to the success of this procedure.

UTERINE DISTENDING MEDIUM

Dextran 70, 32% in 10% glucose (Hyskon) is preferred over CO_2 or 5% to 10% glucose. The viscosity and flow characteristics of Hyskon are helpful in clearing the blood, mucus, and endometrial debris out of the tubal ostia (Fig. 34-1). Hyskon suppresses minor bleeding problems, which sometimes occur when hysteroscopy is continued over the 30- to 45-minute period often required for this technique.

ASPIRATION

Aspiration of the uterine cavity contents of blood, mucus, small clots, and polypoid fragments is often essential to finding tubal ostia as a preliminary step in the procedure. A typical view on first visualizing the cavity is shown in Figure 34-2. The aspirator, as developed by Erb (Fig. 34-3), is simple, and consists of a 75-cm length of 2-mm polysulfone tubing attached to a standard 30-ml syringe by a Tuohy-Borst fitting. The tubing is inserted through the operating channel of the hysteroscope and the operator directs the tip selectively around the uterine cavity as the assistant produces suction with the attached syringe. The tip is seen approaching a polypoid fragment of endometrium (Fig. 34-4) and then aspirating it (Fig. 34-5). Mucus, blood, and bubbles (Fig. 34-6) can also be aspirated. If prolonged aspiration causes uterine bleeding, the aspiration should be stopped and Hyskon pressure increased until the field clears.

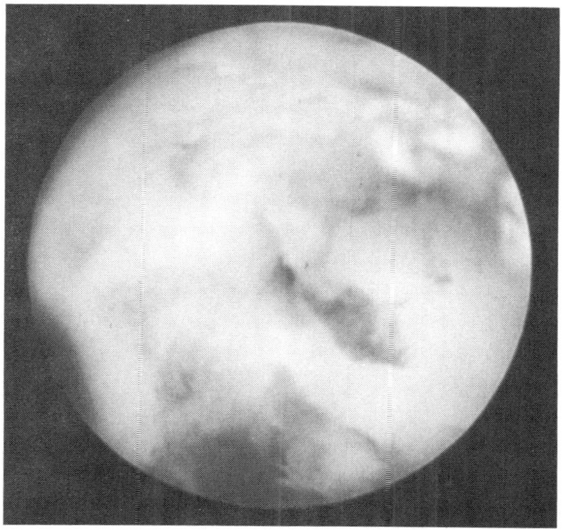

FIG. 34-1. Bloody mucus flowing out of cornual tubal ostium.

METHYLENE BLUE TESTS

Occasionally artifacts in the endometrium appear to be tubal ostia. These are noted particularly if the procedure is done late in the menstrual cycle or early in the postpartum period, or in nursing mothers. When an ostium or two seem apparent in the cornual area of the cavity but flow does not seem clear, or perfusion is not satisfactory, results of the methylene blue tests may be helpful in proper identification.

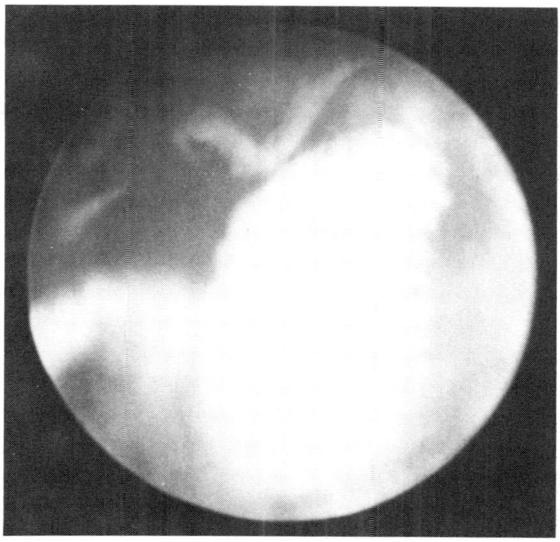

FIG. 34-2. Typical first view through hysteroscope with fragment of endometrium and mucus in the cavity.

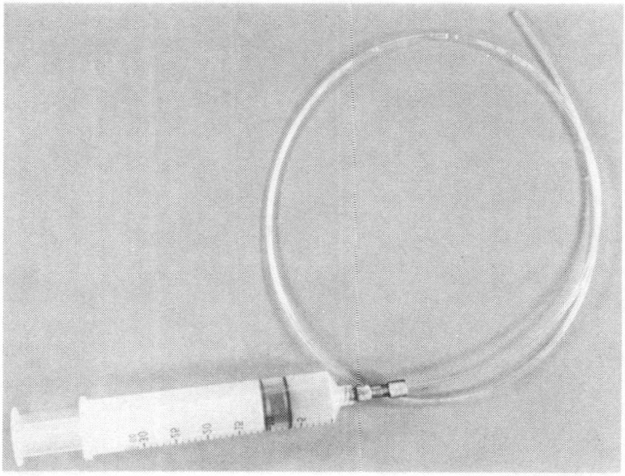

FIG. 34-3. Aspirator, consisting of 75 cm of 2-mm polysulfone tubing with Tuohy-Borst connection to standard 30-ml plastic syringe.

The methylene tap test (Fig. 34-7) is performed by the operator holding the tip of the guide close to the tubal ostium and continuing the flow of Hyskon. Then the assistant taps a small amount (0.1 ml to 0.3 ml) of dilute methylene blue into the flowing Hyskon. It will not diffuse into the Hyskon but will flow separately into the fallopian tube (Fig. 34-8).

Once the obturator tip is placed in the tubal opening, the methylene push test is done. This test is most important to the success of the procedure. Rarely does an improperly formed plug result when a good push test is obtained before the plug is formed. The test is done by the assistant pushing firmly on the guide syringe and expelling 0.5 ml to 1.0 ml of methylene blue into

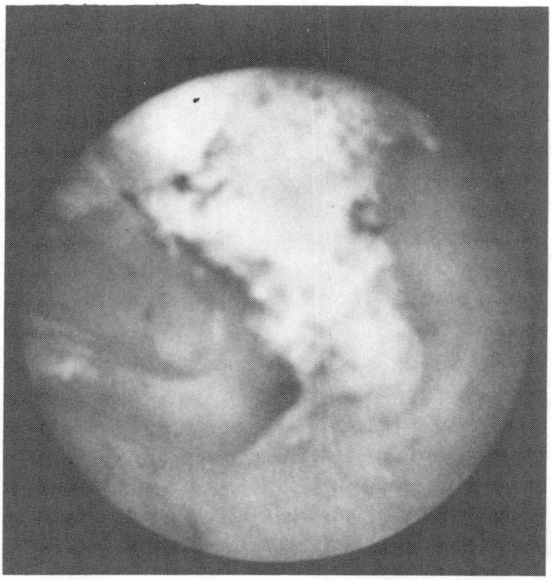

FIG. 34-4. Aspirator tip seen approaching polypoid fragment of endometrium.

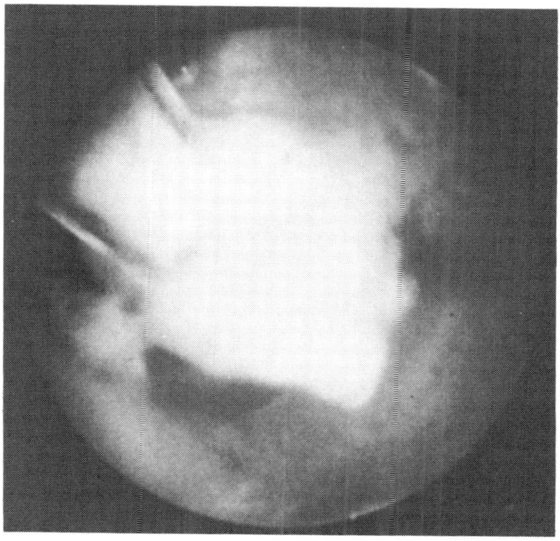

FIG. 34-5. Aspirating fragment of endometrium.

the tube (Fig. 34-9). If no resistance is felt and there is no reflux of methylene blue back into the uterine cavity (Fig. 34-10), proper axis with a tight seal has been obtained (Fig. 34-11), and tubal patency is ensured. Occlusion of the tube without a proper push test should not be done.

METHOD OF TUBAL PERFUSION

Aids in obtaining proper tubal perfusion can be categorized into two groups: instruments and medications.

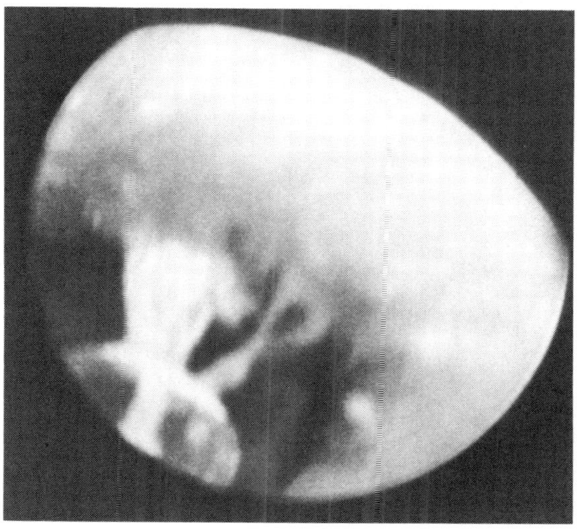

FIG. 34-6. Aspirating mucus and blood.

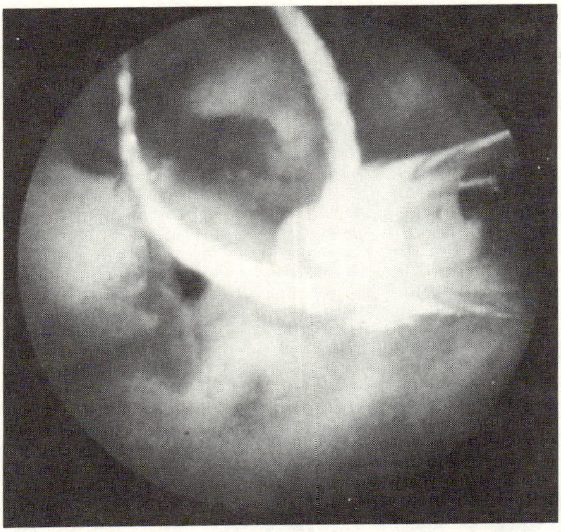

FIG. 34-7. Obturator tip close to tubal ostium in readiness for methylene blue "tap" test.

One modified instrument is a "kink" or memory curve placed in the guide. Some patients seem to have "laterally" placed tubes or may have tubal ostia difficult to obturate because of considerable degrees of uterine retroversion. Lateral tubal ostia are possibly the result of minor degrees of failure of union of the müllerian ducts during embryonic development. These ostia are observed particularly with septate uteri and bicornuate uteri. With severe degrees of uterine retroversion the pubic rami may prohibit proper alignment of the guide with tubal ostia. [In either of these situations, a "kink," or curve,

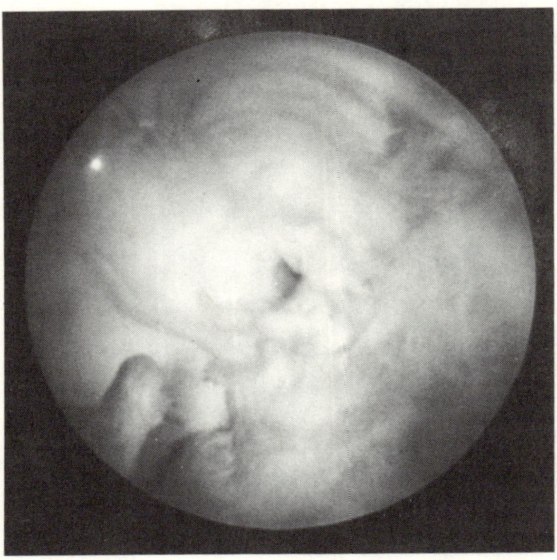

FIG. 34-8. Methylene blue flowing out tube demonstrating proper "tap" test.

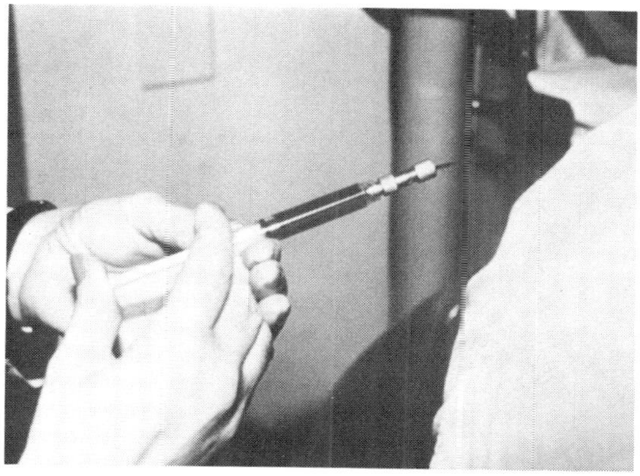

FIG. 34-9. Assistant pushing firmly on syringe for "push" tests.

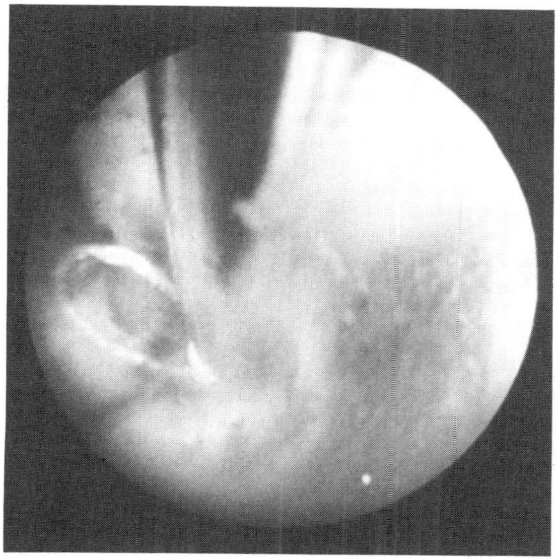

FIG. 34-10. Free flow of methylene blue out of tube and no reflux into cavity.

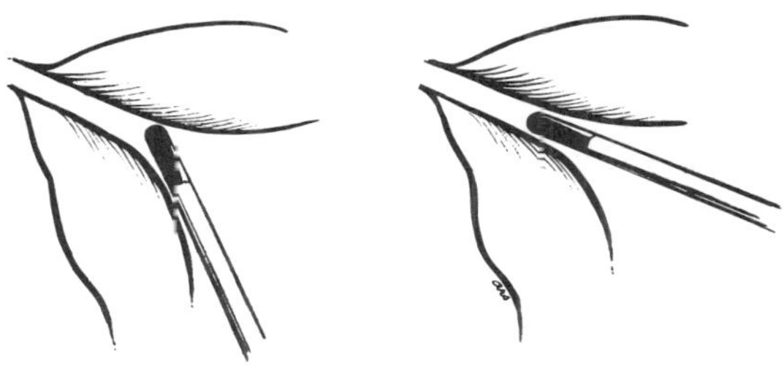

FIG. 34-11. Diagram of parallel and unparallel axes.

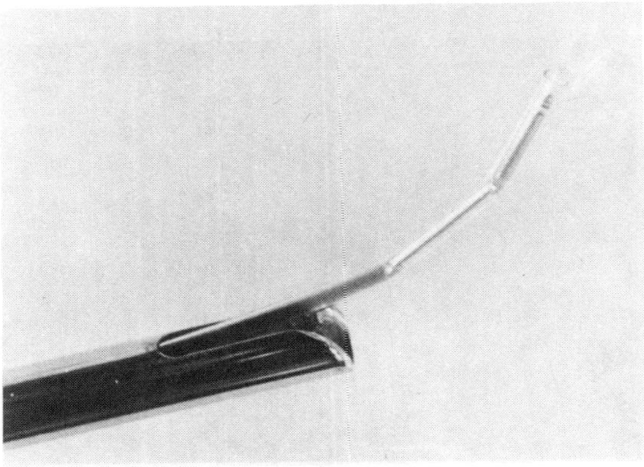

FIG. 34-12. "Kinks" placed in guide at 1-cm intervals to aid in obturating lateral tubal openings.

placed in the guide at approximately 1-cm intervals (Fig. 34-12) will often permit proper axis to be obtained with the tubal ostia (Fig. 34-13)].

Modified obturator tips (Fig. 34-14) have been developed for two purposes. The enlarged cylinders (approximately 3 mm and 4 mm in diameter) and the cone-shaped tip are for large tubal ostia. Enlarged tubal ostia are often encountered in grand multiparous patients and perhaps in patients with some degree of tubal disease. The double length (2 mm × 10 mm) tip was developed for obtaining a parallel axis with minor degrees of lateral tubal ostia.

Medications are directed at trying to relieve tubal spasm. Prostaglandin inhibitors, according to one report, may relax the smooth muscle of the fallopian tubes.[2] We have used sodium naproxen (Anaprox) for many procedures, and it is our impression that this may cause some uterine relaxation

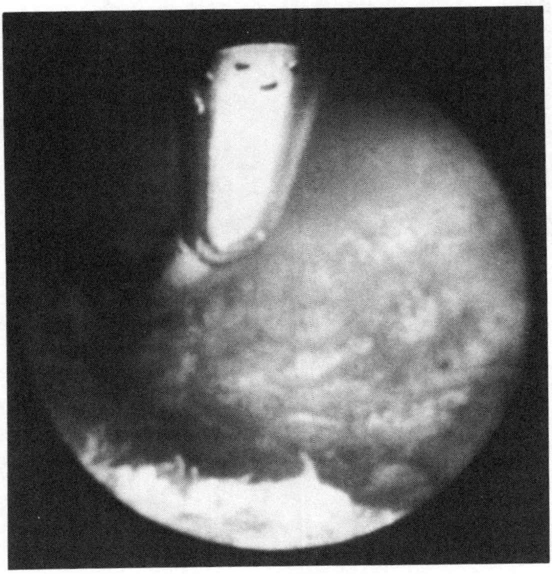

FIG. 34-13. Curved guide placed in lateral tubal opening.

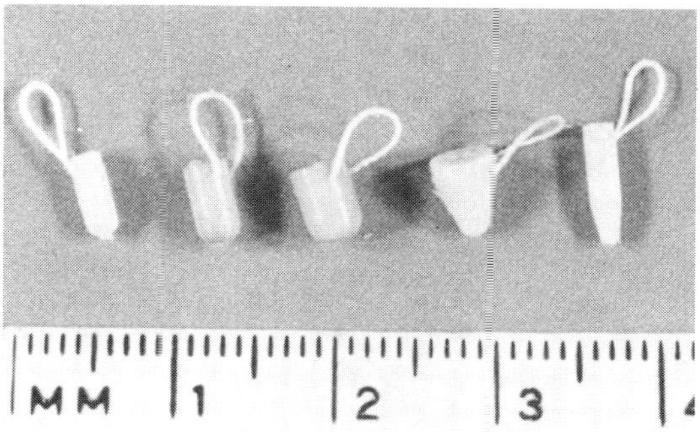

FIG. 34-14. Standard tip approximately 2×5 mm on left and four modified tips.

and prevent some cramping during the procedure, but tubal spasm can still occur. Tubal spasm is evidenced on attempting to perfuse a tube with a second methylene push test. The standard procedure is to test both fallopian tubes with the methylene push test to ensure obturation and patency in both tubes before occluding either. On returning to occlude the second tube and redoing the push test before occlusion, some resistance may be experienced and slight reflux of methylene blue observed. At this point, one unit (1 mg) glucagon is given intravenously, and waiting 6 to 7 minutes is recommended; then, usually the spasm will be relieved and a proper push test can be obtained.

This procedure failed in 3 of 20 patients. One patient also had 550 mg sodium naproxen 1 hour preoperatively and 5 mg diazepam and 25 mg meperidine intravenously during the procedure, none of which relieved the apparent tubal spasm. An attempt was made to form the plug despite the spasm, but the effort failed and a reflux-type inadequate plug was formed. At the second procedure, the medications mentioned above were repeated, and, again, there was spasm and failure resulted. At the third procedure, with the patient under general anesthesia, the second tube was successfully occluded. This is the only case in which general anesthesia was used. Our experience indicates that while diazepam will help relax the patient and meperidine will relieve painful uterine cramping that is experienced occasionally during the procedure, neither of these drugs will relieve tubal spasm. However, glucagon often seemed to relieve tubal spasm (Table 34-5).

LIMITATIONS

The limitations to the procedure are primarily anatomical. Aside from an occasional myoma that may prohibit tubal obturation, the two more commonly encountered problems are fixed retroversion and tubal disease. Fixed retroversion usually prohibits obturation because the bony pubic arch prevents rigid scopes from achieving proper tubal alignment.

Patients with known tubal disease or history of possible pelvic infection, as with the use of an IUD or in endometriosis, should be evaluated with hysterosalpingograms prior to attempting the procedure. Obviously, the method would be unsuccessful for patients who have gross tubal disease such as hy-

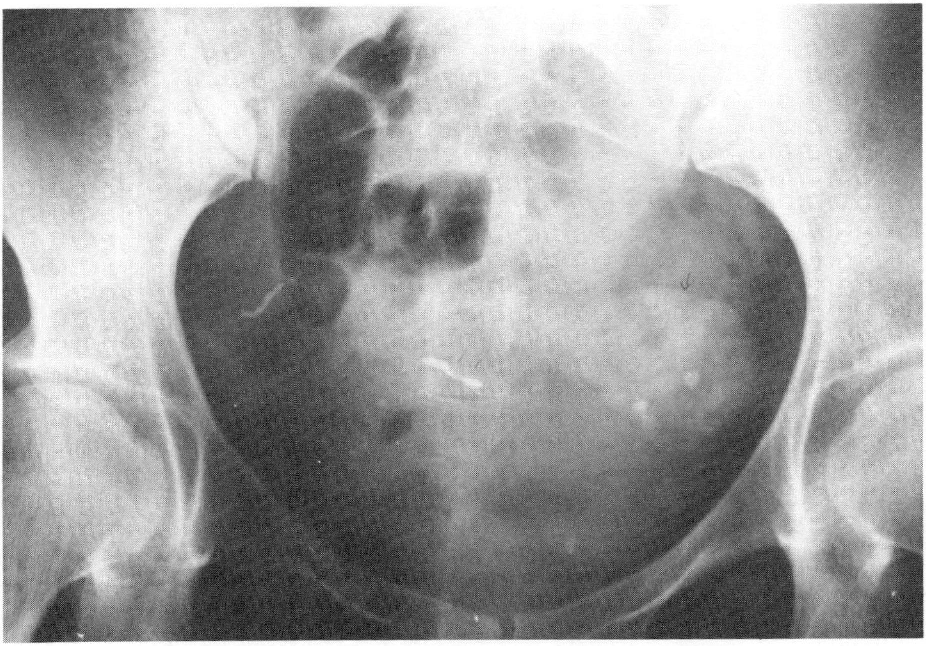

FIG. 34-15. Irregularly shaped interrupted plug in a diseased tube.

drosalpinx or complete occlusion. It is our experience that less obvious damage to the tubes also gives poor results, such as irregularly shaped plugs (Fig. 34-15) and "straight" plugs without bulbous ampullar ends (Fig. 34-16), which are usually expelled by the patient after a few weeks.

Performing the procedure on patients too early during the postabortal or postpartum period can present difficulties. When attempting the procedure before 3 months postabortion or 6 months postpartum, it may be difficult to identify tubal ostia because of the thickened endometrium or persistent venous sinuses. This subinvoluted state may persist for longer periods in nursing mothers. Some difficulty has been experienced here. Extravasation in a patient 4 months postpartum is shown in Figure 34-17. What is probably occlusion of a venous sinus with silicone rubber in a nursing mother 9 months postpartum is shown in Figure 34-18.

COMPLICATIONS

Serious complications other than pregnancy have been very few (Table 34-1). In 965 women treated, 13 pregnancies have occurred to date, all of which have been associated with failure to get proper bilateral plug formation. Of these, there has been only one ectopic pregnancy in a fallopian tube on the side of an improper plug. Most of these pregnancies occurred early in the investigations when knowledge was being gained about proper plug formation and identification.

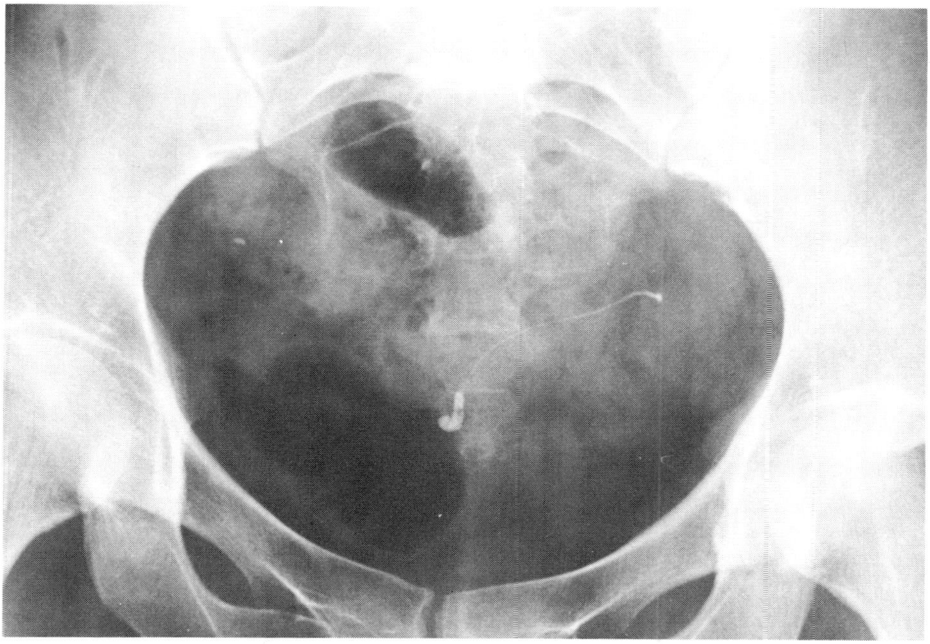

FIG. 34-16. Straight plug with very small bulbous tip in ampulla.

FIG. 34-17. Extravasated plugs in a 4 months' postpartum patient.

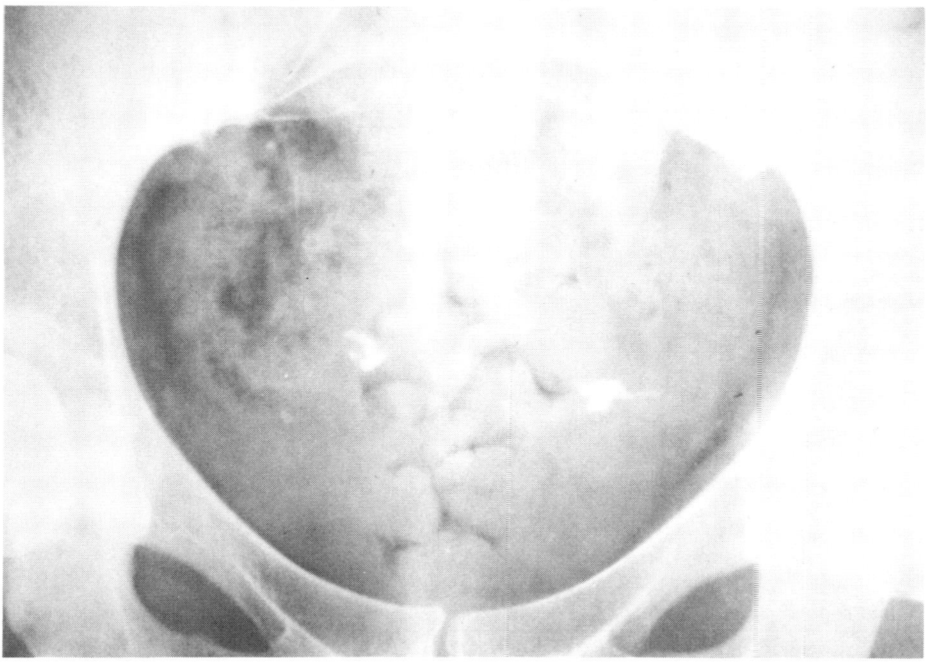

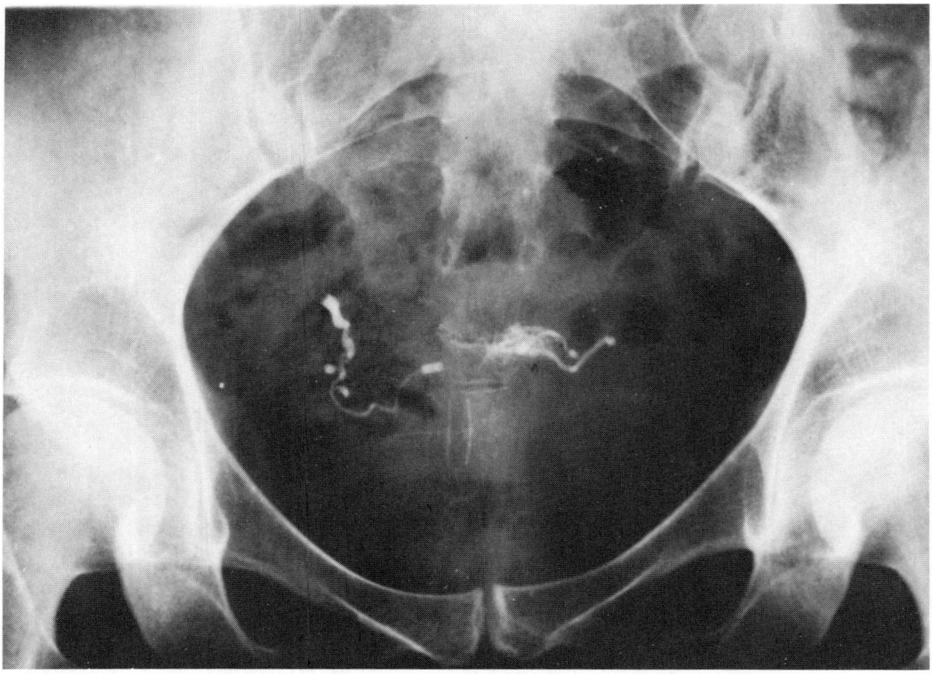

FIG. 34-18. Occlusion of venous sinus in postpartum patient (at 9 months, still nursing).

TABLE 34-1. Complications Following Tubal Occlusion in 965 Women, All Centers, as of April 1, 1982

COMPLICATION	NO. PATIENTS	
Pregnancies	13	(none with normal plugs bilaterally)
Normal plugs bilaterally	0	(pregnancy)
Uterine perforation	5	
Bleeding problems (less than 3%)	28	
Dilation and curettage	4	
Disrupted plugs	2	
Expelled plugs	4	
Separated tips	9	
Severe infection	1	
Chronic pain	3	
Postpartum patients attempted	7	
Unable to identify tubal ostia	1	
Large ostium	1	
Venous occlusions	2	
Diseased tube	1	
Extravasated plugs	1	
Bilateral good plugs	1	

Three patients developed chronic low-grade pelvic pain after having proper plugs in place for 12 to 18 months. One of these patients had associated low-grade fever (<37.8°C [100°F] daily). Two of the patients were studied thoroughly, and no other cause for symptoms could be found. All three patients had the plugs removed, and their symptoms were relieved. The patient with the low-grade fever requested Pomeroy sterilization, which was done. Tissue examination by our pathologist showed chronic foreign body reaction but not infection.

Five uterine perforations have occurred, two of them with the guide assembly. There were no serious sequelae, and the perforations were treated with observation only.

Minor bleeding problems occurred on occasion (less than 3%), and most patients could be successfully treated medically. Four patients required dilation and curettage. Pathology showed normal endometrium in two women and chronic endometritis in two women. In two of the patients, the plugs were disrupted by the curette. All patients had relief of symptoms. It is recommended that all patients requiring dilation and curettage with plugs in place should have a hysteroscopy prior to the curettage for diagnosis and accurate location of the obturator tips and retrieval loops prior to curettage.

One patient had an instillation of the plugs after a history of pelvic inflammatory disease. This patient's complete blood cell count and sedimentation rate were normal, and a hysterosalpingogram showed no reaction, prior to the instillation. However, 48 hours after the instillation the patient had an acute exacerbation of pelvic inflammatory disease with sepsis and a need for hospitalization and triple chemotherapy. The patient responded well and is doing well at the present time.

To date, only two plugs have been expelled intact through the fimbriated end of the tube. Three improperly formed plugs secondary to tubal disease, as mentioned above, have been expelled through the cornual end. At the 24-month follow-up roentgenographic examination, tip separation, due to breaking of the formed intraluminal segment close to the obturator tips, has occurred. This has been found in 9 of 67 patients evaluated at 24 months so far. We felt this occurred because of a defect in the original plug formation, as shown in Figure 34-19. None of these patients has become pregnant. Studies on design of equipment are presently being undertaken to correct this problem.

RESULTS

The total number of patients requesting the procedure, the successful results, and the total number of patients eliminated for various anatomical reasons are shown in Table 34-2. Of the patients treated thus far, 82% have had successful bilateral occlusion of their tubes.

The total number of women-months of use with proper plugs without pregnancy is shown in Table 34-3, along with the number of patients who have used the method for 6 months or more. To date there have been no pregnancies when proper plug formation was achieved.

The percentage of good plug formation bilaterally in one series is shown in Table 34-4, and the results with glucagon administration are presented in Table 34-5.

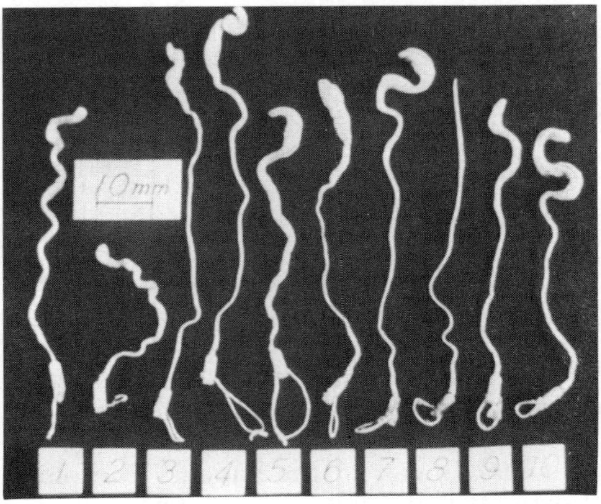

FIG. 34-19. Plugs demonstrating poor connections on No. 5 and No. 8, probably accounting for late separation.

TABLE 34-2. Total Number of Patients in the Series, All Centers, as of April 1, 1982

FACTOR	NO. PATIENTS
Patients requesting procedure	1058
Patients eliminated	93
Patients remaining in study	965
Patients with successful bilateral occlusion*	791 (82%)
Patients lost to follow-up	7

*Unacceptable patients were eliminated.

TABLE 34-3. Women-months of Use Without Pregnancy and With Proper Plugs, All Centers, as of April 1, 1982

TIME	TOTAL NO. WOMEN
Total women-months	4525
24 months or more	65
18 months or more	159
12 months or more	279
6 months or more	456

TABLE 34-4. Patients Requiring Second Procedure as of April 1, 1982*

NO. PATIENTS	%
68 patients of 350 required second procedure	16.5
In these 68 patients, good plugs were achieved bilaterally in 42	64.6

*Author's series only.

TABLE 34-5. Glucagon Series as of April 1, 1982*

ACTION	NO. PATIENTS
Glucagon given	20
Spasm considered relieved	17
Proper bilateral plugs	14
Spasm relieved but failure to get good plug	3

*Author's series only.

CONCLUSION

There are now eight centers doing this procedure successfully. Overall results indicate that the method can be effectively taught and has adequate antifertility efficacy. It can be applied successfully to an estimated 90% of properly selected patients.

REFERENCES

1. ERB RA, REED TP: Hysteroscopic oviductal blocking with formed-in-place silicone rubber plugs: I. Method and apparatus. J Reprod Med 23:65, 1979
2. LINDBLOM B, HAMBERGER L: Copper and contractility of the human fallopian tube. Am J Obstet Gynecol 141:399, 1981
3. REED TP, ERB RA: Hysteroscopic oviductal blocking with formed-in-place silicone rubber plugs: II. Clinical studies. J Reprod Med 23:69, 1979
4. REED TP, ERB RA: Tubal occlusion with silicone rubber: An update. J Reprod Med 25:25, 1980

35
Discussion: Tubal Occlusive Devices

ELIZABETH B. CONNELL

GERALD I. ZATUCHNI, MODERATORS

IS THERE ANY EVIDENCE THAT THE TUBAL PLUGS RESEMBLE IUDs IN SUCH CHARACTERISTICS AS "WANDERING," MIGRATING THROUGH THE MYOMETRIUM, OR CAUSING LEUKOCYTOSIS?

No hematologic study has been done with the uterotubal junction (UTJ) blocking device to provide an answer about whether it would cause a mild leukocytosis. The local effect of the device involved some minimal to moderate lymphocytic infiltration around the plug and the spines; what happens systemically is not known, but little effect would be predicted.

With the P-block device, investigators have looked for leukocytosis in the endometrium and have not found an increased number of round cells or leukocytes. The irritation is minimal, which with the IUD would be a problem, because leukocytosis is necessary for a good effect. But with the P-block the effect is achieved without any leukocytosis.

Thus far, in all of the animal studies and limited human studies, no perforation of the uterus has occurred with any of the tubal blocking devices.

WHEN ONE PLUG IS LOST AND THE TUBE IS FOUND TO BE PATENT, DOES THE PATIENT NEED TO UNDERGO A SECOND HYSTEROSCOPIC PROCEDURE FOR REMOVAL OF THE OTHER PLUG?

Obviously, yes. The patients participating in the study know that this may be necessary and are willing to take the chance. Often, rather than removing the remaining plug, the procedure is repeated to place a new plug on the other side.

Panelists: Jan Brundin, Jay M. Cooper, Robert A. Erb, Abdol H. Hosseinian, Theodore Reed, III. *Discussants:* Nancy J. Alexander, William Droegemueller, Enrique Guiloff, Harrith M. Hasson, Lourens J. D. Zaneveld

DOES PERMEABILITY OF THE FALLOPIAN TUBES MEAN POSSIBILE FERTILITY?

It most patients it probably does. In fact, some of the patients with tubes that were thought not to be permeable became pregnant. If there is some leakage around the plug, there is a chance of pregnancy.

HOW MUCH DOES THE P-BLOCK EXPAND?

By adding more or less nylon 6, the swelling factor can be increased or decreased. The present P-block plugs have an expansion factor of 2.5, but the plug could easily be designed to have an expansion factor of 3.0. This means that it is very soft and it is compressible by the oviduct, so that it always has an intimate contact with the epithelial lining, whether the tube is 1 mm or 3 mm in diameter. It is well known that the tubal diameter changes with the hormonal phases, so to warrant a complete occlusion, the device should be compressible but always trying to distend outward toward the epithelial lining.

IN THE NEWER DESIGN, THE P-BLOCK PLUG HAS TWO WINGS; IS INCREASED RETENTION THE PURPOSE OF THE SECOND WING? ALSO, IS THIS PLUG MORE DIFFICULT TO REMOVE?

The second set of wings was necessary because in one woman who became pregnant, the whole hydrogelic body had slid off the nylon-6 skeleton, and a second set of wings was needed. This other set of wings has nothing to do with the retention of the P-block; it serves only to keep the hydrogelic body on the nylon-6 skeleton.

CAN THE HYSTEROSCOPICALLY PLACED PLUG METHOD BE CONSIDERED A NONSURGICAL PROCEDURE, CONSIDERING THAT ANESTHESIA IS REQUIRED?

With placement of the UTJ blocking device, the patient has a paracervical block prior to the procedure, but an anesthesiologist does not need to be present in the operating room. As with the P-block, the procedure could be done in a clinic and with time will be done as an outpatient procedure, with local or no anesthesia.

Although the placement of tubal plugs could be considered a surgical procedure, the invasiveness is limited and the peritoneal cavity is not invaded. Hence, the term *nonsurgical* in the present discussion means the patient's perception that no surgical incision or cutting is required. Thus, even though hysteroscopy might have to be used with a paracervical block, in the mind of the patient, it is still a nonsurgical approach.

WHAT IS THE STATUS OF RESEARCH ON THE "STEERABLE" HYSTEROSCOPE?

A "steerable" hysteroscope was being developed under the auspices of the National Institutes of Health, but work seems to have stopped on the project. The implantation of plugs in the tubes could be greatly facilitated with such a hysteroscope. An instrument company is presently designing a "steerable" hysteroscope, for use in placing the UTJ blocking device.

WHAT IS THE STATUS OF CRYOSURGERY AS A TUBAL OCCLUDING METHOD?

For the past 8 or 10 years, investigators have been looking at cryosurgery of the endometrium, and specifically for the past 5 or 6 years, they have looked at cryosurgery of the cornu, not the interstitial part of the tube, for tubal occlusion. The most recent report was published about 4 years ago.

The technique has always been studied in women prior to hysterectomy, and the interval between cryonecrosis and subsequent surgery has varied but has been, in general, somewhere between 4 and 10 weeks.

During the past 4 years, in one series 120 cryosurgery procedures were done, with the majority of procedures employing nitrous oxide. Although obstruction of the cornu occurred in a minority of cases, the maximum necrotic isotherm of nitrous oxide was not sufficient to produce adequate necrosis. No matter how the freeze-thaw cycles were varied, some basalis epithelium regenerated.

About a year and a half ago, the equipment was redesigned to use liquid nitrogen. With this approach, of 31 cases (18 of a single freeze-thaw cycle and 13 with multiple short freeze-thaw cycles) the operation could be performed without difficulty with the use of paracervical block anesthesia. The patients did not discern the active freezing cycle, and the pain was analogous to an IUD insertion. There were no difficulties in consistently placing the large probe in the target area of the cornu, and the observation was confirmed by serial histologic sections of that area. With liquid nitrogen, coagulation necrosis was consistently produced in the target area and, in fact, probably produced too well.

Obstruction was achieved with single freeze-thaw cycles; in some cases there was abrupt sloughing, but obstruction was inconsistent, owing to regeneration of tubal epithelium and muscle, which grew downward from the interstitial portion of the tube through the granulation tissue. The goal is cornual obstruction, but when coagulation necrosis is produced in that area, this peculiar regenerative phenomenon occurs. With the nitrous oxide, however, that has not been seen.

The investigators have tried another approach, producing a smaller area of coagulation necrosis but with multiple short freeze-thaw cycles of less than 30 seconds as the active freeze cycle, for three cycles, done under the same setting. The tissue is frozen for 30 seconds, thawed for 30 seconds, and then refrozen. With the shorter cycles, the granulation tissue grows across the area before the tubal epithelium has an opportunity to grow down and recanalize the area. This is producing much more consistent closure. The coagulation necrosis has a depth of 5 mm, and there is obstruction over 2 mm to 3 mm of the cornu.

Because only 13 such procedures have been done, the investigators will not be ready to expand this to a clinical trial for another year or two. They are optimistic, however, that they will be able to develop a single protocol for treating all women requesting cryosurgical tubal occlusion.

CONTRIBUTING AUTHORS

Alfonso Balbontin Bernales, M.D.
Chapter 10
Department of Obstetrics and Gynecology
Universidad Austral de Chile
Valdivia, Chile

David A. Blake, Ph.D.
Chapters 6, 7, 15
Associate Professor, Department of Gynecology/Obstetrics and Pharmacology
The Johns Hopkins University School of Medicine
Baltimore, Maryland

Lee Bolduc
Chapter 24
BioNexus, Inc.
Raleigh, North Carolina

Manoel Bomfim de Souza Filho, M.D.
Chapters 24, 27
Associate Professor
Federal University of Bahia
Maternidade Climerio de Oliveira
Salvador, Bahia, Brazil

Jan Brundin, M.D., Ph.D.
Chapter 31
Associate Professor, Department of Obstetrics and Gynecology
Karolinska Institute
Danderyd, Sweden

Mo-Ye Chen, M.D.
Chapter 19
The Second Affiliated Hospital, Zhongshan Medical College
Guangzhou (Canton), Guangdong, China

Xue-Huang Chen, M.B.
Chapters 18, 19
The Second Affiliated Hospital, Zhongshan Medical College
Guangzhou (Canton), Guangdong, China

Lynda Painter Cole, M.A.
Chapters 9, 10
Project Leader, Department of Research
International Fertility Research Program
Research Triangle Park, North Carolina

Jay M. Cooper, M.D.
Chapter 33
Chairman, Department of Obstetrics and Gynecology
Phoenix Baptist Medical Center
Phoenix, Arizona

Elsimar M. Coutinho, M.D.
Chapter 25
Professor
Federal University of Bahia
Maternidade Climerio de Oliveira
Salvador, Bahia, Brazil

Donald R. Cowsar, Ph.D.
Chapter 14
Director, Applied Sciences Department
Southern Research Institute
Birmingham, Alabama

Maria C. DiBlasi, B.A.
Chapters 6, 7
Department of Obstetrics and Gynecology
The Johns Hopkins University School of Medicine
Baltimore, Maryland

Norman H. Dubin, Ph.D.
Chapters 6, 7, 8, 15
Associate Professor, Department of Gynecology and Obstetrics
The Johns Hopkins University School of Medicine
Baltimore, Maryland

Richard L. Dunn, Ph.D.
Chapter 14
Head, Polymer Division
Southern Research Institute
Birmingham, Alabama

Carlton A. Eddy, Ph.D.
Chapter 2
Associate Professor, Department of Obstetrics and Gynecology
The University of Texas Health Science Center at San Antonio
San Antonio, Texas

David Edelman, Ph.D.
Chapter 9
Director of Research
International Fertility Research Program
Research Triangle Park, North Carolina

Robert A. Erb, Ph.D.
Chapter 32
Institute Fellow
Franklin Research Center
Philadelphia, Pennsylvania

Ramesh B. Ghodgaonkar, B.Pharm.
Chapter 6
Research Assistant, Department of Gynecology and Obstetrics
The Johns Hopkins University School of Medicine
Baltimore, Maryland

Alfredo Goldsmith, M.D., M.P.H.
Chapter 13
Assistant Professor, Department of Obstetrics and Gynecology
Head, Research Project Development, Program for Applied Research on Fertility Regulation
Northwestern University Medical School
Chicago, Illinois

Rene Guzman-Serani, M.D.
Chapters 10, 27
Professor, Instituto de Obstetricia y Ginecologia
Universidad Austral de Chile
Santiago, Chile

Abdol H. Hosseinian, M.D.
Chapter 30
Professor and Chairman, Division of Reproductive Endocrinology
Department of Obstetrics and Gynecology
Cook County Hospital, The Chicago Medical School
Chicago, Illinois

Richard M. Houck, M.D.
Chapter 23
Phoenix Baptist Medical Center
Phoenix, Arizona

Mohammed T.M. Jiffrey, Ph.D.
Chapter 6
Fellow, Department of Obstetrics and Gynecology
The Johns Hopkins University School of Medicine
Baltimore, Maryland

Theodore M. King, M.D., Ph.D.
Chapters 6, 7, 15
Professor and Director, Department of Gynecology and Obstetrics
The Johns Hopkins University School of Medicine
Baltimore, Maryland

Robert E. Krall, Ph.D.
Chapter 21
Director of Chemical Research
BioNexus, Inc.
Raleigh, North Carolina

Leonard E. Laufe, M.D.
Chapters 8, 12
Professor
Department of Obstetrics and Gynecology
University of Texas
San Antonio, Texas

Danny H. Lewis, Ph.D.
Chapter 14
Stolle Research and Development Corporation
Birmingham, Alabama

Wilson A. Morales, M.D.
Chapter 30
Department of Obstetrics and Gynecology
Cook County Hospital
Chicago, Illinois

Nargesh D. Motashaw, M.D.
Chapters 25, 27
Professor, Department of Obstetrics and Gynecology
King Edward Memorial Hospital
Bombay, Maharashtra State, India

Robert S. Neuwirth, M.D.
Chapters 21, 22, 23, 27, 28
Director, Department of Obstetrics and Gynecology
The St. Luke's–Roosevelt Hospital Center
New York, New York

Per Agnar Nilsen, M.D.
Chapter 27
Professor, Department of Gynecology
Aker Sykehus
Oslo, Norway

Tim H. Parmley, M.D.
Chapters 6, 7, 8, 15
Assistant Professor, Department of Gynecology/Obstetrics and Pathology
The Johns Hopkins University School of Medicine
Baltimore, Maryland

Carl J. Pauerstein, M.D.
Chapter 2
Professor and Chairman, Department of Obstetrics and Gynecology
The University of Texas Health Science Center at San Antonio
San Antonio, Texas

Pei Li Qian
Chapter 17
Department of Pharmacology
Institute of Pharmaceutical Industry of Shanghai
Shanghai, China

Theodore P. Reed, III, M.D.
Chapter 34
Chief of Gynecology
Lankenau Hospital
Philadelphia, Pennsylvania

Ralph M. Richart, M.D.
Chapters 3, 21, 22, 23, 27, 28
Professor of Pathology
Director, Division of Obstetrics/Gynecology and Pathology
Columbia–Presbyterian Medical Center
New York, New York

Jacques E. Rioux, M.D., M.P.H.
Chapter 28
Professor, Department of Obstetrics and Gynecology
Laval University Medical School
Sainte–Foy, Quebec, Canada

Mirta Rivera
Chapter 9
Midwife
Hospital Sotero del Rio
Santiago, Chile

Susan C.M. Scrimshaw, Ph.D.
Chapter 4
Associate Professor of Public Health
University of California at Los Angeles
Los Angeles, California

Rochelle N. Shain, Ph.D.
Chapter 4
Assistant Professor, Department of Obstetrics and Gynecology
The University of Texas Health Science Center at San Antonio
San Antonio, Texas

James D. Shelton, M.D., M.P.H.
Chapter 1
Medical Epidemiologist, Research Division
Office of Population
Agency for International Development
Washington, D.C.

J. Joseph Speidel, M.D.
Chapter 1
Deputy Director, Office of Population
Agency for International Development
Washington, D.C.

John Standberg, D.V.M., Ph.D.
Chapter 8
Associate Professor, Department of Pathology
The Johns Hopkins University School of Medicine
Baltimore, Maryland

Gail Stetten, Ph.D.
Chapter 7
Assistant Professor, Department of Gynecology and Obstetrics
The Johns Hopkins University School of Medicine
Baltimore, Maryland

Wiktor Szczedrin, M.D.
Chapter 26
Chief of Department, Servicio de Planificacion Familiar
Maternidad "Concepcion Palacios"
Caracas, Venezuela

Rohin B. Talati, M.D.
Chapter 25
Clinical Assistant, Department of Obstetrics and Gynecology
Parsee General Hospital
Bombay, Maharashtra State, India

Shueh Ping Tien, B.S., M.D.
Chapter 17
Instructor, Department of Obstetrics and Gynecology
Xin Hua Hospital, Shanghai Second Medical College
Shanghai, China

Robert G. Wheeler, Met. Eng.
Chapters 11, 12
Biomedical Engineer
International Fertility Research Program
Research Triangle Park, North Carolina

Yu-Hau Wu, M.D.
Chapter 17
Instructor, Department of Obstetrics and Gynecology
Xin Hua Hospital, Shanghai Second Medical College
Shanghai, China

Lian-Cheng Xing, M.D.
Chapter 19
Department of Pathology
The Second Affiliated Hospital, Zhongshan Medical College
Guangzhou (Canton), Guangdong, China

Lourens J.D. Zaneveld, D.V.M., Ph.D.
Chapter 13
Department of Physiology and Biophysics
University of Illinois at the Medical Center
Chicago, Illinois

Hui-Guo Zheng, M.D.
Chapter 18, 19
Professor and Chief, Department of Obstetrics and Gynecology
The Second Affiliated Hospital, Zhongshan Medical College
Guangzhou (Canton), Guangdong, China

Itic Zighelboim, M.D.
Chapters 26, 27
Chief del Servicio de Fertilidad
Maternidad "Concepcion Palacios"
Caracas, Venezuela

Jaime Zipper, M.D.
Chapter 9
Hospital Sotero del Rio
Santiago, Chile

WORKSHOP PARTICIPANTS

Nancy J. Alexander, Ph.D.
Scientist
Oregon Regional Primate Research Center
Beaverton, Oregon

Bert Amdahl
President and Chief Executive Officer
BioNexus, Inc.
Raleigh, North Carolina

Ruben A. Apelo, M.D.
Project Director
JFMH Comprehensive Family Planning Center
Manila, Philippines

Rohit V. Bhatt, M.D.
Professor and Head, Department of Obstetrics and Gynecology
Medical College and S.S.G. Hospital
Baroda, India

David A. Blake, Ph.D.
Associate Professor, Department of Gynecology/Obstetrics and Pharmacology
The Johns Hopkins University School of Medicine
Baltimore, Maryland

Lee Bolduc
Vice President
BioNexus, Inc.
Raleigh, North Carolina

Manoel Bomfim de Souza Filho, M.D.
Associate Professor
Federal University of Bahia
Maternidad Climerio de Oliveira
Salvador, Bahia, Brazil

Jan Brundin, M.D., Ph.D.
Associate Professor, Department of Obstetrics and Gynecology
Karolinska Institute
Danderyd, Sweden

Lynda Painter Cole, M.A.
Project Leader, Department of Research
International Fertility Research Program
Research Triangle Park, North Carolina

Elizabeth B. Connell, M.D.
Department of Gynecology and Obstetrics
Emory University School of Medicine
Atlanta, Georgia

Jay M. Cooper, M.D.
Chairman, Department of Obstetrics and Gynecology
Phoenix Baptist Medical Center
Phoenix, Arizona

Philip A. Corfman, M.D.
Director, Center for Population Research
National Institute of Child Health and Human Development
Bethesda, Maryland

Elsimar M. Coutinho, M.D.
Professor
Federal University of Bahia
Maternidad Climerio de Oliveira
Salvador, Bahia, Brazil

Nicholas Dodd, M.D.
Policy Officer, Policy and Evaluation Division
United Nations Fund for Population Activities
New York, New York

William Droegemueller, M.D.
Professor and Chairman, Department of Obstetrics and Gynecology
University of North Carolina
Chapel Hill, North Carolina

Norman H. Dubin, Ph.D.
Associate Professor, Department of Gynecology and Obstetrics
The Johns Hopkins University School of Medicine
Baltimore, Maryland

Richard L. Dunn, Ph.D.
Head, Polymer Division
Southern Research Institute
Birmingham, Alabama

David Edelman, Ph.D.
Director of Research
International Fertility Research Program
Research Triangle Park, North Carolina

Amy D. Engineer, M.D.
Emeritus Professor, Department of Obstetrics and Gynecology
King George Medical College
Lucknow, India

Robert A. Erb, Ph.D.
Institute Fellow
Franklin Research Center
Philadelphia, Pennsylvania

Michael Free, Ph.D.
Technical Officer
Program for the Introduction and Adaptation of Contraceptive Technology
Seattle, Washington

Jorge Jose Garcia, M.D.
Representative for Latin America and Caribbean
International Development Research Center
Santiago, Chile

Alfredo Goldsmith, M.D., M.P.H.
Assistant Professor, Department of Obstetrics and Gynecology
Head, Research Program Development
Program for Applied Research on Fertility Regulation
Northwestern University Medical School
Chicago, Illinois

Enrique Guiloff, M.D.
Professor
Universidad de Chile
Santiago, Chile

Rene Guzman–Serani, M.D.
Professor, Instituto de Obstetricia y Ginecologia
Universidad Austral de Chile
Valdivia, Chile

Harrith M. Hasson, M.D.
Associate Professor, Department of Obstetrics and Gynecology
Rush Medical College of Chicago
Chicago, Illinois

Abdol H. Hosseinian, M.D.
Professor and Chairman, Division of Reproductive Endocrinology
Department of Obstetrics and Gynecology
Cook County Hospital, The Chicago Medical School
Chicago, Illinois

Douglas Huber, M.D.
Medical Director
Association for Voluntary Sterilization, Inc.
New York, New York

Andrew M. Kaunitz, M.D.
Senior Resident, Department of Obstetrics and Gynecology
Northwestern University Medical School
Chicago, Illinois

Theodore M. King, M.D., Ph.D.
Professor and Director, Department of Gynecology and Obstetrics
The Johns Hopkins University School of Medicine
Baltimore, Maryland

Michael Klitsch
Associate Editor
Family Planning Perspectives
New York, New York

Robert E. Krall, Ph.D.
Director of Chemical Research
BioNexus, Inc.
Raleigh, North Carolina

Miriam H. Labbok, M.D., M.P.H.
Assistant Professor, Department of Population Dynamics
The Johns Hopkins University School of Hygiene and Public Health
Baltimore, Maryland

Leonard E. Laufe, M.D.
Professor
Department of Obstetrics and Gynecology
University of Texas
San Antonio, Texas

John Lim, M.D.
Department of Obstetrics and Gynecology
Princess Margaret Hospital
Kowloon, Hong Kong

Hugo Maia, Jr., M.D.
Federal University of Bahia
Maternidad Climerio de Oliveira
Salvador, Bahia, Brazil

Suman Mehta, M.D.
Senior Research Officer
Indian Council of Medical Research
New Delhi, India

Nargesh D. Motashaw, M.D.
Professor, Department of Obstetrics and Gynecology
King Edward Memorial Hospital
Bombay, Maharashtra State, India

Dean L. Moyer, M.D.
Professor of Pathology
University of Southern California School of Medicine
Sherman Oaks, California

Robert S. Neuwirth, M.D.
Director, Department of Obstetrics and Gynecology
The St. Luke's–Roosevelt Hospital Center
New York, New York

Per Agnar Nilsen, M.D.
Professor
Oslo Kommune
Oslo, Norway

Tim H. Parmley, M.D.
Assistant Professor, Department of Gynecology/Obstetrics and Pathology
The Johns Hopkins University School of Medicine
Baltimore, Maryland

Carl J. Pauerstein, M.D.
Professor and Chairman, Department of Obstetrics and Gynecology
The University of Texas Health Science Center at San Antonio
San Antonio, Texas

Malcolm Potts, M.B., B.Chir., Ph.D.
Executive Director
International Fertility Research Program
Research Triangle Park, North Carolina

Rodolfo Quinones, M.D.
Medical Advisor
Instituto de Seguridad y Servicios Sociales de los Trabajadores del Estado
Mexico City, Mexico

Theodore P. Reed, III, M.D.
Chief of Gynecology
Lankenau Hospital
Philadelphia, Pennsylvania

Ralph M. Richart, M.D.
Professor of Pathology
Director, Division of Obstetrics/Gynecology and Pathology
Columbia–Presbyterian Medical Center
New York, New York

Jacques E. Rioux, M.D., M.P.H.
Professor, Department of Obstetrics and Gynecology
Laval University Medical School
Sainte–Foy, Quebec, Canada

Guillermo Rosa, M.D.
Instructor
Universidad Austral de Chile
Valdivia, Chile

John J. Sciarra, M.D., Ph.D.
Professor and Chairman, Department of Obstetrics and Gynecology
Director, Program for Applied Research on Fertility Regulation
Northwestern University Medical School
Chicago, Illinois

Susan C.M. Scrimshaw, Ph.D.
Associate Professor of Public Health
University of California at Los Angeles
Los Angeles, California

Rochelle N. Shain, Ph.D.
Assistant Professor, Department of Obstetrics and Gynecology
The University of Texas Health Science Center at San Antonio
San Antonio, Texas

James D. Shelton, M.D. M.P.H.
Medical Epidemiologist, Research Division
Office of Population
Agency for International Development
Washington, D.C.

Aquiles J. Sobrero, M.D.
Professor, Department of Obstetrics and Gynecology
Northwestern University Medical School
Chicago, Illinois

William Stewart, M.D.
Director, Clinical Research in Obstetrics and Gynecology
G.D. Searle Company
Chicago, Illinois

Shueh-Ping Tien, B.S., M.D.
Professor and Chairman, Department of Obstetrics and Gynecology
Xin-Hua Hospital, Shanghai Second Medical College
Shanghai, China

Rafael Valle, M.D.
Associate Professor, Department of Obstetrics and Gynecology
Northwestern University Medical School
Chicago, Illinois

Robert G. Wheeler, Met. Eng.
Biomedical Engineer
International Fertility Research Program
Research Triangle Park, North Carolina

Earle W. Wilson, M.D.
Special Program of Research in Human Reproduction
World Health Organization
Geneva, Switzerland

Lillian Yin, Ph.D.
Director, Division of Obstetrics/Gynecology and Radiology Devices
Bureau of Medical Devices
Food and Drug Administration
Silver Spring, Maryland

Lourens J.D. Zaneveld, D.V.M., Ph.D.
Department of Physiology and Biophysics
University of Illinois at the Medical Center
Chicago, Illinois

Gerald I. Zatuchni, M.D., M.Sc.
Professor, Department of Obstetrics and Gynecology
Director of Technical Assistance
Program for Applied Research on Fertility Regulation
Northwestern University Medical School
Chicago, Illinois

Hui-Guo Zheng, M.D.
Professor and Chief, Department of Obstetrics and Gynecology
The Second Affiliated Hospital, Zhongshan Medical College
Guangzhou (Canton), Guangdong, China

Itic Zighelboim, M.D.
Chief del Servicio de Fertilidad
Maternidad "Concepcion Palacios"
Caracas, Venezuela

Jaime Zipper, M.D.
Hospital Sotero del Rio
Santiago, Chile

INDEX

Index

Numbers followed by an "f" indicate a figure; the letter "t" following a page number indicates tabular material.